T0210194

Herbs & Natural Supplements

An evidence-based guide

4TH EDITION
VOLUME 1

Lesley Braun
PhD, BPharm, DipAppSciNat

Associate Professor of Integrative Medicine (Hon) National Institute of Complementary Medicine, University of Western Sydney, NSW Senior Research Fellow (Hon), Monash/Alfred Psychiatric Research Centre, Melbourne, VIC, Australia

Marc Cohen
MBBS(Hons), PhD, BMedSc(Hons), FAMAC, FICAE

Professor of Health Sciences, School of Health Sciences, RMIT University, Melbourne, VIC, Australia

ELSEVIER

ELSEVIER

Elsevier Australia. ACN 001 002 357
(a division of Reed International Books Australia Pty Ltd)
Tower 1, 475 Victoria Avenue, Chatswood, NSW 2067

Knowledge and best practice in this field are constantly changing. As new research and experience broaden our understanding, changes in research methods, professional practices, or medical treatment may become necessary.

Practitioners and researchers must always rely on their own experience and knowledge in evaluating and using any information, methods, compounds, or experiments described herein. In using such information or methods they should be mindful of their own safety and the safety of others, including parties for whom they have a professional responsibility.

With respect to any drug or pharmaceutical products identified, readers are advised to check the most current information provided (i) on procedures featured or (ii) by the manufacturer of each product to be administered, to verify the recommended dose or formula, the method and duration of administration, and contraindications. It is the responsibility of practitioners, relying on their own experience and knowledge of their patients, to make diagnoses, to determine dosages and the best treatment for each individual patient, and to take all appropriate safety precautions.

To the fullest extent of the law, neither the Publisher nor the authors, contributors, or editors, assume any liability for any injury and/or damage to persons or property as a matter of product liability, negligence or otherwise, or from any use or operation of any methods, products, instructions, or ideas contained in the material herein.

National Library of Australia Cataloguing-in-Publication Data

---

Braun, Lesley, author.

Herbs and natural supplements : an evidence-based guide.
Volume 1 / Lesley Braun, Marc Cohen.
Fourth edition.

9780729541718 (paperback)

Herbs–Therapeutic use–Textbooks.
Dietary supplements–Textbooks.
Alternative medicine–Textbooks.

Cohen, Marc, author.

615.321

Content Strategist: Larissa Norrie
Senior Content Development Specialist: Neli Bryant
Project Managers: Devendran Kannan and ShriVidhya Shankar
Edited by Margaret Trudgeon & Liz Williams
Proofread by Tim Learner
Cover and internal design by Tania Gomes
Index by Robert Swanson
Typeset by Toppan Best-set Premedia Limited
Printed in Malaysia by Papercraft.

Herbs & Natural Supplements

An evidence-based guide

4TH EDITION

VOLUME 1

CONTENTS

ORGANISATION OF THIS BOOK

This fourth edition of *Herbs and Natural Supplements: an evidence-based guide* is organised into four sections. The first volume provides a basic introduction to complementary medicine in general and then, more specifically, to herbal medicine, clinical nutrition, aromatherapy and food as medicine. It is hoped that many of your general questions will be answered here. In this first volume, we have also included the chapters relating to clinical practice and explore the relatively new fields of integrative medicine and wellness as it relates to health. These areas are gaining popularity around the globe and complementary medicine philosophy and treatments are often an integral part of the approach. We have also included chapters with a focus on safety because the wise clinical use of all interventions must be based on a benefit versus risk assessment. There are general chapters discussing the safety of herbs and natural supplements and drug interactions, and then specific chapters focusing on safety in pregnancy, before surgery and for people undertaking treatment for cancer. These topics are discussed in both a theoretical and a practical way to clarify the key concerns and produce some general guidelines that can be used to inform practice.

The second part of this volume consists of ready-reference appendices, the largest of which is a table outlining the interactions possible between the complementary medicines reviewed and pharmaceutical drugs. Although investigation into this area is still in its infancy, we have provided a brief explanation for each possible interaction and a general recommendation based on what is currently known or suspected. It is intended as a guide only, to be used to inform practice when clinicians take a medical and medication history; obviously it should be interpreted within the individual patient's context. It is anticipated that this section will continue to change in future editions as more clinical studies are published and theoretical predictions are tested.

The second volume comprises of 132 evidence-based reviews of some of the most popular herbs and natural supplements available over the counter. Exhaustive reviews of the peer-reviewed literature have been undertaken by the author team to update, modify and expand information from the previous edition. Common names, chemical components, main actions, clinical uses, dosage range and safety issues are included for each herbal medicine. For nutritional supplements, background information and pharmacokinetics, food sources, deficiency signs and symptoms and the new Australian and New Zealand recommended daily intakes (RDIs) are also included where appropriate. Although technical language is frequently used, there is also a summary in non-technical language (Practice Points/Patient Counselling) and answers to key questions patients may have about the product (Patients' FAQs). A Historical note is included where appropriate and occasionally there are also Clinical note boxes that provide further information.

ACKNOWLEDGMENTS

Each edition of *Herbs and Natural Supplements* is bigger than the last and has required even more effort to produce. This is certainly true of this, our fourth edition, which has been expanded to two volumes and is now also available as an eBook.

The increase in size is chiefly due to the enormous amount of new material we have uncovered and felt important enough to include in this completely revised edition. Between Medline, Science Direct and the Cochrane database, there are tens of thousands of peer-reviewed articles that are now available to help us uncover the potential of herbs and natural supplements.

Identifying, interpreting, collating and synthesizing this information is an important and challenging task. For this edition, we significantly expanded our contributor team and searched for people with a range of backgrounds, training and skills. Some contributors are research academics with an expertise in complementary medicine; others are university lecturers working at the interface with students, whereas others are clinicians that bring a real-world perspective to the task. As always, I believe the author team to be among the brightest and most talented technical CM writers in the country. Their dedication, tenacity and enthusiasm have been integral to this project and I am privileged to have them on the team.

On a personal note, undertaking such a major project as this book means many hours dedicated to working in the home office, away from family and friends. It also means mentally retreating from everyday life as thoughts about the book and the issues raised, permeate nearly everything.

I'd like to thank my husband Gary, who is my biggest support, greatest teacher and best friend. His understanding and patience are always given without a second thought and forever appreciated. My three daughters Sarah, Lori and Jaimie are wonderful, warm and intelligent people who have found a genuine interest in health and helping others. I am so proud and thank you for your understanding and support during my busy and distracted writing periods.

I'd also like to thank all my parents Shana and Fred Green, Judy Braun for their emotional and hands-on support; my late grandfather Leon Kustin and father-in-law Emil Braun, who continue to serve as reminders to me to have courage and persevere; and the rest of my wonderful extended family and friends who accept that I'm off the radar every now and again, working on another book.

I'd like to make a special mention of my late father, Magenesta, who passed away between editions. Without him I would not have finished my pharmacy degree or started my life long journey into natural medicine - you have been my mentor and guide from the beginning.

I'd like to thank associate editors Liza Oates, Rachel Arthur, Gina Fox, Evelin Tiralongo, Louise Zylan and Brad McEwan for helping to guide the newer contributors with their patience, experience and wisdom. I'd like to thank returning contributors Ondine Spitzer, Leah Hechtman, Emily Bradley, Trisha Dunning and Surinder Baines for their continued commitment and professionalism and Marc Cohen for your unwavering vision. We also have a large number of new contributors who have been important additions to the author team; without you, this book simply would not have been possible — thank you.

I'd like to thank the team at Elsevier, especially Neli Bryant, for her energy and co-ordination, and my inspiring work colleagues at The Alfred Hospital (especially Prof Frank Rosenfeldt), Monash University (esp. Prof Paul Komesaroff), National Institute of Complementary Medicine (esp Prof Alan Bensoussan) and most recently, Blackmores (esp Christine Holgate and Marcus Blackmore) and the wonderful Blackmores Institute.

Finally, thank you to all the health care professionals that have told me they use this book every day to guide their clinical practice. Knowing this helps make the difficult journey easier and is an important reminder of why our work is important, because the information within helps improve people's lives through you.

ABOUT THE AUTHORS

Lesley Braun, PhD, BPharm, DipAppSciNat
Associate Professor of Integrative Medicine (Hon)
National Institute of Complementary Medicine,
University of Western Sydney, NSW, Senior
Research Fellow (Hon), Monash/Alfred Psychiatric Research Centre, Melbourne, VIC, Australia

Dr Lesley Braun is a registered pharmacist
and naturopath. She holds a PhD from RMIT
University, Melbourne, in which she investigated the integration of complementary medicine into hospitals in Victoria. Dr Braun is an
Adjunct Associate Professor of Integrative Medicine at the National Institute of Complementary Medicine (NICM) at the University of
Western Sydney. NICM provides leadership
and support for strategically directed research
into complementary medicine and translation
of evidence into clinical practice and relevant
policy to benefit the health of all Australians.

Dr Braun serves on the Australian Therapeutic Goods Advisory Council, which oversees
the implementation of TGA reforms and provides general strategic guidance to the TGA,
advice on relationships and communication with
stakeholders. She is also on the executive for
the Complementary and Integrative Therapies
interest group of the Clinical Oncology Society
of Australia and is an advisory board member
to the Australasian Integrative Medicine Association. As of 2014, she is also Director of
Blackmore's Institute, the academic and professional arm of Blackmores, which entails engaging with a broad range of academics, government
and industry bodies and overseeing a comprehensive academic and research program.

Since 1996 Lesley has authored numerous
chapters for books and more than 100 articles,
and since 2000 has written regular columns for
the *Australian Journal of Pharmacy* and *Journal of
Complementary Medicine*. She lectures to medical
students at Monash University and to chiropractic students at RMIT University, and is
regularly invited to present at national and
international conferences about evidence-based
complementary medicine, drug interactions,
complementary medicine safety and her own
clinical research.

Her role as the main author of *Herbs and
Natural Supplements: an evidence-based guide* represents a continuation of a life-long goal to
integrate evidence-based complementary medicine into standard practice and improve patient
outcomes safely and effectively.

**Marc Cohen, MBBS(Hons), PhD, BMedSc
(Hons), FAMAC, FICAE**
Professor of Health Sciences, School of Health
Sciences, RMIT University, Melbourne, VIC,
Australia

Professor Marc Cohen is one of Australia's
pioneers of integrative and holistic medicine
who has made significant impacts on education, research, clinical practice and policy. He
is a medical doctor and Professor of Health
Sciences at RMIT University, where he leads
postgraduate wellness programs and supervises
research into wellness and holistic health,
including research on yoga, meditation, nutrition, herbal medicine, acupuncture, lifestyle
and the health impact of pesticides, organic
food and detoxification. Professor Cohen sits
on the board of a number of national and
international associations, including the Australasian Integrative Medicine Association, the
Global Spa and Wellness Summit and the Australasian Spa and Wellness Association, as well
as serving on the editorial boards of several
international peer-reviewed journals. Professor
Cohen has published more than 80 peer-reviewed journal articles and co-edited *Understanding the Global Spa Industry*, along with
more than 10 other books on holistic approaches
to health. He is a frequent speaker at many
national and international conferences where
he delivers inspiring, informative and uplifting
presentations. His impact on the field has been
recognised by four consecutive RMIT Media
Star Awards, as well as the inaugural Award for
Leadership and Collaboration from the National
Institute of Complementary Medicine.

CONTRIBUTORS

Phil Dowling, MA(LiveFoodNut), Naturopathic Practitioner, BA(Econ), BHSc, DipNat, Dip Herb
Senior Head, Faculty of Naturopathy and Nutrition, Wellpark College of Natural Therapies, Auckland, New Zealand
Chapters updated: Chapter 1 Introduction to complementary medicine

Leah Hechtman, PhD(candidate), MSciMed(RHHG), BHSc(Nat), ND
Director and Clinician, The Natural Health and Fertility Centre
PhD candidate — University of Sydney, Department of Obstetrics, Gynaecology and Neonatology, Faculty of Medicine, President, National Herbalists Association of Australia, NSW, Australia
Chapter updated: Chapter 11 Herbs and natural supplements in pregnancy

Liza Oates, PhD, GCert Evid-based CompMed, BHSc(Nat)
Course co-ordinator 'Food as Medicine' and 'Wellness Practices & Perspectives', Postgraduate Wellness Program, RMIT University, Vic, Australia
Naturopathic Clinical Supervisor, Southern School of Natural Therapies and Endeavour College of Natural Health
Teaching Associate, Department of General Practice, Monash University
Chapter updated: Chapter 5 Introduction to food as medicine

Tanya Wells, B.Sc.(Hons), BHSc(Nat), GCertHealthProfEd, Memberships: MNHAA AMAIMA AMCOSA
Integrative Medicine Naturopath, Lecturer Synergy Health — Consulting, Seminars and Training — Drug–Herb/Nutrient Interaction Seminars for Medical and Nursing Practitioners, Vic, Australia
Chapter updated: Chapter 10 Cancer and the safety of complementary medicines

REVIEWERS

Sandy Davidson, MPH(USYD), DipNat, AdvDipNat, DipNutr; Membership: DRM
Associate Program Leader — Nutritional Medicine, Endeavour College of Natural Health

Myfanwy Graham, MPharm
Associate Lecturer, School of Biomedical Sciences and Pharmacy, Faculty of Health and Medicine, University of Newcastle, NSW, Australia

Elizabeth MacGregor, MEd(HighEd), BHSc(Nat)
Naturopathic Practitioner, Senior Lecturer of Naturopathic Medicine, Endeavour College, Perth, WA, Australia

Karen Wallace, BHSc(Nat), BBus(HAdm), MANTA
Naturopathic Practitioner, Lecturer, Endeavour College of Natural Health, Perth, WA, Australia

PREFACE

Welcome to the fourth edition of *Herbs and Natural Supplements: an evidence based guide*. Due to the exponential growth in the peer-reviewed literature, we have had to expand our team of contributors significantly since the last edition. We have contributions from experts with a range of backgrounds such as nutrition and naturopathy, herbal medicine, pharmacy, dietetics and medicine and also a number of research active academics and university lecturers.

I started writing the first edition, together with Prof Marc Cohen, nearly 10 years ago, and it is very heartening to see the enormous growth in the evidence base that has occurred since that time. We now have far more information available in the peer-reviewed literature about key active components in herbal medicines, pharmacological activity in vivo and clinical trials. In particular, the complexity of herbal medicines has become more evident as nearly all have multiple mechanisms of action and we have well and truly moved beyond using solely traditional evidence to guide their use. Unfortunately, some authors of meta-analyses still continue to pool information from studies that have tested different plant parts and even species. This is like lumping apples and oranges together, and thereby compromises the usefulness of these reviews. However, overall reporting in herbal medicine studies has improved and where possible, we state the extract used, dose and administration form to help guide you in your practice.

The area of drug-herb interactions was of particular concern in the early-mid 2000s and there is now far more information about interactions that are clinically relevant. You will notice that we place most importance on drug interactions that have been demonstrated in vivo because in vitro testing has led us all astray in the past with false positives.

Probably the biggest growth area has been in nutritional science and research. In this edition, the fish oil, vitamin D and probiotic monographs in particular have expanded significantly. They are among the most popular supplements being bought in retail stores today. Fish oils are being intensively investigated for health conditions beyond cardiovascular disease, and there is work being done in mental health, neurological diseases, neonates and children and even cancer. Unfortunately, some researchers still use olive oil as a placebo, which is unfortunate because this is not an inert substance and could be compromising results. Vitamin D is also being investigated for conditions unrelated to the musculoskeletal system, and population studies are indicating low vitamin D status is rife. Probiotics has been another area to explode with new information about potential effects beyond the gastrointestinal tract. The effect of the microbiome on multiple diseases is only starting to be understood and the role of pre- and probiotics in influencing it is slowly being uncovered. In contrast, there have been relatively fewer studies published on vitamins E and C than in the past.

Our team of contributors have systematically searched the main medical databases, using primary literature where possible, to capture, collate and synthesise the best and most relevant information for busy clinicians. We used Medline, Science Direct and the Cochrane database as a starting point to identify articles published since our last edition. This means having access to over 24 million peer-reviewed articles. Despite our best efforts, no doubt we will have missed something. This is due to the intense research activity underway and almost weekly publication of new information making it extremely difficult to keep up.

In this book, we report on positive, negative and inconclusive results and try to put forward theories as to why results are inconsistent. I think that in the future, we will better understand these differences. In particular, I wonder how much individual genetics is playing a role which we have not yet fully explored at this time. I also think there will be a time in the near future when personalised optimal nutrition will be developed and the one-size-fits all evidence based approach, which uses averages and bell shaped curves, will be seen as a blunt instrument of the past.

We have tried our best to capture and present the available information in such a way that is useful to clinicians. I hope that this book will help expand your practice by unlocking the potential of natural medicines and safely guide your patients to use them appropriately.

CHAPTER 1

INTRODUCTION TO COMPLEMENTARY MEDICINE

The practice of medicine aims to reduce human suffering through the treatment and prevention of disease, and has been part of every human society and civilisation throughout history. Although medicine has a single aim, over the ages many different practices and techniques have evolved to achieve this. We are currently living at a time when the wisdom of many different cultures and philosophies is widely available to us. Despite the existence of a wide range of therapies, medicine in the Western world has been largely institutionalised and dominated by the scientific biomedical model that centres on treating disease with drugs and surgery. In more recent times a new model has emerged; it attempts to integrate some of those therapies and medicines that are not based on the biomedical model and that have been previously termed 'alternative'. In integrative medicine, as some have called it, 'alternative medicine' is viewed as complementary to the existing system and practitioners seek to improve and enlarge the scope of the existing biomedical model.

WHAT IS COMPLEMENTARY MEDICINE?

The definition of complementary and alternative medicine (CAM) has been the subject of some debate. In 1995 the following definition was formulated at a conference held by the National Institutes of Health's Office of Alternative Medicine in the USA, with the aim of producing a definition that has the broadest and most consistent applicability and that excludes bias and partisanship:

> Complementary and alternative medicine (CAM) is a broad domain of healing resources that encompasses all health systems, modalities, and practices and their accompanying theories and beliefs, other than those intrinsic to the politically dominant health system of a particular society or culture in a given historical period. CAM includes all such practices and ideas self-defined by their users as preventing or treating illness or promoting health and well-being.
>
> **National Institutes of Health Panel on Definition and Description 1997**

Like many definitions produced by committees, this one seems a little unsatisfying. Simply dividing interventions into those that are part of the politically dominant health system and those that are not does not provide useful insight. This classification is also subject to regional political differences that may be unrelated to healthcare.

Rather than focus on political acceptance as the basis for defining alternative and complementary medicine, a discussion paper by the Australian Medical Council addresses 'unorthodox therapies' and states that 'the practices they embrace are by definition unscientific and of unproven efficacy until proved otherwise (in which case they become part of mainstream medicine)' (Australian Medical Council 1999).

The division of therapies into unorthodox and mainstream based on scientific merit is a little simplistic, and open to subjective interpretation. Similarly, the divide between complementary and conventional medicine can no longer be based on differences in scientific support as some herbals have high-level evidence yet remain classified as complementary (such as St Johns wort). On the other hand, some complementary medicines, such as fish oils, are now embraced by medical doctors and specialists and it remains to be seen how long they will continue to be called complementary.

When defining therapies on political or scientific grounds, further confusion is added because of the amount of time it takes to gain wide acceptance. For example, even though scientific evidence in support of acupuncture has been accumulating since the discovery of endogenous opioids in the mid-1970s, it is well accepted in countries such as China, and government rebates via Medicare have been available for acupuncture for nearly two decades, this therapy is still not universally accepted as mainstream in Australia and New Zealand.

Over the last few decades there has been a move away from calling complementary medicine 'unorthodox' or 'unconventional' or 'fringe' medicine as more scientific research has been conducted and there has been greater integration of many complementary medicine modalities and specific treatments into interdisciplinary medical clinics, hospitals, pharmacies and many allied health clinics. In fact, for many treatments traditionally thought of as complementary, such as massage, yoga, meditation and acupuncture, the broad acceptance of their usefulness by medical practitioners really challenges whether they can be called 'complementary' at all.

The range of therapies traditionally described as complementary is vast and includes treatments based on traditional philosophies, manual techniques, medicinal systems, mind–body techniques and bioenergetic principles (Table 1.1). These techniques vary widely with respect to levels of efficacy, cost, safety and scientific validation, yet they often share common principles, including the concept of supporting the body's homeostatic systems, as well as acknowledging the role of lifestyle practices, personal creativity, group sharing, the mind–body connection and the role of spiritual practice in health.

COMPLEMENTARY MEDICINE IN AUSTRALIA

Complementary medicine (CM) in the form of herbal medicine, clinical nutrition, bodywork therapies and mind-body techniques has existed in Australia for generations. Over the last three decades, public support for CM has grown to the point where it is highly unusual to find someone who has not taken a herbal or natural supplement, visited a massage therapist or tried meditation or yoga.

TABLE 1.1 THE RANGE OF COMPLEMENTARY THERAPIES		
PHILOSOPHICAL SYSTEMS	**MEDICINAL**	**BIOENERGETIC**
Ayurvedic Yoga Traditional Chinese medicine Shamanic healing Naturopathy	Herbal therapies Homeopathy Diet modification Nutritional supplementation Aromatherapy	Magnetism Pulsed electromagnetic fields Qi gong Reiki Therapeutic touch
MIND–BODY	**MANUAL**	
Meditation Hypnosis Self-help/support groups Biofeedback Prayer/spiritual healing	Chiropractic Massage Reflexology Shiatsu Osteopathy	

In 2000 it was estimated that about 50% of the Australian population took a 'natural supplement', about 20% formally saw a complementary medicine practitioner and public spending on complementary medicines (A$2.3 billion in 2000) was more than four times patients' contributions for all pharmaceutical medications (MacLennan & Taylor 2002). A follow-up survey performed in 2004 found that although spending on complementary medicines had decreased to A$1.8 billion, there was a slight increase in the number of people taking natural supplements, and visits to complementary medicine practitioners rose to 26.5% (MacLennan et al 2006). More recent statistics reveal that up to 70% of the Australian population has used complementary medicine in a number of different forms (Xue et al 2007). Data from the Australian Bureau of Statistics (ABS) indicates that in the 10 years leading up to 2006, the number of people visiting CM practitioners within a 2-week period rose from approximately 500,000 to 750,000, and over the same period there was an 80% increase in the number of people employed as CM practitioners. The most commonly consulted CM practitioners were chiropractors, naturopaths and acupuncturists (ABS 2004–05, ABS 2008).

CM is used by children, adults and older people across the age spectrum. It is used by people with cancer, HIV/AIDs, musculoskeletal pain, cardiovascular disease, diabetes and many other conditions, indicating that its use is broad and not chiefly the domain of the 'worried well'.

One of the main reasons people choose CM is to manage chronic disease, improve wellbeing and as a preventive healthcare approach (Braun et al 2010, Brownie 2006, MacLennan et al 2006). In 2010, a national survey of over 1100 pharmacy customers found that 72% of them were using complementary medicine products and rated them as effective or effective enough. Additionally, over 50% of all customers thought pharmacies should employ naturopaths (Braun et al 2010). This signifies that much of the general public recognises the usefulness of naturopaths and don't see the artificial 'us' and 'them' divide that used to exist. Another national survey of 479 naturopaths and Western herbalists found that 24% had worked in a community pharmacy in the past and some had their own herbal tinctures and

private consulting space in this setting (Braun et al 2011).

GREATER ACCEPTANCE

Signs of greater acceptance of various complementary practices are also evident among conventional medicine practitioners. This is signified by the Australian Medical Association's (AMA) formal position statement on complementary medicine recognising 'that evidence-based aspects of Complementary Medicine are part of the repertoire of patient care and may have a role in mainstream medical practice'. This statement was endorsed by the Royal Australian College of General Practitioners (RACGP). The Australian Medical Students Association (AMSA) has over 17,000 members and also holds a position advocating for the education of CMs in medical programs across Australia, insofar as it is important for students to understand commonly-used CM practices to ensure a holistic approach to patient management and wellbeing. It also goes on to to state that 'At present the medical curriculum of most Australian Universities does not facilitate adequate opportunities for medical students to gain an appropriate awareness of CMs' (AMSA 2014).

According to a Melbourne-based survey, over 70% of doctors, surgeons, anaesthetists and pharmacists ($n = 127$) at a Victorian public teaching hospital rated the following complementary medicine practices as effective: acupuncture, yoga, meditation, massage (Braun 2007). A similar finding was reported for Australian general practitioners (GPs) who thought acupuncture, meditation, yoga, hypnosis and massage were highly effective (Cohen et al 2005). In fact, surveys have estimated that 30–40% of Australian GPs practise a complementary therapy and more than 75% formally refer their patients for such therapies (Cohen et al 2005, Hall 2000, Pirotta et al 2000). It is also estimated that more than 80% of GPs think it appropriate to practise therapies such as hypnosis, meditation and acupuncture and that most GPs desire further training in various complementary therapies (Cohen et al 2005, Pirotta et al 2000).

The interest of GPs in CM is supported by the forming of links between the Australasian Integrative Medicine Association and the Royal Australian College of General Practitioners with the release of a joint position paper on complementary medicine (RACGP/AIMA 2005). Further academic support globally is evident by the proliferation of peer-reviewed journals documenting the growing body of rigorous research in the field.

Despite this, there will always be detractors who take an emotional stance and define complementary medicine as 'quackery' or 'pseudoscience'. An in-depth look through the peer-reviewed literature, and certainly wading through the two volumes of this book, will make it obvious that many herbs and natural supplements have demonstrated pharmacological actions and are clinically effective, often with far fewer side effects than their pharmaceutical counterparts. Similar to conventional medicine, some studies are rigorous whereas others suffer from poor methodology; however, the evidence base is growing and more research is being published daily. The notion that CM is entirely based on anecdote and unscientific is out of step with the evidence and embarrasses the holder of such an outdated view. This begs the question as to why some groups continue to push this idea, an issue that was recently explored by numerous academics in Australia.

Starting in 2011, a group called 'The Friends of Science in Medicine' (FSM) undertook a campaign to condemn complementary medicine and push for universities to stop teaching any complementary medicine content, chiefly by labelling it as 'pseudoscientific' and suggesting that it would discredit genuine scientific pursuits (MacLennan & Morrison 2012). By April 2012, the focus on university education had broadened to include clinical practice and the legitimacy of complementary medicine in Australian society. Flatt (2013) reports that in multiple interviews the FSM 'express incredulity at the willingness of the public to engage with "nonsensical" medicine and disbelief at the potential for intelligent people to suspend their normal judgement to pursue complementary medicine healthcare'. There are also continuous assertions by FSM representatives in the media that complementary medicine is un-testable using scientific processes and therefore cannot be evidence-based.

A response by Myers et al (2012) makes the point that removing CM programs from universities is short-sighted, will not have a significant impact on the demand for clinical services and may in fact decrease the educational rigour of these courses, to the detriment of patients (Myers et al 2012). Additionally, when the issue is viewed from a sociological perspective, the activities of FSM say much less about good science and much more about control and power. Komesaroff (2014) agrees and stated in *The Conversation* that there is a current tendency in Australia that may have crossed the line from reasoned discussion to the inappropriate use of power and authority.

FSM took on many different activities including a persistent letter-writing campaign to university vice-chancellors, articles in the professional medical press, internet postings and numerous media interviews. Responses also emerged from researchers and academics, professional associations and practitioners. In particular, associations argued that emotive reasoning based on anecdote was being used by FSM together with inaccurate definitions and out-dated information (National Herbalists Association of Australia 2012, Australian Traditional Medicine Society 2012). Some academics also argued that the depiction of CM by FSM was power-based and actually did nothing to advance science which should aim to explore new ways of thinking and enquiry. Komesaroff et al (2012) went even further, stating that medicine and science must strongly oppose the intolerance and censorship advocated by FSM and that the group was no friend of science at all.

Flatt (2013) undertook a critical analysis of 13 separate media events that took place in early 2012 and found that FSM tried to represent CM through a strategy of rhetoric and argumentation that contradicts the literature. The discourse used was symbolic and derived from a power-based ideological perspective that formed the basis for promoting exclusion of complementary medicine from university education and primary health care.

Despite the obviously emotive nature of their appeal and lack of research undertaken by FSM to portray complementary medicine accurately, there have been some overt and also less obvious responses by university authorities to either discontinue providing CM education or stop supporting CM research.

While the universities have been the main target of FSM, the Australian public has largely ignored their plea and continued to use CM and consult with practitioners.

WHY IS IT STILL POPULAR?

There appear to be many reasons for the popularity of complementary medicine. Certainly, conventional Western medicine does not have a monopoly on cure and, despite its effectiveness in treating trauma and acute disease, when it comes to chronic illness there are many people in the community who continue to suffer. The public is also demanding greater autonomy and involvement in their own healthcare, and wants to prevent or slow down ageing and achieve higher levels of functioning. Additionally, the exponential increase in scientific studies being published on complementary medicine therapies has no doubt added to the public's interest and confidence in its use. Finally, in medical practice, what are often called 'health outcomes' are actually 'illness outcomes'. Many medical practitioners are trained to detect and treat episodes of illness and often become interested in people only when they become unwell and then lose interest when they become well again. Some of these 'well' people are interested in preventing future disease, or are not feeling quite as well as they would like to. CM practitioners have a focus on health promotion and wellness in addition to providing symptomatic and curative treatment and may also be filling the gap left by medical doctors.

Despite its popularity and general acceptance, in practice it seems that there are two distinct healthcare systems operating in parallel, and collaboration is still in its infancy. It is estimated that of the patients who go to complementary practitioners, more than 57% do not inform their doctor they are doing so (MacLennan et al 2006). This lack of communication is potentially hazardous, as it raises the possibility of treatment interactions; this is even more significant when it is considered that in the USA more than 80% of people seeking complementary treatment for 'serious medical conditions' were found to be receiving treatment from a medical doctor for the same condition (Eisenberg et al 1993, 1998).

COMPLEMENTARY MEDICINE IN NEW ZEALAND

Complementary medicine has been practised in New Zealand since the 19th century (Duke 2005). In 1908, the *Quackery Prevention Act* was enacted to prevent the sale of dubious medicines or medical devices and represents an early attempt to regulate the practice of CM. At the time, what is now termed CAM had achieved a level of acceptance among the medical profession; however, a division began to emerge between medical and complementary practices because of the Act.

Over the past decade, studies have indicated that conventional medical practitioners in New Zealand practise some form of complementary therapy or refer their patients to CM practitioners (Duke 2005). One study of 226 GPs in Wellington suggested that they saw their role as ranging from comprehensive provider of both conventional and complementary medicine to selective practitioner of some options (Hadley 1988). Of these GPs, 24% had received CM training, 54% wanted further training in a complementary therapy and 27% currently practised at least one therapy. The study also found that acupuncture, hypnosis and chiropractic were the most popular therapies among this group.

CM received a further boost when in 1992 the Australasian Integrative Medicine Association (AIMA) was set up in Australia by doctors to enable them to work with medical practitioners, medical students and complementary therapists in order to achieve their aims of integrated practice (AIMA 2014). Since AIMA came to New Zealand 10 years ago CM has benefited greatly from doctors affiliated to AIMA with several AIMA doctors forming good links with naturopaths and other CM practitioners.

In June 2001, the Ministerial Advisory Committee on Complementary and Alternative Health (MACCAH) was established in order to advise the New Zealand Minister of Health. Policies regarding regulation, consumer information needs, research evidence and efficacy and integration were investigated, together with a range of strategies to allow CM to contribute to the mainstream objectives of the New Zealand Health Strategy (MACCAH 2004).

Currently, the New Zealand Charter of Health Professionals estimates that there are 10,000 CM practitioners nationally. The 2002–03 New Zealand Health Survey ($n = 12,000$) indicated that approximately 24% of adults had visited a CM practitioner over the 12-month study period (MACCAH 2004). Massage therapists, chiropractors, osteopaths, homeopaths and naturopaths were the most commonly consulted CM practitioners. The survey found that 32.5% of people seeing CM practitioners did so for the treatment of a chronic condition, long-term illness or disability, while 33% also saw a GP for the same condition. A belief that CM practitioners can provide help with conditions that other health-care professionals are unable to treat was the main driving force behind their choice. Most referrals came from friends; however, 12% reported that they had been referred to the service by a medical doctor.

The 2002–03 health survey also revealed interesting data about those who chose to visit a CM practitioner. In a survey-related study (Pledger et al 2010) it was concluded that CAM users are more likely to be middle-aged, rich, well-educated, female and of European descent, with a greater likelihood of having 'hard to treat' conditions. The conclusion goes on to say they will generally be less well, but will actively try to stay healthy. Additionally, they will tend to use more health services, and seek information about their health and medicines.

More recent data derived from the New Zealand census of 2006 (Statistics New Zealand 2006) and 2013 (Statistics New Zealand 2013) indicate a general continued growth in the numbers of CM practitioners. In particular, figures reveal that between 2006 and 2013 the number of acupuncturists rose from 252 to 489, naturopaths from 435 to 492 and complementary health therapists from 654 to 804. The creation of degree courses in acupuncture, massage and naturopathy has signalled a positive trend in CM in the last few years and gives a good reflection of where future progress is likely to be achieved. Contrary to the general progress, homeopath numbers fell from 102 to 78 over the period, possibly reflecting the poor publicity that continues to affect homoeopathy worldwide.

Further evidence of the support for CM among doctors came in March 2011 when the Medical Council of New Zealand (MCNZ) released a statement on CM to advise doctors of their required standards of practice with their patients who use CM (Medical Council of New Zealand 2014). The council stated it did not oppose CM use, provided benefits had been demonstrated to the patients and that they have made an informed choice. The council added that CM therapies can adversely impact on conventional medical care, so practitioners need to be aware and record their patient's use of CM to allow it to be taken into account when providing conventional care. Further, if a patient is making a choice between conventional medicine or CM, the doctor should present the information in a way that a patient would expect to learn of the options available, including risks, benefits and costs.

The general expansion in the use of CM practitioners in New Zealand is well summarised in a study by Gilbey (2009), who investigated CM use and concluded:

> It is clear from my brief investigation that the CAM industry in New Zealand is thriving and that our love affair with all things alternative is growing stronger over time. What is more, the increasingly high profile of CM may create yet more momentum to the industry and even raise the possibility that CM is viewed more as an alternative to orthodox treatment, than a complement (p. 113).

CM use is likely to continue to grow in New Zealand for the foreseeable future, particularly in the fields of naturopathy, herbalism, acupuncture and massage.

THE MEDICAL SPECTRUM

The range of available therapies is vast, but there are common benchmarks for all — reducing human suffering and improving health and quality of life. On this criterion, it is possible to classify all medicine into good and bad, with good medicine defined as safe, first and foremost, effective, practical and, ideally, evidence-based, while bad medicine is defined as harmful and/or ineffective.

Additionally, the different therapies can be seen to exist across a spectrum with multiple dimensions, such as safety, efficacy, practicality, availability, utility and cost-effectiveness. At one end of this spectrum is the science of medicine, which aims to understand and combat the disease process from a pathophysiological perspective. Therapies using this approach are often at the core of mainstream medicine, require practitioner intervention, target a specific organ, system, tissue or biochemical process and are usually subsidised by the public purse. At the opposite end is the art of medicine, which aims to support the body's homeostatic processes to facilitate healing and enhance the subjective sensation of wellness. Therapies using this approach often involve philosophical systems with a spiritual dimension, are highly individualised, consider the whole person and may require significant patient involvement and cost. When considering the different dimensions of medical practice, it becomes clear that best practice should incorporate both approaches, combining the art and science of medicine.

Health and disease can also be considered to inhabit opposite ends of an illness–wellness spectrum, with health being classified into three broad areas — ill-health, average health and enhanced health (Figure 1.1) (see also Chapter 12). In the past, Western medicine has traditionally focused on helping people move from ill-health to average health and has viewed the absence of disease as an ideal goal. In relatively recent times, preventive treatment has also been incorporated into medical management, in an attempt to reduce the incidence or exacerbation of disease states. By comparison, CM has always maintained a focus on preventive approaches and moving people from average health to a state of enhanced health. In Eastern medicine there is a concept of a 'perfect health' state, in which a person is totally balanced and 'at one with the universe', and hence in a state of perpetual bliss or 'nirvana'.

INTEGRATIVE AND HOLISTIC MEDICINE

When complementary and conventional approaches to medicine are combined, their practice is often called holistic or integrative medicine (see Chapter 6). This combined approach aims to achieve a balance between art and science, theory and practice, mind and body and prevention and cure. The practice of integrative medicine is highly individualised and focuses on *how* medicine is practised rather than the use of any particular modalities. It embraces a philosophy that adheres to certain principles, such as the BEECH principles:

B **B**alance between complementary aspects

E **E**mpowerment and self-healing

E **E**vidence-based care supporting the concept 'First, do no harm'

C **C**ollaboration between practitioner and patient, and between different practitioners

H **H**olism and the recognition that health is multidimensional.

Integrative medicine focuses on patient self-healing and empowerment through education and health promotion, and aims for a collaborative approach through a partnership model. Overall, an evidence-based, patient-centred care approach is adopted that includes the fundamental principle of *primum non nocere* or 'First, do no harm'. This approach considers the best available evidence on safety and efficacy, and recognises that each person is an individual whose health involves physical, psychological, social, spiritual and environmental dimensions. Integrative medicine also recognises that optimal healthcare requires a multidisciplinary approach, with each discipline having its own defined strengths, weaknesses and limitations.

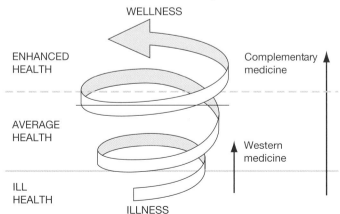

FIGURE 1.1 Conceptualisation of the spectrum of health

Besides the use of disease-specific treatments, integrative medicine also incorporates general health-enhancing and supportive interventions to improve wellbeing. This may include stress management techniques, such as meditation and relaxation training; exercise programs to improve physical activity; dietary recommendations to improve nutritional status; and education to provide a greater sense of control and understanding of illness and health. These interventions form the pillars of a holistic approach to healthcare and can be summarised by the SENSE approach:

S   **S**tress management
E   **E**xercise
N   **N**utrition
S   **S**ocial and spiritual interaction
E   **E**ducation

HERBAL MEDICINES AND NATURAL SUPPLEMENTS

Since the beginning of time, humans have sought to ease pain, heal sickness and improve energy levels by using various substances as medicines. These attempts began by using things found in the local environment, such as plants, minerals and animal parts, and has now evolved to include many previously unknown chemical entities, such as vitamins, minerals and phytochemicals. Today, an unprecedented range of herbal and natural supplements and functional foods is available.

As with all treatments, the benefits of using a medicine, changing a diet or making lifestyle changes must be weighed against the potential for doing harm: that is, the risk of using/taking/doing something and causing harm, or of not using/taking/doing it and causing harm (Table 1.2). Adverse effects from the use of natural supplements can result from an inherent property of the substance itself, inappropriate use, product adulteration or contamination not related to the substance but found within the preparation and interactions with other substances or preexisting medical conditions.

These issues are discussed in greater depth in the following chapters.

PRODUCT QUALITY AND REGULATION

Risk assessments are a key factor in the decision to use any intervention. Australia has an international best-practice, risk-based, regulatory system for both complementary and prescription medicines. This system is regulated by the Therapeutic Goods Administration (TGA), which aims to ensure safety, quality and truth in the labelling of therapeutic goods available to the Australian public. The TGA acts to control the supply of therapeutic goods, including complementary medicines, through three main processes — regulation of manufacturers, and pre- and post-marketing assessment and surveillance. These elements are supported by penalties for breaches of regulations.

The TGA acts to ensure that all therapeutic goods sold in Australia, including herbs and natural supplements as well as prescription medicines, are manufactured according to good manufacturing practice. It licenses manufacturers and conducts regular inspections to audit their compliance. High-risk products, such as prescription medicines, or low-risk products with high-level claims, are individually evaluated for safety, quality and efficacy in the pre-market period and are entered into the Australian Register of Therapeutic Goods (ARTG) as *registered* goods, thereby carrying an 'AUST R' number on their labels. Low-risk products, such as most herbs and natural supplements, are evaluated only for safety and quality in the pre-market period and are *listed* on the ARTG, carrying an identifying 'AUST L' number on their label. Audits of the

TABLE 1.2 REASONS FOR USING HERBAL MEDICINES AND NATURAL SUPPLEMENTS	
Efficacy	When they will alleviate symptoms of disease, reduce exacerbation or present a cure.
Safety	When they present a safer treatment option than other therapies.
Cost	When they provide cost-effective treatment options.
Adjunct	If the efficacy and/or safety of other interventions can be improved with adjunctive use.
Prevention	When they provide safe prevention strategies in at-risk populations.
Enhance health	If they give a sense of improved wellbeing and quality of life.
Enlists	They involve patients in their own healthcare.

evidence held by sponsoring companies for AUST L products occur in the post-market period.

Listed products are awarded low-risk status based on a number of controls, including assessment of the scientific evidence, the presence of label advisory information, dosage limits, mode of administration, restriction on the use of particular plant parts or other preparation restrictions and container type. These products are able to carry a wide range of low- and medium-level medicinal claims, which must be supported by the appropriate level of evidence (Table 1.3). It should be noted that the levels of evidence designated by the TGA are slightly different from the levels designated by the National Health and Medical Research Council (NHMRC 1999), because the TGA acknowledges evidence from traditional use, accepting that, if a substance has been used with good effect and apparent safety for three generations, it may be considered safer than a newly created substance that has never existed in nature (TGA 2001).

In addition to regulating manufacturing and the control over label claims, the TGA also conducts post-marketing surveillance such as:

- monitoring of adverse drug reactions
- targeted and random laboratory testing of products and ingredients
- audits of good manufacturing practice
- an effective co-regulatory approach to controlling advertising of therapeutic goods.

The regulation of complementary medicine products specifically is conducted by the Office of Complementary Medicine as part of the Therapeutic Goods Administration.

The Advisory Committee on Complementary Medicine (ACCM) is a ministerially appointed committee that advises the Office of Complementary Medicine within the TGA about matters relating to complementary medicine products.

Although Australia employs the same rigorous system for maintaining the quality of herbs and natural supplements as for prescription pharmaceuticals, this is not the case in many other countries. The problem of poor product quality has become a major concern in some Asian countries, where authorities have undertaken random sampling of suspected herbal products to determine whether adulteration has occurred. Huang et al (1997) report one survey in Taiwan where 2609 herbal samples were collected by eight major general hospitals. Analysis with thin-layer chromatography found an average of 23.7% of samples to be adulterated with chemical substances not stated on the label. Of these, more than half (52.8%) contained two or more adulterants (Awang 1996, Huang et al 1997).

Government actions: the PAN Pharmaceuticals recall in Australia

On 28 April 2003 the TGA suspended the licence of Pan Pharmaceuticals, Australia's largest manufacturer of herbal, mineral and nutritional supplements at the time, and ordered the immediate withdrawal of hundreds of products it had manufactured. The company was accused of substituting ingredients, manipulating test results and having substandard manufacturing processes. The TGA was first alerted to possible manufacturing problems when dozens of adverse reaction reports were lodged relating to a pharmaceutical motion sickness tablet known as Travacalm. After some investigation, it was found that manufacture of this product was substandard and doses of the active ingredient varied enormously from that stated on the label.

Although the original product in question was a pharmaceutical drug, over the next few months media attention remained focused on natural medicine products, with some commentators seizing the opportunity to call into question the value of CAM in general. As a result, the federal government set up an expert committee to examine the role of complementary medicines in the healthcare system, including the supply of safe, high-quality complementary medicines, quality, use of and timely access to these medicines, and the maintenance of a responsible and viable complementary medicines industry. The terms of reference set for this committee were very broad, not unlike those of the White House Commission on Complementary Medicine. The recommendations made by the expert committee, which covered the regulation of complementary medicines and complementary healthcare practitioners, research and the information and education needs of healthcare practitioners and

TABLE 1.3 LEVELS OF EVIDENCE USED BY THE AUSTRALIAN TGA	
LEVEL OF EVIDENCE	TYPE OF EVIDENCE REQUIRED
High-level scientific evidence	Evidence obtained from a systematic review of all relevant RCTs, without significant variations in the direction or degree of results. *OR* Evidence obtained from at least one properly designed randomised, controlled (preferably multicentre), double-blind trial. It is preferable to have data from at least two trials independent of each other, but in some cases, one large well-conducted trial may suffice (advice should be sought from the TGA in such cases).
Medium-level scientific evidence	Evidence obtained from well-designed controlled trials without randomisation. In the case of a homeopathic preparation, evidence from a well-designed, controlled homeopathic proving. *OR* Evidence obtained from well-designed analytical studies, preferably from more than one centre or research group, including epidemiological cohort and case–control studies. *OR* Evidence obtained from multiple time series with or without intervention, including within-country and between-country population studies. *Note:* In practice, the sources of most medium-level evidence will be peer-reviewed published papers and evidence-based reference texts. However, other evidence that meets the requirements, including independently reviewed unpublished evidence, may also be acceptable. Websites evaluating peer-reviewed published evidence may be a source of suitable evidence.
Low-level or general scientific evidence	Descriptive studies, case series or reports of relevant expert committees. Texts, such as TGA-approved pharmacopoeias or monographs, or other evidence-based reference texts, may be included in this level. Evidence derived from non-human data, such as in vitro studies and animal studies, and non-clinical studies, such as biochemical, nutritional and microbiological studies, does not stand alone and may be used only as supporting evidence.
Traditional evidence	Three or more generations of recorded use of a substance for a specific health-related or medicinal purpose that are documented by at least one of the following: TGA-approved pharmacopoeia TGA-approved monograph three independent written histories of use in the classical or traditional medical literature availability through any country's government public dispensaries authenticated evidence of use from an oral tradition; modern texts that accurately report the classical or traditional literature may be used to support claims.

Source: TGA 2001

consumers to improve community confidence in, and the viability of, the complementary medicines industry, can be viewed online (TGA 2013), along with the government's response to these recommendations.

National Institute of Complementary Medicine

Following recommendations from this committee, and in recognition of the growing importance of complementary medicine in the Australian health system, the Federal Government and NSW state government established the National Institute for Complementary Medicine (NICM) in 2007, based at the University of Western Sydney. Its role is to provide leadership and support for complementary medicine research and the translation of evidence into clinical practice and policy, as well as to build research capacity and foster collaborations among researchers from different disciplines (see NICM 2014). NICM was provided with A$4.8 million for 2 years to achieve these goals. As part of its role in developing Australia's complementary medicine research capacity, NICM established three NICM collaborative research centres after a competitive submission process. Despite significant government support during the first few years of its existence, NICM now has to rely largely on philanthropic and industry support to meet its goals. Under the directorship of Professor Alan Benoussan, NICM now has the largest concentration of complementary medicine research academics in Australia and in 2013 was the only complementary medicine research department to be ranked as 'better than international best practice' by national university criteria (NICM 2014).

The establishment of NICM coincided with the National Health and Medical Research Council (NHMRC) making complementary medicine a priority area for research in 2008 with over A$5 million of funding being allocated to CM research. This encouraged interdisciplinary collaboration, as many established researchers from other disciplines have become involved in funded projects in different areas of CM. Since then, NHMRC funding for complementary medicine research has declined considerably, with many in the complementary medicine research sector frustrated by the relative lack of funding opportunities provided by the government. This is particularly disappointing as complementary medicine continues to enjoy great popularity by the Australian public and both complementary medicine and general practitioners want to use scientific evidence to guide their practice.

The US government has probably made the greatest impact in regards to providing opportunities for complementary medicine research largely due to the establishment of the National Centre for Complementary and Alternative Medicine (NCCAM) as part of the National Institute of Health, with US$121 million in funding allocated in 2008 (NCCAM 2014). Complementary medicine also seems to be on the US policy agenda: the recent Senate Committee on Integrative Care: A Pathway to a Healthier Nation received testimony from leaders of integrative medicine (US Senate Committee 2014).

EVIDENCE-BASED COMPLEMENTARY MEDICINE — THE BURGEONING SCIENTIFIC EVIDENCE BASE

In complementary medicine, as with all medicine, knowledge was originally held by practitioners and based on careful observations collected over time in what we could call today longitudinal case series. Eventually, practitioners wrote down their findings and some produced textbooks, such as the famous Persian academic and physician Avicenna, who listed the traditional uses and actions of many herbs and natural ingredients in the Canon of Medicine (al-Qanun fi al-tib) (Hosseinzadeh & Nassiri-Asl 2013). Education and practice was based on apprenticeships, peer-group discussions and meetings. Now, with the advent of scientific research methodologies, electronic databases and other repositories of information, the amount of available information has exploded. These traditional sources of information guided the practice of medicine for centuries, in the absence of better quality information. Over the last century, scientific evidence and research methodologies in pharmaceutical science have changed dramatically, with much scientific investigation becoming laboratory-based in an effort to identify or create pharmacologically active molecules that may prevent or treat disease. Additionally, large-scale randomised studies have been performed, using larger patient numbers than ever seen before in history. Governments and industry have spent untold billions of dollars in this endeavour, which has helped to uncover many important insights about disease, novel treatments and safety issues.

In comparison to conventional medicine, CM continues to draw on traditional evidence, whereas scientific investigation is still an emerging field. This is largely due to extremely poor government funding or attention and the lack of incentives to attract millions of industry dollars into research. There is also a lack of opportunities for CM practitioners to pursue higher degree education and research, thereby under-utilising a workforce with a genuine interest in this field.

As a result, there are far fewer large-scale multicentre studies investigating complementary medicines and it is simply not possible to expect that many unpatentable CM treatments will have achieved the same level of investigation as pharmaceutical drug therapies. A more realistic expectation is that many treatments remain under-investigated and rely on a series of smaller studies backed up by preclinical tests or traditional evidence to provide a rationale for their use in practice. Importantly, lack of scientific evidence does not indicate negative evidence but may indicate that further research is required. This is particularly imperative when preclinical research and traditional evidence align.

Regardless of these significant hurdles, numerous CM-specific databases have been established in the last decade to capture research findings and disseminate information. There has also been an exponential growth in the number of Medline-indexed articles being published which relate to treatments and recommendations used by CM practitioners. Scientific research conferences, such as those convened by the International Society for Complementary Medicine Research (ISCMR) and the Consortium of Academic Integrative Medicine Centres in North America, stimulate the conduct of research and scientific enquiry, provide opportunities for international collaborations and dissemination of findings to a broader academic audience (ISCMR 2014, Consortium of Academic Integrative Medicine Centers in North America 2014).

Forty-five databases for CM information were identified in a 2010 review published in Health Information and Libraries Journal (Boehm et al 2010). Of these, eleven databases focused on herbal therapies (206,456 entries), nine on Chinese medicine (606,664 entries) and eight contained information about a vast number of CM modalities (780,270 entries). Furthermore, three acupuncture databases were identified (48,000 entries) and two dietary supplement databases (764,894 entries). Fourteen databases originated in the USA, seven from the UK, six from Germany, four from China, three each from Australia and India. The amount of time the databases had been in existence ranged from four to 53 years and English was the main language in 42 of 45 databases, while two were available in German.

WHERE IS THE SCIENTIFIC EVIDENCE CREATED?

IN VITRO STUDIES

In vitro testing generally looks at fundamental biological and biochemical processes and can provide important information about biochemical pathways, as well as pharmacokinetic data. Although in vitro tests are helpful, caution should be taken when extrapolating results from them, as these may not accurately reflect the biological effects seen in the human body.

An example of this is St John's wort. In vitro tests have found that St John's wort inhibits several cytochrome P450 isoenzymes (Budzinski et al 2000, Obach 2000). Clinical tests, however, show that the herb actually has enzyme inducer activity, which is the opposite finding to that of the in vitro tests (Durr et al 2000, Roby et al 2000, Ruschitzka et al 2000).

Anomalies such as this are not restricted to herbal preparations, but have been observed in regular drug-testing. Thus, while in vitro evidence may be useful, the most accurate method for determining biological activity of a substance is to test it directly on humans (Wienkers 2002).

IN VIVO STUDIES

Studies conducted in animals are able to examine dietary manipulations or administration of experimental agents in specific diseases and deficiency states, and to determine the effects on organ systems and physiological functions. These studies allow for a more rigorous investigation of pharmacological activity than in vitro testing. However, in vivo studies can never be more than suggestive when attempting to assess clinical significance because of interspecies differences. Additionally, the relevance of the dose used must be considered, and extrapolation to clinical relevance in humans is not always accurate.

HUMAN STUDIES

Studies conducted in humans range from anecdotal reports or individual case series, to case–control and cohort studies, and randomised placebo-controlled trials of specific interventions for particular diseases, as well as meta-analyses and systematic reviews of RCTs.

Case reports

Case reports supply informative and realistic information within a clinical setting involving the relevant patient population. Rather than providing definitive information, case reports are merely an investigative starting point for determining clinical relevance.

Extrapolating information from case reports presents some unique challenges and may lead to an overestimation of significance when confounders are not identified and considered carefully. Some of the confounding influences that need to be considered include patient factors such as the placebo effect and concomitant illness and/or the administration or interactions of other agents, as well as factors concerning the substance itself, including errors in labelling, herbal substitution, product adulteration and contamination. It is therefore of prime importance that the product be chemically analysed to confirm its contents, especially when an adverse reaction or interaction is reported in this way.

Randomised controlled trials

Randomised controlled trials (RCTs) provide the most solid foundation for clinical decision making. Those trials performed on the population of patients likely to use the therapeutic agent being tested have the highest validity.

The conduct of an RCT is specifically designed to remove possible sources of bias so that the results are as impartial as they can be. The specific nature of RCTs means they cannot answer the general (and non-specific) question as to whether a certain intervention works. An RCT is a specific research tool designed to show whether a specific (active) intervention improves clearly defined outcomes for a specific group of patients suffering from a particular medical condition better than a comparative intervention. These trials are generally defined by four parameters designated by the mnemonic PICO:

P a specifically-defined patient **P**opulation
I a well-defined **I**ntervention
C a suitable **C**omparative intervention (often a placebo)
O specific **O**utcome measures.

Although RCTs provide solid evidence, it must be realised that these trials do not always accurately reflect real life, because they are set in a controlled, experimental context with strict inclusion and exclusion criteria and standardised interventions and outcomes. Furthermore, individual variation still occurs, and it is imperative that a study has sufficient statistical power (largely determined by sample size) to be able to detect a clinically relevant result.

Systematic reviews and meta-analyses

When more than one randomised trial has been conducted to answer a particular question, it is possible to statistically combine their results and perform an analysis using the summary statistics from each study as data points. Such a meta-analysis requires that studies use similar measures. By accumulating the results of multiple studies a meta-analysis can provide greater statistical power and therefore a more accurate representation of the relationship under investigation than the individual studies.

Systematic reviews also provide a way of reviewing and summarising the result of multiple RCTs. These reviews attempt to identify all the individual RCTs conducted for an intervention. After systematically examining the methodology and results of each study, they provide a summary of the results and then reach an overall conclusion. Because systematic reviews rely on the results of RCTs, they must be updated regularly as new RCTs are constantly being published.

THE COCHRANE COLLABORATION

The Cochrane Collaboration is an international, not-for-profit collaborative effort that aims to produce up-to-date systematic reviews of all RCTs for both conventional and complementary therapies. The Cochrane Collaboration takes its name from doctor and humanitarian Archie Cochrane (1906–1988), who strongly advocated the production of critical summaries of research evidence as a way of creating 'evidence-based medicine'.

A systematic review assembles all the RCTs on a given health topic and uses explicit methods to minimise bias (systematic errors) and random error (simple mistakes). It then critically reviews the evidence and summarises the results to determine the safety and effectiveness of an intervention. The Collaboration publishes its systematic reviews quarterly in the Cochrane Library, which are freely available through the National Institute of Clinical Studies.

The Cochrane Consumer Network aims to help healthcare consumers make sense of medical research. Its website provides useful information about research jargon and styles, explains how to tell a good study from a bad one and provides help in finding and understanding health and medical research results.

WHOLE SYSTEM PRACTICE RESEARCH

While it is tantalising to undertake scientific research with one clearly defined treatment, this does not reflect real-world practice. CM practice in particular consists of whole systems or disciplines of health care (such as naturopathy, Western herbal medicine, Ayurvedic medicine and Chinese medicine) which utilise a range of modalities (interventions), including diet and lifestyle recommendations, nutritional supplements, herbal medicines, massage and relaxation techniques. These different interventions are used together after individualised assessment and not usually in singular form.

Clinical research with single entity treatments is very useful, but is also limited because all the key components of the practitioner's management plan working together to create an outcome have not been explored. This is easily understood when considering an obesity case whereby a multi-faceted management plan is required to promote weight-loss and the testing of one component does not demonstrate the full effects of a combined approach.

Assessing the efficacy of whole systems is more complex than assessing the efficacy of single modalities or treatments with RCTs. Realistically, RCTs may have powerful internal validity but poor external validity, meaning they don't necessarily have relevance in real-life practice. Pragmatic trials and observational studies can have good external validity, as individualised treatments can be applied in real world settings to reflect everyday practice. Qualitative research methods, which employ patient interviews and focus groups among other methodologies, provide the opportunity to explore the meaning that patients ascribe to an intervention or system and allow better understanding about whether it is clinically effective for them (Verhoef et al 2005).

ASSESSING EVIDENCE

There are many dimensions to consider when assessing evidence from clinical studies. Thus, it is important not only to consider the level of evidence, but to determine the quality of the study (how well the investigators carried out the particular study design), as well as the certainty (statistical precision) of the results. Furthermore, it is important to assess whether the outcome measures and the size of the observed effect are clinically relevant. More specifically, in regards to herbal medicines, it is important to be certain that the test substance contained the suspected/known active constituents, and with all studies, that inert substances are used as placebos. In regards to nutritional studies, it would be helpful to understand volunteers' baseline status, conduct diet intake surveys alongside the study to help determine the most likely responders and whether dietary intake is a potential confounder and ensure adequate bioavailability of supplements before testing. These dimensions are considered by the NHMRC (2000) and are summarised in Table 1.4.

LIMITATIONS OF EVIDENCE

The rational use of medicines has recently moved towards 'evidence-based care' and recognises that this relies on the conscientious,

TABLE 1.4 DIMENSIONS OF EVIDENCE		
TYPE OF EVIDENCE		**DEFINITION**
Strength of evidence	Level	The study design used, as an indicator of the degree to which bias has been eliminated by design.
	Quality	The methods used by investigators to minimise bias within the study design.
	Statistical precision	The *P*-value or, alternatively, the precision of the estimate of the effect (as indicated by the confidence interval). It reflects the degree of certainty about the existence of a true effect.
Size of effect		The distance of the study estimate from the 'null' value and the inclusion of only clinically important effects in the confidence interval.
Relevance of evidence		The usefulness of the evidence in clinical practice, particularly the appropriateness of the outcome measures.

Source: NHMRC 2000

explicit and judicious use of the *best available evidence* in making decisions about the care of individual patients (Sackett et al 1996). An evidence-based approach recognises different levels of evidence and that the most rigorous types are not always available. In the light of this, many clinical questions cannot be answered by reference to well-conducted trials and require additional information, such as that obtained from experience and historical use.

RCTs have been commonly performed only since the 1950s and are complex and costly processes that require large investments of time and money, as well as access to specialised infrastructure and technical and clinical skills. These hurdles are often even higher for herbs and natural supplements than for pharmaceutical medicines, because the lack of patent protection for these products means there is little incentive for companies to invest millions of dollars in research when they cannot obtain a commercial advantage from the results. The relative lack of funding also means that very few research centres are dedicated to exploring this field and few dedicated researchers with the necessary skills are available. Inevitably, there is a smaller scientific evidence base for herbal and natural substances than for synthetic pharmaceuticals.

There are several other serious limitations to the sole use of existing scientific evidence, as most are based on statistics that aim to produce results that can be applied to populations of people rather than individuals. Additionally, they are based on averages and probabilities, which also fail to account for individual factors. Thus, despite some recent studies that have attempted to address these issues through novel methodological approaches, the application of scientific evidence is often extremely limited when assessing the effectiveness of individualised therapy.

A further problem arises when trying to make decisions about health rather than disease. Most clinical trials are interested in studying movement across the line that separates 'defined disease' from 'average health' (see Fig 1.1, p. 7). While it is possible to define the particular disease in question through reference to objective parameters, such as biochemical and/ or physiological variables, as well as to specific patterns of symptoms, defining optimal health and wellbeing is not as easy. Optimal or enhanced health is a subjective and highly individual state that does not lend itself easily to scientific scrutiny. It is therefore difficult to provide scientific evidence for measures designed to move people from 'average health' towards 'enhanced health' or 'optimal health'.

APPLYING EVIDENCE

Despite the publication of the NHMRC and TGA guidelines for assessing scientific evidence, applying evidence in clinical practice can be extremely complex. Not only does evidence take many different forms, it can also be applied to answer many different types of questions, such as whether a particular therapy works in theory (a question of efficacy) or in clinical practice (a question of effectiveness), as well as whether the use of a therapy is safe and/or cost-effective. Furthermore, there is the question of how a therapy actually works: it is common for evidence to suggest that a therapy is beneficial, even though the mechanism of action remains unknown or, if it is known, for questions about whether the therapy provides clinical benefit to remain unanswered.

The complexity of applying evidence to clinical decision making is compounded by the tens of thousands of studies published every year, with varying degrees of clinical relevance and methodological rigour. Evaluating this evidence can be very confusing, as the results of studies are not always obvious, and their relevance to a particular clinical situation is not always clear. There may also be conflicting results and ongoing controversies in which even the experts disagree. Furthermore, it can be difficult to determine the independence of the information provided, as many influences may be involved: for example, governments, regulatory authorities, commercial interests, such as the pharmaceutical, natural medicine and food industries, disease advocacy and consumer groups, the personal interests of the individual researchers and the editorial board and publication bias.

FINDING EVIDENCE

Obtaining and assessing the available evidence can be both difficult and time-consuming for the busy clinician. Although general medical information is freely available on the internet and via electronic bibliographical databases, fees may need to be paid to access specialised resources for CAM. Additionally, the information available varies considerably in its scope, quality and practicality.

Collections of original research with bibliographical data and abstracts include services such as Medline, Embase, Science Direct and ProQuest. Other databases, such as Herbmed, MicroMedex and the Natural Medicines Comprehensive Database, provide summaries of current research for numerous herbal and natural medicines. Other collections, such as the Cochrane Collaboration Library, attempt to produce the most authoritative guide to medical research by providing only systematic reviews of RCTs.

Although databases that provide references to original research are extremely useful, there is a definite need for more summarised and critically reviewed material. This need is met to a certain extent by the publication of review articles in textbooks such as the German Commission E Monographs, or by commercially available databases, such as Integrative Medicine Gateway, Natural Medicines Comprehensive Database and the Natural Standard Database.

MISLEADING HEADLINES

Unfortunately, many health professionals do not have ready access to research papers or are too busy to be able to read through full reports and therefore rely on short summaries to provide information. As in the popular press, the medical press is prone to creating sensational headlines to attract interest, but this can lead to inaccurate assumptions. A good example is the case of an apparent coma state brought on by the combination of the herbal medicine kava kava and the benzodiazepine alprazolam. The case was reported with the headline 'Coma from the health food store: interaction between kava and alprazolam' (Almeida & Grimsley 1996). A closer look at the report reveals that the patient described was lethargic and disoriented, but at no time comatose. Additionally, he was also taking cimetidine, a CYP450 inhibitor that can affect alprazolam metabolism, resulting in raised serum levels and symptoms of lethargy. An interaction with kava kava is unlikely.

FACTORS TO CONSIDER IN DECISION MAKING

As previously discussed, scientific evidence provides useful and important information; however, it must be combined with several other important factors in clinical practice to be truly effective for the individual patient. An expanded

NPS REVIEW OF COMPLEMENTARY MEDICINE INFORMATION RESOURCES

In 2008 the National Prescribing Service (NPS) in Australia commissioned a review of complementary medicine information resources. It aimed to identify high-quality resources that could be recommended for use by Australian health professionals and consumers. A list of 52 information resources from reputable sources was tested against broad criteria encompassing currency, coverage, transparency and content quality to produce a short list of 26 electronic resources. These final resources were evaluated for technical quality, content quality and clinical utility, producing a final list of nine resources.

The second edition of this book was included in the final list of highest-quality resources, a feat of which the authors are particularly proud, as it was the only resource not to be linked to an online database. A summary of the report can be obtained from the NPS website.

approach, often discussed as 'evidence-based patient-centred care', is becoming more widely adopted, the chief principles of which are in unison with the integrative medicine approach to incorporating evidence into clinical practice. The key principles may be summarised by the PEACE mnemonic:

P acknowledgment and respect for the **P**ersonal preferences of both the practitioner and the patient

E the strength of the available scientific **E**vidence

A the range of possible **A**lternatives

C the associated **C**osts and risks versus the potential benefits of a proposed treatment

E aspects of **E**xpedience, such as availability, accessibility and immediacy of treatment.

It is easy to become overwhelmed when reviewing the vast range of therapeutic options available, the complexities of accessing and appraising the different types of scientific evidence and the other factors that must be considered when making choices about treatment options. This evidence-based book is an attempt to provide some guidance through the current maze of information and evidence. Certainly, more information is needed: in an ideal world every therapy would have clear evidence to support or refute its use in different conditions, and this information would be freely available and without inherent bias. However, that time is still far away, and clinical decision making remains both a subtle art and an inexact science, where there is always room for more information, research and debate.

REFERENCES

ABS (Australian Bureau of Statistics). National Health Survey 2004–05. ABS cat no. 4364. Available: http://www.ausstats.abs.gov.au/ 10 June 2014.

ABS (Australian Bureau of Statistics). Census of Population and Housing. Australian Social Trends, 2008. ABS cat no 4102. Available: http://www.abs.gov.au/ 10 June 2014.

Almeida JC, Grimsley EW. Coma from the health food store: interaction between kava and alprazolam. Ann Intern Med 125.11 (1996): 940–941.

AMSA (Australian Medical Students Association). The orange book: The advocacy platform of the Australian Medical Students Association (2014). Available: http://media.amsa.org.au.s3.amazonaws.com/policy/orange_book/Orange_book_1ed_Dec2013.pdf 9 June 2014.

Australasian Integrative Medicine Association (AIMA). website. Available: http://www.aima.net.nz/about-aima/ 9 June 2014.

Australian Medical Council. Undergraduate medical education and unorthodox medical practice, unpublished discussion paper, 1999.

Australian Traditional Medicine Society (ATMS). Professor Dwyer's ignorance is on display again (2012). Available: http://www.atms.com.au/professor-dwyers-ignorance-on-display-again/ 9 June 2014.

Awang DV. Siberian ginseng toxicity may be case of mistaken identity. Can Med Assoc J 155.9 (1996): 1237.

Boehm K, Raak C, Vollmar HC, Ostermann T. An overview of 45 published database resources for complementary and alternative medicine. Health Info Libr J 27.2 (2010): 93–105.

Braun L. The integration of complementary medicine in Victorian hospitals — a focus on surgery and safety (2007) RMIT. PhD thesis.

Braun LA, Spitzer O, Tiralongo E, Wilkinson JM et al. The prevalence and experience of Australian naturopaths and Western herbalists working within community pharmacies. BMC Complement Altern Med 11.41(2011).

Braun LA, Tiralongo E, Wilkinson JM et al. Perceptions, use and attitudes of pharmacy customers on complementary medicines and pharmacy practice. BMC Complement Altern Med 10.38 (2010).

Brownie, S. Predictors of dietary and health supplement use in older Australians. Aust J Adv Nurs 23.3 (2006): 26–32.

Budzinski JW et al. An in vitro evaluation of human cytochrome P450 3A4 inhibition by selected commercial herbal extracts and tinctures. Phytomedicine 7.4 (2000): 273–282.

Cochrane Collaboration 2014. Available: http://www.cochrane.org 12 June 2014.

Cochrane Consumer Network 2014. Available: http://consumers.cochrane.org/ 12 June 2014.

Cohen MM, Penman S, Pirotta M et al. The integration of complementary therapies in Australian general practice: Results of a national survey. J Altern Complement Med 11.6 (2005): 995–1004.

Consortium of Academic Integrative Medicine Centers in North America. Website (2014) Available: http://www.imconsortium.org/

Duke K. A century of CAM in New Zealand: a struggle for recognition. Complement Ther Clin Pract 11.1 (2005): 11–116.

Durr D et al. St John's wort induces intestinal P-glycoprotein/MDR1 and intestinal and hepatic CYP3A4. Clin Pharmacol Ther 68.6 (2000): 598–604.

Eisenberg DM et al. Unconventional medicine in the United States. Prevalence, costs, and patterns of use. N Engl J Med 328.4 (1993): 246–252.

Eisenberg DM et al. Trends in alternative medicine use in the United States, 1990–1997: results of a follow-up national survey. JAMA 280.18 (1998): 1569–1575.

Flatt J. Critical discourse analysis of rhetoric against complementary medicine. Creative Approaches to Research 6.2 (2013): 57–70.

Gilbey A. Ninety years' growth of New Zealand complementary and alternative medicine. NZ Med J 122.1291(2009): 111–113.

Hadley CM. Complementary medicine and the general practitioner: a survey of general practitioners in the Wellington area. NZ Med J 101.857 (1988): 766–768.

Hall KCB. Complementary therapies and the general practitioner: a survey of Perth GPs. Aust Fam Physician 29.6 (2000): 602–606.

Hosseinzadeh H, Nassiri-Asl M. Avicenna's (Ibn Sina) the Canon of Medicine and saffron (Crocus sativus): a review. Phytother Res 27.4(2013): 475–483.

Huang WF et al. Adulteration by synthetic therapeutic substances of traditional Chinese medicines in Taiwan. J Clin Pharmacol 37.4 (1997): 344–350.

ISCMR (International Society for Complementary Medicine Research. Website. (2014) Available: http://www.iscmr.org/ 10 June 2014.

Komesaroff P. Complementary vs western medicine — both have a role in universities. Available: http://theconversation.com/complementary-vs-western-medicine-both-have-a-role-in-universities-8232 9 June 2014.

Komesaroff PA, Moore A, Kerridge IH. Medicine and science must oppose intolerance and censorship. Med J Aust 197.2 (2012): 82–83.

MACCAH (Ministerial Advisory Committee on Complementary and Alternative Health). Complementary and alternative health care in New Zealand: Advice to the Minister of Health. Wellington: MACCAM, 2004. Available: http://www.newhealth.govt.nz/maccah.htm 3 August 2006.

MacLennan AWD & Taylor A. The escalating cost and prevalence of alternative medicine. Prev Med 35.2 (2002): 166–173.

MacLennan AH et al. The continuing use of complementary and alternative medicine in South Australia: costs and beliefs in 2004. Med J Aust 184.1 (2006): 27–31.

MacLennan AH, Myers SP & Taylor AW. The continuing use of complementary and alternative medicine in South Australia: costs and beliefs in 2004. Med J Aust 184.1 (2006): 27–31.

MacLennan A & Morrison R. Tertiary education institutions should not offer pseudoscientific medical courses. Med J Aust 196.4 (2012): 225–226.

Medical Council of New Zealand. Statement on complementary and alternative medicine. Available: http://www.mcnz.org.nz/assets/News-and-Publications/Statements/Complementary-and-alternative-medicine.pdf 9 June 2014.

Myers S P, Xue CC, Cohen MM, et al. The legitimacy of academic complementary medicine. Med J Aust, 197.2 (2012): 69–70.

NCCAM (National Center for Complementary and Alternative Medicine). website (2014) Available: http://nccam.nih.gov/ 10 June 2014.

National Herbalists Association of Australia. (2012). Response to Friends of Science in Medicine. Available: http://www.nhaa.org.au/index.php?option=com_content&view=article&id=481:response-to-friends-of-science-in-medicine&catid=107:nhaa-news&Itemid=273[not online]

National Institute of Clinical Studies website. Available: www.nicsl.com.au/cochrane/index.asp 12 June 2014.

NICM (The National Institute of Complementary Medicine) website. (2014) Available: http://www.nicm.edu.au/ 10 June 2014

National Institutes of Health Panel on Definition and Description. Defining and describing complementary and alternative medicine. Altern Ther Health Med 3.2 (1997): 49–57.

NHMRC (National Health and Medical Research Council). A guide to the development, implementation and evaluation of clinical practice guidelines. NHMRC, Canberra (1999).

NHMRC (National Health and Medical Research Council). How to use the evidence: assessment and application of scientific evidence. NHMRC, Canberra (2000).

National Prescribing Service (NPS). MedicineWise. 2014. Available: www.nps.org.au 12 June 2014.

Obach RS. Inhibition of human cytochrome P450 enzymes by constituents of St John's Wort, an herbal preparation used in the treatment of depression. J Pharmacol Exp Ther 294.1 (2000): 88–95.

Pirotta MC et al. Complementary therapies: have they become mainstream in general practice? Med J Aust 172 (2000): 105–109.

Pledger MJ, Cumming J, Burnett M. Health service use amongst users of complementary and alternative medicine. NZ Med J 123.1312 (2010): 26–35.

RACGP/AIMA (Royal Australian College of General Practitioners & Australasian Integrative Medicine Association). RACGP/AIMA joint position statement on complementary medicine (2005). Available: www.racgp.org.au

Roby CA et al. St John's wort: effect on CYP3A4 activity. Clin Pharmacol Ther 67.5 (2000): 451–457.

Ruschitzka F et al. Acute heart transplant rejection due to Saint John's wort. Lancet 355.9203 (2000): 548–549.

Sackett DLR et al. Evidence based medicine: what it is and what it isn't. BMJ 312.7023 (1996): 71–72.

Statistics New Zealand. Census 2006. Available: http://www.stats.govt.nz/searchresults.aspx?q=occupations 9 June 2014

Statistics New Zealand. Census 2013. Available:
http://www.stats.govt.nz/searchresults.aspx?q=occupations
9 June 2014

TGA (Therapeutic Goods Administration). Guidelines for levels and kinds
of evidence to support indications and claims for non-registrable
medicines including complementary medicines, and other listable
medicines. (2001) TGA, Canberra.

TGA (Therapeutic Goods Administration). Australian regulatory guidelines
for complementary medicines. (2013) Available http://www.tga.gov.au/
industry/cm-argcm.htm#.U5a9Xyh7p6Y 10 June 2014.

US Senate Committee (US Senate Committee on Health, Education,
Labor & Pensions). Integrative care: A pathway to a healthier nation.

Available: http://www.help.senate.gov/hearings/hearing/?id=03629575-
0924-cb2e-13cb-68a8065ababb 9 June 2014.

Verhoef MJ, Lewith G, Ritenbaugh C, et al. Complementary and
alternative medicine whole systems research: beyond identification of
inadequacies of the RCT. Complement Ther Med, 13.3 (2005):
206–212.

Wienkers LC. Factors confounding the successful extrapolation of in vitro
CYP3A inhibition information to the in vivo condition. Eur J Pharm
Sci 15.3 (2002): 239–242.

Xue CC et al. Complementary and alternative medicine use in Australia:
a national population-based survey. J Altern Complement Med 13.6
(2007): 643–650.

CHAPTER 2

INTRODUCTION TO HERBAL MEDICINE

Herbal medicine, also known as phytomedicine, can be broadly defined as both the science and the art of using botanical medicines to prevent and treat illness, and the study and investigation of these medicines. The term 'phytotherapy' is used to describe the therapeutic application of herbal medicines and was first coined by the French physician Henri Leclerc (1870–1955), who published numerous essays on the use of medicinal plants (Weiss 1988).

Phytotherapy can be considered one of the oldest forms of medicine. Since the dawn of time, plants have been used by people of all races, religions and cultures to sustain life and alter the course of disease. Over this time, the medicinal use of plants has evolved along two parallel paths, with the comparatively recent evolution of modern medicine. One path involves the accumulation of empirical knowledge over centuries. Gathered through careful observation of nature and disease, and from cumulative experiences of informed trial and error, the empirical knowledge base for herbal medicines is large and diverse. For example, the *Rig veda*, a text from India, and the Egyptian papyri *Antiquarium* both date from 3000 BC and contain extensive lists of medicinal plants used to treat illness (Berman et al 1999). In South America, the use of herbal medicine has also been documented, such as in the *Badianus* manuscript, a text written by the Aztecs (Walcott 1940). Their use of herbs, such as datura and passionflower, has been adopted in modern European and American pharmacopoeias. Native Americans were particularly knowledgeable about the botanical medicines in their environment. It has been estimated that more than 200 medicines used by one or more Indian nations have been incorporated into the US Pharmacopoeia or National Formulary (Vogel 1970).

Two of the most prominent historical figures in European herbal medicine were Dioscorides and Galen, who were physicians in ancient Greece. Dioscorides was a Greek army surgeon in the service of the Roman emperor Nero (54–68 AD). He is best known for his *De materia medica*, which describes more than 600 herbs and their uses. Today this work is considered to be the first book ever written about medical botany as an applied science. Galen (131–201 AD) not only wrote several dozen books on pharmacy, but also developed an elaborate system of herbal polypharmacy in which herbal combinations were devised to produce more specific results. The modern term 'galenicals' is still used to describe herbal simples.

Alongside the 'empirical knowledge' approach a second path developed, which involved a more theoretical and formalised method of diagnosis and treatment. The resulting 'healthcare' systems were complex and often used herbal medicines as an important part of a more comprehensive approach to treatment that also included dietary control, lifestyle changes and spiritual practice. This approach reached its peak in the East with traditional Chinese medicine and Ayurvedic medicine in India.

Although contemporary clinical practice of herbal medicine still relies heavily on traditional wisdom, this knowledge is now being re-examined with the aid of modern analytical methods and scientific methodology. The use of science to establish an evidence base in modern healthcare is changing the way herbalism is being practised and who is using herbs. An emphasis on phytochemistry and an assessment of risk are inherent features of contemporary research into herbs. While these are important gains in knowledge about the actions and uses of herbs, there is an accompanying shift in the practice of herbal medicine, with less emphasis on the importance of traditional and empirical knowledge, which in time may lead to a loss of the paradigm of holistic and individualised care (Evans 2008). Whether this improves patient outcomes remains to be seen.

HERBS, DRUGS AND PHYTOCHEMICALS

Most pharmaceutical medicines contain a single, highly purified, often artificially produced substance that has a well-known (and occasionally specifically designed) chemical structure that can be patented and owned by the company that developed it. The dosage of these chemicals can also be precisely calculated down to the microgram and can usually be characterised by a very clear pharmacokinetic profile. Additionally, pharmaceutical drugs tend to have a generally agreed upon mechanism of action and series of indications that guide their use within the Western medical model.

As most of these drugs do not exist in nature, they must go through extensive testing to ensure efficacy and safety. New drugs are assessed in test-tube and animal studies for their potential to cause cancer, fetal malformations and other toxic effects, and are ultimately tested on humans to further define the safety profile, pharmacokinetics and drug effectiveness in a targeted disease (Wierenga & Eaton 2003). This process is very costly and requires the application of highly specialised knowledge and infrastructure, as well as many years of concentrated effort. It is estimated that the development of a new drug requires the investment of approximately US$800 million, but it is also extremely lucrative (Di Masi & Grabowski 2003).

PHARMACOGNOSY

In 2001 and 2002, approximately one-quarter of the best-selling drugs worldwide were natural products or derived from natural products. Research on natural products further accounted for approximately 48% of the new chemical entities reported from 1981 to 2002.

Modern drug discovery from medicinal plants has evolved to become a sophisticated process that includes numerous fields of enquiry and various methods of analysis. Typically, the process begins with a botanist, ethnobotanist, ethnopharmacologist or plant ecologist collecting and identifying plants based on the biological activity suggested by their traditional use. Additionally, plants are randomly selected for inclusion in screening programs based on molecular targets identified through the human genome project (Balunas & Kinghorn 2005).

Pharmacognosy is the term used to refer to the study of botanical supplements and herbal remedies, as well as to the search for single-compound drugs from plants. Increasingly, pharmaceutical medicines and preclinical research into herbal medicines are focused on identifying suitable chemical entities that may form the basis for novel treatments (Balunas & Kinghorn 2005).

CHEMICAL COMPLEXITY

In contrast to pharmaceutical drugs, which are based on single molecules that may or may not be derived from natural substances, herbal medicines are chemically complex and may contain many hundreds or even thousands of different 'phytochemicals', including various macro- and micro-nutrients such as fats, carbohydrates and proteins, enzymes, vitamins and minerals. A group of important secondary metabolites are also present, which are generally chemicals used to defend against herbivores, pathogens, insect attack and microbial decomposition, or which are produced in response to injury or infection, or used for signalling and growth regulation. It is these compounds, such as tannins, isoflavones, saponins, flavonoids, glycosides, coumarins, bitters, phyto-oestrogens etc, that are often responsible for the therapeutic properties of herbal medicines (Mills & Bone 2001).

As the secondary metabolites largely dictate a herb's pharmacological nature, a knowledge of herbal chemistry is essential to understand a herb's use and provide valuable insight into its clinical effects. It is sometimes tempting to take the modern reductionist approach and predict the pharmacological activity of a herbal medicine from an understanding of the effects of one key constituent or chemical group; however, this is unlikely to be entirely accurate. In practice, the overall pharmacological activity and safety of each herb is the result of the interaction of numerous constituents, some of which have demonstrated pharmacological effects, rather than the effect of a single active ingredient.

An example of this is the herb *Paullinia cupana*, commonly known as guarana. As there are limited clinical studies on guarana, it is often reported that the herb owes its pharmacological activity to one key constituent, caffeine, which may be present in concentrations as high as 10%. Studies referring to the isolate caffeine provide some clues about the effects of guarana, but are not entirely accurate, as other important constituents are also present in the remaining 90%. This has been borne out recently in clinical studies of low-caffeine-containing guarana preparations, which still demonstrated significant effects on cognitive function.

Because of the range of phytochemicals present in plants, herbal medicines often include many different active substances with different pharmacokinetics that work at different sites with different mechanisms of action. Herbal medicines therefore potentially have multiple pharmacological actions and many different clinical indications. Furthermore, in addition to the active ingredients, herbs may also contain substances that act to inhibit or promote the active properties, and/or potential unwanted side effects of the active agents. Thus, although specific components may not be active themselves, they may influence the activity of other components by altering their solubility, absorption, distribution or half-life.

For instance, berberine is a constituent of herbs such as goldenseal and barberry and exhibits numerous activities in vitro; however,

in vivo, it has poor bioavailability (Pan et al 2002). Berberine has been shown to upregulate the expression and function of the drug transporter P-glycoprotein (P-gp) (Lin et al 1999), thereby reducing the absorption of P-gp substrates. Studies with the P-gp inhibitor cyclosporin have shown that it increases berberine absorption six-fold, as it counteracts the inducing effect of berberine (Pan et al 2002). P-gp inhibitors are also found in nature, such as the virtually ubiquitous quercetin, and when they are present in the same herb competing effects on P-gp expression and function will occur.

The herb St John's wort provides yet another example. The extraction method used in Germany in the product's commercial manufacture was modified in the late 1990s, resulting in higher concentrations of hyperforin than previously obtained (Madabushi et al 2006). Since then, numerous reports and studies have identified pharmacokinetic drug interactions with St John's wort, based on its ability to induce cytochromes and P-gp. It is now well established that hyperforin is the key constituent responsible for these unwanted effects, and St John's wort preparations manufactured with this newer extraction method, such as LI 160, can put people at risk of interactions. Meanwhile, studies with low-hyperforin preparations, such as Ze117, have found that it fails to induce the same interactions (Madabushi et al 2006). Unfortunately, this distinction between St John's wort preparations is not well known, and many references and texts fail to mention this important point.

As these examples and many others in this book demonstrate, each herb is chemically complex and produces a pharmacological effect based on the total sum of actions produced by a myriad of constituents that may be acting in synergy. This complexity complicates the ability to test herbal medicines as they are most commonly used (that is, in their more natural states) and in combination with other herbal medicines.

SYNERGISTIC INTERACTIONS

The concept of synergistic interactions is another fundamental difference between herbs and drugs and explains how a single herb may have a number of seemingly unrelated mechanisms of actions and be indicated for a variety of conditions. Intra-herbal interactions between active and apparently non-active constituents also mean that tests performed with single, isolated constituents will not accurately represent the actions and safety of the entire herbal medicine. As such, these tests provide limited information. By and large, it is suspected that it is the intra-herbal interactions that give herbs a broad therapeutic range and very good tolerability.

St John's wort, popularised as a useful treatment for depression, is also an excellent example of intra-herbal interaction. It contains many different constituents, such as hypericin and pseudohypericin, flavonoids such as quercetin and rutin, vitamins C and A, phenolics such as hyperforin, sterols and an essential oil. Although many of the herb's pharmacological activities appear to be attributable to hypericin and hyperforin, it is now known that the flavonoid content also contributes to its antidepressant activity. In other words, the antidepressant effects identified for isolated hypericin or hyperforin are greater when the whole herb is used.

In practice, synergistic interactions are used in another important way — herbal polypharmacy. This is the combining of different herbal medicines within the same treatment for a more specific outcome, and is similar to the method Galen described centuries ago. In Chinese medicine the concept of synergistic interactions has reached a great level of sophistication, with Chinese formulas containing as many as 20 different herbs. In that system, the herb possessing the primary action of the formula is considered the 'emperor herb', while 'minister herbs' support the primary action and 'assistant herbs' modify the formula according to the needs of the individual. Finally 'messenger herbs' are used to aid absorption or reduce side effects of the formula. The practice is also common in Ayurvedic medicine and, in fact, in all traditional systems of herbal practice. Although it may be common in conventional medicine to give certain drugs specifically to reduce the side effects of other drugs, such as the administration of antiemetics and laxatives together with opiates, generally the giving of multiple drugs in combination is discouraged. In contrast, in herbal medicine this practice is often considered essential to provide both safety and the best effects.

KEY CONSTITUENT GROUPS

To better understand a herb's mechanisms of action, pharmacokinetics, pharmacodynamics, interactions and side effects, a basic knowledge of the key constituent groups is helpful. Here is a brief outline of the main constituent groups found in popular herbal medicines.

FLAVONOIDS

Flavonoids are plant pigments that are largely responsible for the colour of flowers, fruits and berries. There are many different types of flavonoids, including flavones, flavonols, isoflavones and flavins. They are generally antiinflammatory, antioxidant and anti-allergic, and may decrease capillary fragility. Herbs that are well known for their flavonoid content are ginkgo (*Ginkgo biloba*), St Mary's thistle (*Silybum marianum*) and calendula (*Calendula officinale*).

Flavanols may be further oxidised to yield anthrocyanins. These bluish/purplish compounds contribute to the colour of blueberries and red grapes. They are greatly revered for their antioxidant and anti-inflammatory properties.

TANNINS

Tannins are astringent and often taste bitter. They can be divided into two groups, hydrolysable tannins and non-hydrolysable tannins (sometimes called condensed tannins or proanthocyanidins). Tannins have the ability to stabilise proteins and were used historically to tan or preserve animal hides. In herbal medicine, tannins are valued for their ability to dry and tone tissue. Some plants with appreciable levels of tannins include witch hazel (*Hamamelis virginiana*), oak bark (*Quercus robor*) and lady's mantle (*Alchemilla vulgaris*).

COUMARINS

Coumarins have a limited distribution in plants and may be either naturally present or synthesised by the plant in response to a bacteria or fungus (Heinrich et al 2004). They are a heterogeneous group, and thus different compounds have various effects on the body. For example, some coumarins demonstrate antispasmodic activity (for example, scopeletin from *Viburnum* spp), others anticoagulant activity (for example dicoumarol from sweet clover), and others anti-oedema effects (for example, coumarins from clivers and red clover).

ALKALOIDS

Alkaloids are so named for their alkaline properties. This group of phytochemicals has contributed much to modern medicine, and more than 10,000 have been isolated (Evans 2002). Consequently, they are perhaps the best-known constituent group. There are many different types of alkaloids with many different therapeutic properties; however, they commonly contain nitrogen, usually in a heterocyclic ring. Below is a brief outline of the main subgroups:

- **Pyridine, piperidine & pyrrolizidine alkaloids.** Nicotine (*Nicotiana tabacum*) is perhaps the best-known example of the pyridine class. The very poisonous piperidine alkaloid coniine is isolated from hemlock (*Conium maculatum*) and the pyrrolizidine alkaloid senecionine is the reason comfrey (*Symphytum officinale*) was withdrawn from sale in Australia due to concerns over hepatotoxicity.

- **Phenylalkylamine alkaloids.** This group of alkaloids differ in that nitrogen is not part of the heterocyclic ring. The most commonly known example is ephedrine, a central nervous system stimulant, bronchodilator and vasoconstrictive agent from *Ephedra sinica*.

- **Quinoline alkaloids.** The antimalarial quinine from *Cinchona* spp belongs in this category. Quinine was used in the synthetic production of many antimalarial drugs against *Plasmodium falciparum*. Interestingly, *Plasmodium* has become resistant to the synthesised medications such as chloroquinine, but not to naturally occurring quinine (Heinrich et al 2004).

- **Isoquinoline alkaloids.** Opium, from *Papaver somniferum*, contains over 30 alkaloids, including morphine, codeine, thebaine, papaverine and noscapine. Morphine is well known for its pain-relieving effects. Other examples are the protoberberines, consisting of berberine, berbamine and hydrastine. Golden seal (*Hydrastis canadensis*) contains berberine and hydrastine; barberry (*Berberis vulgaris*) contains berberine and berbamine; and oregon mountain grape (*Mahonia aquifolium*) contains all three. They are strongly antibacterial.

- **Indole alkaloids.** Examples include reserpine from *Rauwolfia serpentina*, which in the past has been used for hypertension; however, its use has largely been discontinued due to toxic side effects. The anti-cancer agents vincristine and vinblastine, from *Cantharanthus roseus*, are other notable examples.

- **Tropane alkaloids.** Hyoscyamine, from *Atropa belladonna*, is an anticholinergic agent. It has also been used to dilate the pupil of the eye for optical examinations.

- **Xanthine alkaloids.** These are the most widely known and used alkaloids, and include caffeine from tea (*Camellia sinensis*), coffee (*Coffea arabica*) and chocolate (*Theobroma cacao*), which is known to be beneficial to health in small amounts and detrimental in large amounts. Cocoa also contains theobromine and tea contains theophylline and theobromine, both of which are purine alkaloids.

TERPENES

Terpenes are widespread in the plant kingdom. There are many different types:

- **Monoterpene hydrocarbons.** Monoterpenes have a 10-carbon structure. They are major constituents of volatile oils and often have antimicrobial properties. Examples include limonene (lemon, caraway, peppermint and thyme) and alpha-pinene (rosemary, lemon, fennel and eucalyptus).

- **Sesquiterpene hydrocarbons.** Sesquiterpenes have a 15-carbon structure. They are also major constituents of volatile oils and are broadly antimicrobial and insecticidal. Subclasses include alcohols (linalool from lavender, menthol from peppermint), phenols (linalool from lavender), phenols (thymol from thyme, carvacrol from oregano), aldehydes (citronella from citronella), ketones (menthone from peppermint, thujone from wormwood), ethers (anethole from fennel) and esters (methyl salicylate from wintergreen).

- **Diterpene hydrocarbons.** Diterpenes have on average a 20-carbon structure and so are much denser molecules, with higher boiling points, than other hydrocarbons. They are often associated with volatile oils (oleoresins), gums (gum-resins) or with both (oleo-gum-resins) (Evans 2002). Examples include guaiacum resin obtained from *Guaiacum officinale* and gum-resins from frankincense (*Boswellia serrata*).

GLYCOSIDES

Glycosides are composed of two parts: the glycone (sugar molecule) and the aglycone (non-sugar molecule). The aglycone may be a terpene, a flavonoid or potentially any other natural compound (Heinrich et al 2004). Below are the most common classes:

- **Triterpene glycosides.** These may also be called saponins. They are a diverse group and exert many different effects on the human body. Depending on their structure, they may be anti-inflammatory (aescin from horse chestnut) or expectorant (senegin from snakeroot), or may demonstrate steroidal effects (glycyrrhetic acid from licorice, diosgenin from wild yam).

- **Glucosinolates.** Also called mustard oil glycosides, these important compounds are found in the Brassicaceae family of vegetables, such as broccoli, mustard and horseradish. They are topically mildly irritant and have digestive, circulatory and anticancer properties when ingested.

- **Cardiac glycosides.** These glycosides have a specific action on heart muscle. They are steroidal in structure and are related to steroidal saponins and phytosterols. A number of herbs contain cardioactive glycosides, including lily of the valley (*Convallaria majus*) and foxglove (*Digitalis* spp). Digoxin and digitoxin are naturally occurring compounds in digitalis, and digoxin is commonly used in drug form for heart failure.

- **Anthraquinone glycosides.** These compounds have osmotic and stimulant effects in the lower bowel and therefore have laxative properties. Examples of herbs that contain these compounds include cascara (*Rhamnus purshiana*), senna (*Cassia senna*), aloe (*Aloe vera*) and rhubarb root (*Rheum palmatum*).

CHEMOTHERAPEUTICS VERSUS HERBALISM

In practice, drugs and herbs are prescribed quite differently. Drug prescription is often based on the results obtained from clinical trials that measure the effects in populations and use averages to predict outcomes. Investigation and usage is based on the Western medical model and is replicated in almost identical ways by each practitioner who uses this system. By

---

> **CLINICAL NOTE — GERMAN COMMISSION E**
>
> The German Commission E is a German government regulatory agency composed of scientists, pharmacists, toxicologists, physicians and herbalists. It has produced a series of monographs based on the available scientific evidence, as well as evidence from traditional use, case studies and the experience of modern herbalists. These monographs are considered to provide authoritative information on herbs, as well as approved indications, contraindications, side effects, interactions, doses, and so on.

contrast, the same herb may be understood and prescribed in distinctly different ways by different practitioners, depending on the prescribing system being used, with an emphasis on individual prescribing. For example, in Chinese medicine, a herb such as andrographis (*Andrographis paniculata*) is used to clear 'heat' from the blood, because it is considered to be a 'cold' herb, whereas in Western herbalism, it is used to boost immune function and treat the common cold. Further, traditional herbal practice entails combining a number of herbs into a prescription that is tailored to the individual. This customised approach to herbal prescribing is guided by the underpinning paradigm of herbal practice — holism and vitalism. This philosophical basis is lost when herbs are viewed as vehicles for one or two active components or with the increasing cultural emphasis on self-prescribing.

Not only are herbs described and prescribed differently by different medical systems, the properties of herbal medicines are often defined using unique terms not found in drug pharmacology. These properties have traditionally been classified into herbal actions. Thus herbs that relax the gastrointestinal tract and reduce flatulence may be described as carminatives, or those that stimulate bile flow as cholagogues. These actions may be due to particular chemical constituent groups found within the herb or some other property of the herb. Throughout this book, terms specific to herbal medicine and not generally used in drug pharmacology are explained in *Clinical notes*.

In contrast to pharmaceutical medicine, the evidence available to support herbal medicines originally comes from traditional sources, and scientific investigation has only recently been added. Over the past two to three decades there has been an exponential increase in the amount of scientific research being conducted on herbal medicines, chiefly in Europe and Asia, where there are fewer political, economic and regulatory reasons for rejecting traditional medicines. For some herbs there is now sufficient clinical trial evidence to enable meta-analyses to be performed. For many of the popular herbs available over the counter, clinical trial evidence is now being published that can be used to further clarify and determine their place in practice. For others, research may still be in its infancy, with only in vitro testing or testing in experimental models having been conducted so far. Although a general lack of resources, infrastructure, government funding and financial incentive for companies to invest in non-patentable medicines has slowed down investigation, great public popularity continues to fuel further study. Despite the limitations of randomised controlled trials in evaluating complex interventions characterised by traditional herbal practice (Evans 2008), data collections such as the German Commission E monographs are widely cited as gold-standard references, because they use a combination of traditional and scientific evidence to interpret data and make recommendations.

PRODUCT VARIATION AND STANDARDISATION

The chemical complexity of herbal medicines is compounded by the variation that occurs in their production, which starts with the quality of the original plant material. This may be influenced by the identification methods used (and any misidentification or contamination), genetic variability in the original cultivar and the growing conditions, including the soil type, geographical location, aspect, altitude and climate. Other factors further modify a herb's purity and quality, such as growing techniques (for example, wild harvesting, or organic or conventional farming methods), the timing and method of harvesting, drying, processing and storage, as well as the extraction techniques and solvents used. There are therefore numerous factors that determine the compositional profile of a given herbal extract, and attempts to ensure

batch-to-batch consistency are confounded by the inherent chemical complexity of the herb and the natural variations that occur.

As a consequence, clinical research is never simply done on a herb itself. Rather, research must be done on a particular herbal preparation at a specific dose, and the evidence for the efficacy of herbal preparations must be related back to the preparation used in the research. The results of clinical trials are therefore only relevant to the specific herbal preparation that has been tested, at the specific dosage, dose form and route of administration used in the actual trial and cannot necessarily be used to support the use of other extracts or doses of the same herb. The challenge for manufacturers and clinicians, then, is to reproduce a particular preparation, administer it in the proven doses and achieve the expected result. More commonly in practice, herbs are used in variable ways, with different preparations, at a range of doses, and in combination with other herbs or treatments. It is thus hard to guarantee outcomes, either beneficial or adverse, based solely on controlled clinical trials.

STANDARDISATION

Efforts to ensure batch-to-batch reproducibility of herbal medicines have generated a great deal of controversy, particularly involving the term 'standardisation' or the production of so-called standardised extracts. The lack of an agreed definition and the variety of meanings attributed to these terms make them confusing to both consumers and health professionals. Yet they are still used as the basis for product labelling and promotion, where they are used by suppliers for marketing purposes to imply quality, safety or efficacy.

A commonly used (and some may say abused) definition of the term 'standardised' in relation to herbal extracts relies on measuring a specified concentration of an identified constituent or class of constituents known as 'markers'. Markers are usually stable components of a herb that can easily be identified, analysed and measured, but they may or may not be pharmacologically active. An example of this is seen with *Ginkgo biloba*, which is standardised to contain 24% flavonoid glycosides and 6% terpenoids in commercial herbal products, although the active constituents are largely unknown. Sophisticated laboratory techniques are now used to perform this analysis and measurement. Methods include chromatographic techniques, such as thin layer chromatography and high-performance liquid chromatography, both of which provide a visual characterisation of the presence of different chemical constituents, including 'marker' substances in the herb. The graphs produced from chromatographic testing are referred to as 'fingerprints' and are commonly used to determine the identity of herbal material and the integrity of the extraction process, as well as to measure quantities of individual constituents.

LIMITATIONS

Although it is generally accepted that herbal standardisation is a useful procedure, it does raise many problems and concerns. First, standardisation to non-active constituents does not necessarily reflect potency. Second, the more perplexing issue of identifying the exact active constituents in a herb is still the subject of much debate for many herbs. Lastly, individual chemical isolates do not fit the accepted definition of a herb, so if the concentration of an isolate is significantly altered for standardisation purposes, the final product may not be truly representative of the original herbal medicine and may even be considered to be 'adulterated' if marker substances are added. Furthermore, despite recent attempts to standardise herbal extracts, there are still no official standards, and herbal products can vary widely with regard to their quality and clinical effectiveness (American Herbal Products Association 2003).

Although conventional pharmaceutical thinking is based on milligrams of an active substance, such an approach is not appropriate for herbal medicines, which have many biologically active, often unmeasurable constituents. Because there can be hundreds of constituents in a complex herbal extract, standardisation is not possible by merely ensuring that one or two marker constituents are present in the same quantities from batch to batch. The therapeutic actions of herbal medicines rely on the complex combination and interactions of chemicals in the extract rather than on single constituents, and two total extracts can have very different profiles, despite there being a consistent level of one or two marker substances.

The biological activity of any compound, even a marker compound with demonstrated bioactivity, depends on the composition of the rest of the extract. Other components of the extract, even those with no direct physiological effect, may influence the uptake, distribution, metabolism and excretion of other components. Furthermore, this background matrix may affect the solubility, stability and bioavailability of any given compound (Eisner 2001). Thus the presence of chemical markers alone cannot be used to translate clinical evidence from one extract to another.

True standardisation requires more elegant procedures. The American Herbal Products Association has the following definition: 'Standardization refers to the body of information and controls that ensure product consistency from one batch to the next. This is achieved through minimising the inherent variation of natural product composition through quality assurance practices applied to agricultural and manufacturing processes' (American Herbal Products Association 2003). This definition accords more closely with the approach taken in Europe, where process control is an integral component of standardising herbal medicines. The methodology involves proceeding with the aim of standardising all the inputs and processes involved in making a particular extract, in order to ensure batch-to-batch consistency — from the genetic identity of the seed or plant, through to the agricultural processes employed and climatic factors (temperature, rainfall, sunlight), and finishing with drying, processing, extraction, solvent (or solvents), concentration, manufacture, storage, formulation and packaging of the finished product.

In addition to standardising the amount of certain chemical constituents in a herbal preparation, it is also necessary to have a means of standardising doses. Not only can different batches of the same herb have quite different potencies, there are many different formulations. Commercially available herbal preparations include fresh and dried herbs, teas, tinctures, fluid extracts, tablets, capsules and powders, as well as essential oils. When translating doses between different formulations, the amount of dried herb used to produce a set amount of the particular product is often used to give an indication of dosage strength. However, this may not give an accurate indication of potency; for example, fresh grapes, sultanas, grape juice, wine and sherry may all contain the same equivalent dry weight of grapes, but yield very different products with different biological properties.

Because of the lack of formalised standards and the need to prove 'phytoequivalence' for scientific rigour, it is increasingly common for clinical trials to specify the exact dose and extract used and for this information to be used as a basis for government regulation and for marketing purposes. When standardised extracts have been used in clinical trials, this information is included in each monograph.

HERBAL SAFETY

As with all medicines, a risk–benefit profile should be considered before using any herbal medicine. The vast majority of herbal medicines are generally considered to be safe, whether commercially or domestically produced. Most have a wide therapeutic index and only a few have toxic potential. However, adverse reactions may arise from a number of factors and may or may not be predictable. These include inappropriate usage (for example, dose, indication, time frame, administration route) and idiosyncratic reactions such as allergic responses and anaphylaxis.

In addition to adverse reactions arising from the properties of the herb itself, it is also possible for adverse events to arise from contamination or adulteration of herbal products. Contamination occurs when additional substances are inadvertently included in a herbal product. Contaminants can include toxic substances such as heavy metals, pesticide residues and microorganisms, as well as plant material from species other than the intended species, arising from either misidentification or poor quality control. Adulteration, on the other hand, is the intentional inclusion of foreign substances in herbal products, such as pharmaceutical steroids, NSAIDs or synthetic hormones, and may have very serious consequences. The standard of manufacture of commercial herbal products in Australia is generally very high.

INTERACTIONS WITH PHARMACEUTICAL DRUGS

One safety issue that has become more recognised over the past decade is the potential for

---

REPRESENTING WESTERN HERBALISTS IN AUSTRALIA

In Australia, the knowledge and practice of contemporary herbal medicine has been preserved and nurtured mainly by Western herbalists. In fact, the National Herbalists Association of Australia (NHAA) has represented medical herbalists since 1920. Today, many industry insiders consider NHAA to be the industry standard setter for education in medical herbalism. Clinicians are encouraged to check whether herbal practitioners to whom they refer have undergone accredited courses. Further information can be found by contacting the association or accessing the website www.nhaa.org.au.

---

herbs to interact with pharmaceutical drugs. Evidence has emerged to suggest that some herb–drug interactions may be detrimental and have the potential to cause dangerous outcomes, whereas others may be beneficial when an interaction is manipulated to produce positive results (see Chapters 7 and 8).

The popularity of herbal medicine, and the increasing desire among patients for self-treatment and less use of pharmaceutical drugs, have meant that many medical doctors and pharmacists are now dealing with patients who regularly take these types of medicines. As neither doctors nor pharmacists receive comprehensive herbal training as part of their standard education, a potentially detrimental situation can arise in regard to not only patient safety but also negligence. Practical questions, such as whether a herb works in a particular scenario, or is dangerous in another, or compares favourably to a pharmaceutical drug, or can reasonably be expected to have an effect within a certain time frame, are important facts to know. It is hoped that resources such as this text will enable all health practitioners to ensure the safe and rational use of herbal medicines.

REFERENCES

American Herbal Products Association, Botanical Extracts Committee. Standardization of botanical products: White paper. Silver Spring, MD: American Herbal Products Association, 2003.

Balunas MJ, Kinghorn AD. Drug discovery from medicinal plants. Life Sci 78 (2005): 431–441.

Berman B et al. Essentials of complementary and alternative medicine. Philadelphia: Lippincott Williams & Wilkins, 1999.

Di Masi JH, Grabowski HG. The price of innovation: new estimates of drug development costs. J Health Econ 22 (2003): 151–185.

Eisner S (ed.). Guidance for manufacture and sale of bulk botanical extracts, Silver Spring, MD: Botanical Extracts Committee, American Herbal Products Association, 2001.

Evans WC. Trease and Evans pharmacognosy, 15th edn, Edinburgh: WB Saunders, 2002.

Evans S. Changing the knowledge base in Western herbal medicine. Soc Sci Med 67 (2008): 2098–2106.

Heinrich M et al. Fundamentals of pharmacognosy and phytotherapy. Philadelphia: Churchill Livingstone, 2004.

Lin HL et al. Up-regulation of multidrug resistance transporter expression by berberine in human and murine hepatoma cells. Cancer 85.9 (1999): 1937–1942.

Madabushi R et al. Hyperforin in St. John's wort drug interactions. Eur J Clin Pharmacol 62.3 (2006): 225–233.

Mills S, Bone K. Principles and practice of phytotherapy. London: Churchill Livingstone, 2001.

Pan GY et al. The involvement of P-glycoprotein in berberine absorption. Pharmacol Toxicol 91.4 (2002): 193–197.

Vogel V. American Indian medicine. Normal, OK: University of Oklahoma Press, 1970.

Walcott EE, transl. The Badianus Manuscript: An Aztec Herbal of 1552. Baltimore: Johns Hopkins Press, 1940.

Weiss R. Herbal medicine. Beaconsfield, UK: Beaconsfield Publishers, 1988.

Wierenga D, Eaton RC. Phases of product development. Canberra: Office of Research and Development, Australian Pharmaceutical Manufacturers Association, 2003.

CHAPTER 3

INTRODUCTION TO CLINICAL NUTRITION

Nutrition may be defined as the science of food, its nutrients and substances, and their association with the body in relation to health and disease. In every stage of life nutrition is important and influences clinical practice in many branches of healthcare. Clinical nutrition is the use of this information in the diagnosis, treatment and prevention of disease that may be caused by deficiency, excess or imbalance of nutrients, and in the maintenance of good health.

CONSEQUENCES OF POOR NUTRITION

Nutrition plays a vital role in the health of both individuals and society, with poor nutrition and inadequate intake having a devastating effect. Overall, it has been estimated that more than 60% of all deaths in Australia result from nutrition-related disorders, such as cardiovascular disease, diabetes and cancer (Sydney-Smith 2000).

MORTALITY RISK: CARDIOVASCULAR DISEASE AND CANCER

Atherosclerotic cardiovascular disease is the most common cause of death in most Western countries (Anderson 2003). In Australia, it is the leading cause of death, accounting for 34% of all deaths in 2006. Cardiovascular disease kills one Australian nearly every 10 minutes according to the Australian Heart Foundation website. It is well known that dietary factors such as carbohydrate and fat intake affect several important physiological parameters, along with risk factors, such as hypertension, lipid levels, diabetes and antioxidant status. With the exception of tobacco consumption, diet is probably the most important factor in the aetiology of human cancers, responsible for around one-third of all cases (Ferguson 2002). Diet-related cancers have often been considered to relate to exogenous carcinogens; however, it is increasingly apparent that many carcinogens may be endogenously generated, and that diet plays an important role in modifying this process (Ferguson 1999).

Overeating and poorly balanced meals have also led to significant increases in metabolic syndrome (syndrome X) and obesity, which are now major health concerns. A 2003 review stated that the World Health Organization (WHO) estimates there are 1 billion people around the world who are now overweight or obese, and that 20–25% of the adult population in the USA have metabolic syndrome (Keller & Lemberg 2003).

Although overweight and obesity in adulthood is associated with decreased longevity, and the link with cardiovascular disease is well known, a recent series of meta-analyses revealed statistically significant associations for overweight with the incidence of type II diabetes, all cancers (except oesophageal [female], pancreatic and prostate), asthma, gall-bladder disease, osteoarthritis and chronic back pain (Guh et al 2009). It has further been established that obesity is associated with increased death rates from cancer (Peeters et al 2003). A large prospective study of more than 900,000 people found that a BMI above 40 was associated with a higher combined death rate from all cancers of 52% for obese men and 62% for obese women, compared with people of normal weight (Calle et al 2003). The adverse effects of obesity on health are not limited to adults. Overweight children and adolescents are now being diagnosed with impaired glucose tolerance and type 2 diabetes, and show early signs of insulin resistance syndrome and cardiovascular risk (Goran et al 2003).

A large body of research exists that attempts to isolate the influence of individual food groups and nutrients on morbidity and mortality. Research with macronutrients has found that the consumption of diets rich in plant-derived foods, wholegrains and fish reduces the risk of morbidity and mortality. However, numerous surveys have identified inadequate intakes of these foods in many Australian subpopulations (Barzi et al 2003, He et al 2002, Mozaffarian et al 2003, Rissanen et al 2003,

Slavin 2003). The relative roles of micronutrients, phytochemicals and non-nutrients are still under debate.

FOOD UNDER THE MICROSCOPE

More than 25,000 different bioactive components are thought to occur in the foods consumed by human beings (Milner 2008). These components represent a veritable cocktail of chemicals that includes macronutrients (such as carbohydrates, protein, fat, water and fibre) and micronutrients (such as vitamins and minerals as well as phytochemicals), many of which are health-promoting, plant-based compounds (Table 3.1). Additives, such as preservatives, colourings and flavourings, together with contaminants introduced through farming or processing techniques, may also be present.

Nutrients can be divided into two main subgroups — essential and non-essential. Essential nutrients are those that cannot be synthesised

TABLE 3.1 THE CHEMICAL COMPLEXITY OF FOOD	
NUTRIENTS	
Micronutrients	Vitamins: A, B complex, C, D, E, K, coenzyme Q10 Minerals: iron, iodine, fluoride, zinc, chromium, selenium, manganese, molybdenum and copper Others?
Macronutrients	Carbohydrates: simple and complex Proteins: amino acids Lipids: saturated, monounsaturated and polyunsaturated fatty acids Fibre: soluble and insoluble Water Minerals: sodium, potassium, calcium, magnesium, phosphorus Others?
Phytochemicals	Bioflavonoids, carotenoids, isoflavones, glutathione, lipoic acid, caffeic acid, ferulic acid, lignans, allyl sulfides, indoles
NON-NUTRIENTS	
Food additives: natural or synthetic	Colourings: restore colours lost during processing or alter natural colour Flavourings: alter natural flavours Preservatives: prolong shelf-life by reducing bacterial, mould and yeast growth Thickeners: modify texture and consistency of food Humectants: control moisture levels and keep food moist (mainly used in baked foods) Food acids: used to standardise acid levels between different food batches Antioxidants: used to preserve foods mainly containing fats and oils
Contaminants	Natural contaminants Industrial pollutants Processing contaminants Others?

Source: Wahlqvist et al 1997, Wardlaw et al 1997.

by the human body in sufficient quantities to meet average requirements, such as vitamin C, and therefore must be taken in through the diet. Non-essential nutrients can be synthesised in the body from other compounds, although they may also be ingested in foods.

MACRONUTRIENTS

Macronutrients supply energy and essential nutrients, making up the bulk of food. Carbohydrates, lipids, proteins, water and some minerals comprise this group and are all necessary to sustain life. Some macronutrients are produced in supplement form and are used as therapeutic agents. As a result, a number of these are reviewed in this book.

Carbohydrates

Simple carbohydrates, also known as sugars, are termed 'monosaccharides' because they are the single sugar units that form the basis of all sugar structures. Glucose is a monosaccharide and the primary source of energy for most human cells. Most glucose is not ingested through the diet, but rather synthesised from sucrose (common sugar) in the liver (Wardlaw et al 1997). More complex forms of carbohydrates, such as starches and fibres, are composed of many units of smaller carbohydrates found in grains, vegetables and fruit and are termed 'polysaccharides'. Overall, carbohydrates are important as a fuel. They are considered protein-sparing as they prevent the breakdown of proteins in the muscles, heart and liver into amino acids and ultimately glucose to produce fuel.

Lipids

The term 'lipid' is a generic one used to describe a number of chemicals that share two main characteristics: they are insoluble in water and contain fatty acids. When they are solid at room temperature they are called fats, whereas those that are liquid are called oils. Fatty acids are the simplest form of lipids, and more than 40 different types occur in nature (Wahlqvist et al 1997). Of all the various classes of lipids, only precursors of the omega-3 and omega-6 fatty acids are considered essential, meaning they are necessary in the diet to maintain health. The amount of dietary fat ingested and the ratios between saturated, monounsaturated and polyunsaturated fatty acids are important influences on overall health and disease.

Protein

Protein is formed by linking individual amino acids together, with the order of the amino acid sequence determining the protein's ultimate form and function. Proteins are crucial to the regulation and maintenance of many vital body processes, such as blood clotting and fluid balance, cell repair and hormone and enzyme production.

Amino acids can be divided into two broad groups: essential or non-essential. There are nine essential amino acids that must be ingested through the diet to maintain health. Protein foods that contain all nine essential amino acids are also referred to as complete protein sources (e.g. animal protein). By contrast, almost all plant foods are incomplete protein sources, with the possible exception of spirulina and soy. During times of growth, tissue repair or pronounced catabolism, such as after surgery, the body requires additional protein for efficient new tissue growth to occur. There is also emerging evidence that supplementation with individual amino acids produces a variety of pharmacological effects that can be manipulated to provide therapeutic benefits. Several of these amino acids are reviewed in the monograph section.

Minerals

Some minerals fall into the category of macronutrients because they are required in gram amounts every day, although they do not directly produce energy. These include sodium, potassium, calcium, phosphorus and magnesium.

MICRONUTRIENTS

Micronutrients do not in themselves provide energy or fuel for the body, but they may be involved in the chemical processes required to produce energy from macronutrients.

Vitamins and trace minerals fall into this category and are required to sustain life, typically through their roles as enzymatic co-factors in diverse biochemical processes. Many micronutrients are available in supplement preparations and are reviewed in this book.

Vitamins

Vitamins are organic substances (i.e. they contain a carbon atom) essential for normal growth and functioning of the body. They have been divided into two broad groups: vitamin C and the eight members of the B complex (B$_1$, B$_2$, B$_3$, B$_5$, B$_6$, B$_{12}$, biotin and folic acid) are defined as water-soluble vitamins, whereas vitamins A, D, E and K are fat-soluble. Levels in the body need to be replenished on a regular basis, as only vitamins A, E and B$_{12}$ are stored to any significant extent. Just as a vitamin deficiency causes adverse outcomes, high doses of these supplements can also do so if used inappropriately.

Essential trace minerals
These are minerals required by the body, usually in milligram or microgram amounts. They include iron, iodine, fluoride, zinc, chromium, selenium, manganese, molybdenum and copper. All trace minerals have the potential to be toxic when consumed in high doses.

Phytochemicals
Phytochemicals are components in plant foods that appear to provide significant health benefits, yet are not essential. Considerable research has been undertaken in the past few decades to understand the role they play in maintaining health and preventing certain diseases, such as cancer, but there is still much to learn. Some of the better known phytochemicals include isoflavones (e.g. genistein), bioflavonoids (e.g. procyanidins), carotenoids (e.g. lycopene), glutathione and alpha-lipoic acid. Many of the phytochemicals found in food are also found in medicinal herbs and may partly explain their therapeutic qualities.

FOOD LABELS
According to Nutrition Australia, by law all packaged foods must carry labels that state the following information:
- name of food
- name and business address of manufacturer
- country of origin
- ingredients, listed by weight from greatest to smallest (including added water)
- percentage of the key ingredient or component present in the food product
- warnings about the presence of major allergens in the food, such as nuts, seafood, eggs, gluten and soy
- a nutrition information panel, unless the food is not packaged or the package is too small (e.g. tea bags)
- an expiry date.

For further information about labelling, see Food Standards Australia New Zealand (FSANZ) website.

Currently, more than 35 genetically modified (GM) foods have been approved for sale in Australia and New Zealand (FSANZ 2014), including foods derived from soy, sugar beet, corn, cottonseed oil, canola and potatoes. As from December 2001, labels must also state whether a food contains a GM-derived component or protein introduced through genetic modification.

Additives are listed as either numbers, known as additive codes, or by name. Up-to-date lists of the food additives found in Australian and New Zealand food products can be located on the FSANZ website.

NUTRITIONAL DEFICIENCIES
Malnutrition and other deficiency states, such as kwashiorkor (protein deficiency), scurvy or rickets, are major causes of morbidity and mortality in both developing and developed countries under conditions of deprivation. Malnutrition can occur as a result of alcoholism, medication use, fussy eating, anorexia, small bowel obstruction and numerous other medical conditions.

More specific or individual nutritional deficiencies can be classified as either a 'primary deficiency' or a 'secondary deficiency', according to their aetiology.

PRIMARY DEFICIENCY
Primary deficiency is defined as a state arising from inadequate dietary intake. Although considered to be rare in developed countries, inadequate intake and primary deficiency states are not uncommon, as evidenced by numerous dietary surveys both here and overseas.

Inadequate dietary intake
The Australian National Nutrition Survey (NNS), conducted in 1995, found that approximately 30% of 2–7-year-old children ate no fruit or vegetables. Among 8–11-year-olds, 44% of boys and 38% of girls ate no fruit on the previous day and approximately one in four older children consumed no vegetables. Additionally, neither age group consumed the minimum number of serves of dairy products (Cashel 2000). Later results from the Australian

Institute of Health and Welfare in 1998 reported that approximately one in two Australian children under 12 were not eating fruit or fruit products, and more than one in five consumed no vegetables in a typical day.

The dietary intakes of adults are also far from ideal. The 1995 NNS also found that approximately 44% of adult males and 34% of females did not consume fruit in the 24 hours preceding the survey, and 20% of males and 17% of females did not consume vegetables (Giskes et al 2002).

Interestingly, dietary intakes were influenced by income level, with lower-income adults consuming a smaller variety of fruits and vegetables than their higher-income counterparts. Additional research has consistently identified other groups at risk of poor dietary habits, such as the elderly, institutionalised individuals and the indigenous population.

Surveys of individual vitamin and mineral intakes also identify a number of at-risk subpopulations. Calcium intakes for 1045 randomly selected Australian women (20–92 years), as estimated by questionnaire, showed that 76% of women aged 20–54 years, 87% of older women and 82% of lactating women had intakes below the recommended dietary intake (Pasco et al 2000). Of these, 14% had less than the minimum requirement of 300 mg/day and would, therefore, be in negative calcium balance and at risk of bone loss. The 1997 New Zealand National Nutrition Survey found that 20% of all New Zealanders and one in four women had calcium intakes below the UK estimated average requirements, and 15–20% of women aged 15–18 years were considered to have frank deficiency (Horwath et al 2001).

Surveys in Australia and New Zealand report that many adolescent girls have insufficient dietary intakes of iron and zinc to meet their high physiological requirements for growing body tissues, expanding red cell mass and onset of menarche (Gibson et al 2002).

More recent surveys do not show the situation improving. The 2007 Children's Survey, which assessed vegetable and fruit intakes against the recommendations for children aged 2–16 (1–3 serves fruit; 2–4 serves of vegetables) found a total of 22% of boys and girls aged 4–8 years met the recommended serves of vegetables, but this decreased to 11% of boys and 1%

of girls aged 14–16 years (CSIRO & University of South Australia 2008).

About 9 in 10 children aged 2–13 years met the recommendation for fruit serves compared with only 1 in 4 boys aged 14–16 (25%) and about 1 in 5 girls (19%). This decreased substantially when fruit juice was excluded from the analysis, with only 2% of boys and 1% of girls aged 14–16 years meeting the recommendation

According to a 2012 government publication, 'Australia's Food and Nutrition', more than 9 in 10 (91%) people aged 16 years and over do not consume sufficient serves of vegetables, and about 50% do not consume sufficient serves of fruit (Australian Institute of Health and Welfare 2012). When measures of sufficient serves of fruit and vegetables are combined, only 6% of people consume enough fruit and vegetables on a regular basis.

Evidence of deficiency in Australia and New Zealand

It is a common perception that although dietary intakes are not ideal, vitamin and mineral deficiencies are not a major health concern; however, research has shown that several subpopulations, such as children, pregnant and lactating women, older adults, institutionalised individuals, indigenous peoples and vegetarians, are at real risk.

For example, although severe iodine deficiency is rare in Australia and New Zealand, the Australian Population Health Development Principal Committee reports a high incidence of mild to moderate iodine deficiency in primary school aged children in Australia and New Zealand (APHDPC 2007).

This is of great concern because mild iodine deficiency during childhood and pregnancy has the potential to impair neurological development. One survey of Sydney schoolchildren, healthy adult volunteers, pregnant women and patients with diabetes found that all four groups had urinary iodine excretion values below those set by the WHO for iodine repletion (Li et al 2001). Another survey of 225 children in Tasmania identified evidence of mild iodine deficiency in 25% of boys and 21% of girls (Guttikonda et al 2002). A research group at Monash Medical Centre in Melbourne screened 802 pregnant women and found that 48.4% of Caucasian women had urinary iodine concentrations below 50 micrograms/L compared to 38.4% of Vietnamese women and 40.8% of Indian/Sri Lankan women (Hamrosi et al 2005). These figures are disturbing when one considers that normal levels are over 100 micrograms/L, mild deficiency is diagnosed at 51–100 micrograms/L and moderate to severe deficiency at < 50 micrograms/L (Gunton et al 1999). A study conducted at a Sydney hospital involving 81 women attending a 'high-risk' clinic found moderate to severe iodine deficiency in 19.8% of volunteers and mild iodine deficiency in another 29.6% (Gunton et al 1999).

In Australia and New Zealand, the prevalence of vitamin D deficiency varies, but it is now acknowledged to be much higher than previously thought (Nowson & Margerison 2002). The groups at greatest risk are dark-skinned and veiled women (particularly in pregnancy), their infants and older persons living in residential care. The study by Nowson and Margerison found marginal deficiency in 23% of women, and another frank deficiency in 80% of dark-skinned women in Australia. A study conducted in a large aged-care facility in Auckland identified frank vitamin D deficiency in 49% of elderly participants in midwinter and in 33% in midsummer (Ley et al 1999). Even in studies of 'healthy' adults, vitamin D insufficiency has been found to affect more than 40% of residents in Queensland (Kimlin et al 2007, van der Mei et al 2007) and over 65% of Tasmanians (van der Mei et al 2007).

Barriers to good nutrition

Clearly, living in a developed country is not a guarantee of healthy nutrition. Western first-world countries have a wide range of good-quality foods available at affordable prices, yet healthy eating is not commonplace. There are four key levels of influence on dietary behaviours:

1. individual factors
2. interpersonal factors
3. organisational factors
4. environmental factors.

At each level, barriers to healthy eating behaviours exist. Table 3.2 lists some of the more common barriers. Successful nutritional interventions that aim to modify individuals' eating patterns should help people develop new

TABLE 3.2 INFLUENCES OVER FOOD CHOICES
• Nutritional knowledge
• Religious beliefs and practices
• Family beliefs and practices
• Cultural beliefs and practices
• Ethnicity
• Education
• Occupation
• Peer and social influences
• Advertising
• Emotional factors: e.g. indulging in 'comfort' foods
• Medication: dietary alterations may be necessary; side effects may alter appetite
• Food: flavour, texture, appearance, odour
• Income: food choices based on affordability
• Childhood experiences
• Dental health: e.g. ill-fitting dentures, sensitive teeth
• Availability and convenience: e.g. convenience of fast food
• Muscle weakness or joint pain: problems with shopping and cooking
• Problems chewing and swallowing
• Gastrointestinal problems: e.g. nausea, diarrhoea
• Following a specific diet: e.g. fad diets
• Psychosocial problems: loneliness, depression, confusion, isolation

routines and simple internalised rules that they can use to navigate sensibly through the multitude of food choices and personal influences.

Nutritional intervention is a central component of disease prevention and management. Health professionals play a pivotal role in undertaking nutritional interventions with patients because of their knowledge, access to information and credibility as patient educators.

SECONDARY DEFICIENCY

Secondary deficiency may develop when there is reduced nutrient absorption, or increased metabolism or excretion of any given nutrient.

Of these, malabsorption states are the most common and associated with many diseases such as those characterised by chronic diarrhoea (e.g. Crohn's disease), alterations to gastrointestinal tract architecture (e.g. coeliac disease) and liver cirrhosis. In these cases, malabsorption may be specific to certain nutrients and fats or may be more generalised.

The effects of pharmaceutical medicines on nutritional status must not be forgotten. A significant number of drugs affect appetite, nutrient absorption and synthesis, transport and storage, metabolism and excretion. In fact, some of the side effects of medicines may not be related to the medicine directly, but rather to the nutritional deficiencies that develop with their use over time. These will not always produce clinically significant adverse effects, but when combined with a poor diet, or when several medicines affecting the same nutrients are taken, the risk of deficiency is heightened.

Medicines that can reduce intake of nutrients include those that induce nausea, dyspepsia or decrease appetite, such as non-steroidal anti-inflammatory drugs (NSAIDs), and opioid drugs such as codeine and morphine. Medicines with the potential to reduce nutrient absorption include those that reduce gastric motility (e.g. opioid drugs), greatly increase gastric motility (e.g. metoclopramide), compromise digestive enzyme output and function (e.g. proton pump inhibitors) and bind nutrients, preventing their traversal across gastrointestinal membranes, such as anion exchange resins (e.g. cholestyramine). Certain medicines can also increase nutrient excretion, such as thiazide diuretics, which increase potassium excretion. Others can reduce vitamin biosynthesis, such as statins, which reduce the production of coenzyme Q10.

In each of these cases, either increased nutritional intakes may be required to offset possible depletions, or medicines should not be administered with meals or supplements to reduce the likelihood of more direct interactions.

RDA AND RDI REFERENCE VALUES FOR AUSTRALIA AND NEW ZEALAND

The concept of recommended daily allowances (RDAs) originated in the United States in the 1940s as a basis for setting the poverty threshold and food-stamp allocations for the military and civilian populations during times of war and/or economic depression (Russell 2007). At this time, the first RDAs were determined by observing a healthy population's usual dietary intakes and extrapolating RDAs from this information. Over subsequent decades, scientific research into health and nutrition became more sophisticated, rendering the original concept of RDAs incomplete and in need of modification. The main findings to emerge were as follows:

- Many additional nutrients found in food are important for health, so a longer list of nutrients with recommended levels will be required.

- Nutrient intake recommendations need to be related to a specific use, as requirements will vary for different subpopulations.
- Nutritional intake recommendations need to take into account longer-term disease prevention, not just deficiency prevention.
- Clearer endpoints will be required by which to set adequacy levels.
- Risk assessment of nutrients will be necessary.

In the mid-1990s a new framework was developed to address these issues. It aimed to establish new nutrient intake recommendations to meet a variety of uses and to base nutrient requirements on the reduction of chronic disease risk, with a clear rationale for the endpoints chosen. The new guidelines still contain RDAs, but have been expanded to include three new intake recommendations: estimated average requirements (EARs), adequate daily intake (ADI) and upper level (UL) of intake.

Revisions to the nutrient intake framework occurred all around the world and in 2006 the National Health and Medical Research Council (NHMRC) of Australia published its adjusted nutritional guidelines for the adequate intake of vitamins and minerals (NHMRC 2006). These guidelines were far more comprehensive than previous versions and incorporated some of the initiatives developed in the United States.

The NHMRC guidelines are intended for healthy people and specify requirements based on both gender and age, while assuming average body weights of 76 kg for the adult male and 61 kg for the adult female.

Four key dietary reference value terms are defined here:

1. Estimated average requirement (EAR). A daily nutrient level estimated to meet the needs of 50% of the healthy population in a particular life cycle and gender.

2. Recommended daily intake (RDI). A daily nutrient intake estimated to meet the needs of up to 98% of healthy people in a particular life cycle and gender. This remains the most common benchmark of individual nutrient adequacy.

3. Adequate daily intake (ADI). When RDI cannot be determined, this is based on observed or experimentally derived estimates

of daily nutrient intake to meet the needs of healthy individuals.

4. Upper level (UL) of intake. An estimate of the highest level of regular intake that carries no appreciable risk of adverse health effects to almost all people in the general population. It is meant to apply to all groups of the general population, including sensitive individuals, throughout the life stages.

In some instances, the 2006 RDI values for specific nutrients represented a substantial increase (e.g. iron and folate), whereas others increased only marginally (e.g. calcium) or decreased (e.g. zinc requirements for adult females).

RDI and nutritional deficiencies

Although the RDIs provide a guide to preventing nutrient deficiency signs and symptoms in a 'healthy' population, they are only general recommendations and do not take into account each individual's requirements or specific circumstances. As a result, seemingly adequate food intake can provide false security, owing to a number of factors that influence the nutritional content of food and the way important nutrients are absorbed, utilised and excreted.

Unfavourable cooking and storage conditions can significantly reduce the nutritional content of food before it is consumed, no longer providing the expected vitamins and minerals. Many vitamins and minerals are sensitive to changes in temperature, light and oxygen. Up to 50% of vitamins A, D and E and 100% of vitamin C and folate can be lost during cooking (Wahlqvist et al 1997).

Issues relating to various farming techniques have often been cited as affecting the nutritional content of food and are readily reflected in the variability of resulting mineral composition. A good illustration of this is selenium, which, like most other minerals, enters the food chain through incorporation into plants from the soil. Plants grown in soils with low selenium levels are likely to contain smaller quantities than those grown in selenium-rich soils. Acid soils and complexation with metals, such as iron or aluminium, also reduce plant selenium content.

Beyond the actual quantities of nutrients provided by our food, reduced bioavailability of nutrients can occur as a result of interactions between food constituents. Phytates found in dietary fibre and tannins found in tea (and several herbal medicines) are able to bind to iron, zinc and other minerals, impairing the body's ability to absorb them. Therefore, adequate intake of mineral-rich food does not necessarily prevent deficiency. In addition to this, there are other potential contributors to secondary nutrient deficiencies, such as impaired absorption, compromised or accelerated utilisation and increased excretion of individual nutrients as well as genetic variables.

Serious deficiencies of reference values

Setting nutrient reference values is a complex task, which produces only approximate values. Robert Russell from the Human Nutrition Research Centre on Aging at Tufts University has outlined eight different obstacles that prevent accurate determination of reference values (Russell 2007):

1. Few long-term studies are available, so information is extrapolated from short-term studies (e.g. 1–2 weeks).

2. Little good-quality information is available about individual variability in response to the indicators in question.

3. Most research fails to consider the interaction between nutrients (which may be important for good health).

4. Many databases used when determining reference values provided information from studies that evaluated only dietary intakes and ignored supplemental intakes.

5. Most studies fail to consider the variation in nutrient bioavailability that is influenced by the food matrixes in which the nutrient presents.

6. Little good-quality information is available about children, adolescents and the elderly from which to establish reference values with any degree of certainty.

7. Little good-quality dose-response information is available (i.e. responses to multiple levels of the same nutrient in the same individual).

8. The cause and effect of a nutrient on a specific outcome is sometimes still speculative, as multiple factors may affect an outcome, not simply a single nutrient.

The obstacles outlined here clearly indicate that the scientific basis for many of the reference values is weak. They also indicate that for many nutrients and food components the RDI and UL levels are only approximations that are loosely relevant to the general healthy population, and even less relevant to the individual with comorbidities or special needs. Substantial research would be required to create a set of reference values with greater accuracy and relevance, but even then some values, such as ULs, may never be entirely accurate, as ethical considerations would prevent such research from ever being conducted.

OPTIMAL NUTRITION: A STATE BEYOND RDI

Dietary reference values are based on the concept of nutrient requirement. When considering these, it is important to keep in mind how we define or identify 'adequacy'. Historically, one measure of adequacy has been the dose of nutrient required to prevent the clinical manifestations of the corresponding deficiency. This method has yielded RDI reference values, which prevent overt deficiency presentations in most healthy people but do not guarantee the prevention of a less well-defined suboptimal intake which may over time contribute to other pathology.

There is considerable evidence that some nutrients may have health benefits at intake levels greater than the RDI. Higher intake levels appear to play a role in the prevention of many degenerative diseases such as cancer, cardiovascular disease, macular degeneration and cataract, cognitive decline and Alzheimer's dementia, as well as of developmental conditions such as neural tube defect. The NHMRC guidelines for the adequate intake of vitamins and minerals acknowledge this fact and state that 'there is some evidence that a range of nutrients could have benefits in chronic disease aetiology at levels above the RDI or AI' (NHMRC 2006).This has given rise to a new concept, 'suboptimal nutrition'.

The phrase 'suboptimal nutrition' was first coined by Fairfield and Fletcher in their 2002 systematic review evaluating the evidence indicating that certain nutrients had long-term disease prevention properties (Fairfield et al 2002, Fletcher et al 2002). They defined suboptimal nutrition as a state in which nutritional intake is sufficient to prevent the classical symptoms and signs of deficiency, yet insufficient to significantly reduce the risk of developmental or degenerative diseases. As such, avoiding a state of suboptimal nutrition requires adequate dietary intakes of all key food groups with an emphasis on health-promoting foods, and possibly the use of additional nutritional supplements. Furthermore, the balance between micronutrients or macronutrients is important, such as the ratio of omega-3 to omega-6 fatty acids and of high to low glycaemic carbohydrates.

As a reflection of these new developments, the term 'suggested dietary target' has been adopted by the NHMRC to describe the 'daily average intake from food and beverages for certain nutrients that may help in prevention of chronic disease'. It is a move that recognises food components offer more than just deficiency prevention; however, the general recommendations still relate only to the general healthy population.

Theoretically, it can be imagined that there is a level of intake that could be considered to provide optimal nutrition that is above the RDI yet below the UL levels. Figure 3.1 illustrates a theoretical description of beneficial health effects of a nutrient as a function of level of intake. The solid line in the figure represents risk of inadequacy in preventing nutritional deficiency and the broken line represents the risk of inadequacy in achieving a health benefit, that is, disease risk reduction (Renwick et al 2004). As intake falls below the RDI, the risk of adverse effects due to inadequate intake increases, and as intake increases beyond an optimal level, there is an increased risk of adverse effects due to toxicity. Naturally,

FIGURE 3.1 A theoretical description of beneficial health effects of a nutrient as a function of level of intake (Renwick et al 2004)

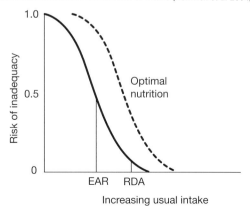

however, such an optimal intake may be highly individualistic, based on the previous discussion of confounding factors.

REDEFINING AN ESSENTIAL NUTRIENT

Clearly the line between essential and non-essential nutrients has blurred as a result of modern scientific inquiry and experimentation (Yates 2005). In the first half of the 20th century, nutrients were termed 'essential' when their removal from the diet caused severe organ dysfunction or death. Since then, modern scientific techniques have enabled us to detect finer gradations of inadequacy well before organic pathology, such as a decline in health status or ability to function optimally, sets in. They have also allowed us to glimpse the potential of nutrients and certain food compounds to prevent genomic mutations, alter metabolic processes and ultimately prevent disease, possibly even extending longevity concomitantly. If we broaden the aim of nutrition beyond prevention of deficiency to include the promotion of wellness and optimal health, many additional nutrients and food components are also likely to be able to be termed 'essential'.

NUTRITIONAL GENOMICS

Nutritional genomics is a field that has emerged alongside the Human Genome Project. It has a unique focus on disease prevention and healthy ageing through the manipulation of gene–diet interactions. Several key scientific domains in nutritional genomics focus on specific areas of this interaction.

Nutrigenomics, also known as nutritional epigenetics, refers to the effect of nutrients and other food components on gene expression and gene regulation, i.e. diet–gene regulation. In contrast, nutrigenetics refers to the genetic makeup of an individual that affects their response to various dietary nutrients and can reveal why different people respond differently to the same nutrient. When understood together, these two emerging fields can help us understand how diet and nutrition affect human health and eventually lead to individualised dietary recommendations to reduce the risk of disease, possibly improve recovery and promote wellness (Gaboon 2011). In other words, from

a clinical perspective, nutritional genomics may help clinicians bridge the gap from overarching public health messages aimed at the broader community to more individualised dietary guidance.

Another concept in nutritional genomics is systems biology, or nutritional engineering. This involves the identification, classification and characterisation of human genetic variants or polymorphisms (mutations) that modify individual responses to nutrients (Fig 3.2) and its application in the manipulation of biological pathways to produce health benefits.

From a public health and research perspective, it is possible that nutritional genomics could play an important role in the conduct and interpretation of clinical trials and epidemiological studies that investigate the associations between diet and/or nutritional supplementation and disease. This knowledge can be used to distinguish between responders and non-responders, and to determine which populations are most likely to benefit from nutritional intervention and which may be at increased risk of harm.

It has further been suggested that there is a need to establish genome-informed nutrient and food-based dietary guidelines for disease prevention and healthy ageing, and better targeted public health nutrition interventions

FIGURE 3.2 Nutrient genome interactions (from Stover and Caudill 2008)

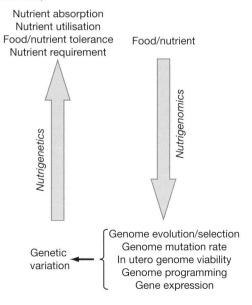

(including micronutrient fortification and supplementation) that maximise benefit and minimise adverse outcomes in genetically diverse human populations (Stover & Caudill 2008).

Whilst a better understanding of an individual's family history and genetic makeup may help inform practice in future, complex disorders, such as cancer, CVD and diabetes, are caused by genetic and environmental factors, and genetic mutations are only partially predictive of risk (Camp & Trujillo 2014). Our understanding of this complicated interplay between genetic variations, diet, lifestyle, environmental and even psychological influences is still far from clear.

The development of nutrigenomics holds great promise for individualised medicine and tailoring nutritional interventions for the individual; however, the science is still developing. The knowledge gained from nutritional genomics requires an evidence-based approach to validate that personalised recommendations result in health benefits to individuals and do not cause harm (Camp & Trujillo 2014). In addition, as with all emerging areas, ethical, legal and social issues need to be addressed, particularly with respect to how the public may access nutrigenetic tests and associated nutritional and lifestyle advice. There are five key areas identified by international experts in the context of both basic nutrigenomics research and its clinical and commercial uses:

1. health claims benefits arising from nutrigenomics
2. managing nutrigenomic information
3. delivery methods of nutrigenomics services
4. nutrigenomics products
5. equitable accessibility to nutrigenomics (Gaboon 2011).

NUTRITIONAL DEFICIENCY, GENOME DAMAGE AND CLINICAL PRACTICE

There is overwhelming evidence that several micronutrients (vitamins and minerals) are required as co-factors for enzymes or as part of the structure of proteins (metalloenzymes) involved in DNA synthesis and repair, prevention of oxidative damage to DNA as well as maintenance methylation of DNA. The main point is that genome damage caused by moderate micronutrient deficiency is of the same order of magnitude as the genome damage levels caused by exposure to significant doses of environmental genotoxins, such as chemical carcinogens, ultraviolet radiation and ionising radiation (Fenech 2008). For example, deficiency of vitamins B_{12}, folic acid, B_6, C, E or iron or zinc appears to damage DNA in the same way as radiation, by causing single- and double-strand breaks, oxidative lesions or both. Half of the population may be deficient in at least one of these micronutrients (Ames 2004). If moderate deficiency in just one micronutrient can cause significant DNA damage, it is possible that multiple moderate deficiencies may have additive or synergistic effects on genome stability.

Current research indicates the amount of micronutrients that appear to be protective against genome damage varies greatly between foods, and careful choice is needed to design dietary patterns optimised for genome health maintenance. Because dietary choices vary between individuals, several interventional options are required, and nutritional supplements may be necessary to fill in gaps not met by food intake, or to elevate intake levels beyond dietary intake to influence key metabolic pathways.

As the field of nutritional genomics matures, healthcare practitioners will have the opportunity to make genetically individualised dietary recommendations aimed at improving human health and preventing disease (Milner 2008). It is possible to envisage preventive medicine being practised in 'genome health clinics', where clinicians would diagnose and nutritionally prevent the most fundamental initiating cause of developmental and degenerative disease — genome damage itself (Fenech 2008).

NUTRITIONAL SUPPLEMENTATION

Nutritional supplements have traditionally been recommended only in cases of established deficiency; however, scientific evidence is accumulating to suggest they may be an important extension of healthy eating and necessary to achieve a level of health and disease prevention beyond what is possible through diet alone. As a consequence, many conservative medical bodies are being forced to reassess their long-established views.

SAFETY ISSUES

Nutritional supplements can be viewed as medicines that have both subtherapeutic and toxic doses, as well as the potential to induce adverse reactions and interactions.

Adverse reactions and interactions

The same subpopulations that have been identified to be at greater risk of adverse reactions to pharmaceutical medicines may be used for the safety assessment of nutritional supplements. These groups are the elderly, atopic patients, people with compromised liver or kidney function, anxiety or depression or serious illness, and those already taking many medicines. In clinical practice, the risk-versus-benefit decision of recommending a supplement or not is always considered and should be discussed with patients. In many cases, the risk of experiencing a minor adverse reaction that is short-lived and not serious may be an acceptable risk, whereas the risk of a more serious adverse reaction is not.

Toxicity

If a toxic dose is defined as one that is capable of causing death or a serious adverse reaction, then only a few nutrients are of special concern. In everyday practice, vitamins A, D and B_6 require special attention, as do the minerals iron, zinc, copper and selenium. Obviously, effects are dose-related and, in some cases, the doses are so large that they cannot practically be achieved in real life (see Appendix 6).

Natural versus synthetic

It is often asked whether natural and synthetic vitamins differ, and whether one is superior to and safer than the other. At this stage, very little research has been conducted to compare natural and synthetic forms, but some investigation into vitamin E has been undertaken.

The biological activity of vitamin E is based on the 'fetal resorption–gestation' method in rats. Using this test, the minimum amount of vitamin E required to sustain fetal growth in pregnant rats is determined. In the case of D-alpha tocopherol (RRR-alpha), which is considered to be the natural form, the highest activity is observed and therefore valued at 100%, whereas the biological activity of other vitamin E isomers has been estimated to be as low as 21% (Acuff et al 1998). Studies in humans have indicated that natural vitamin E has roughly twice the bioavailability of synthetic vitamin E; however, whether this also means that it has greater efficacy has yet to be clarified (Burton et al 1998).

It has also been speculated that the natural beta-carotene used in supplements, which is derived from algae and contains a mixture of carotenoids, may be safer and possibly more effective than synthetic beta-carotene.

RATIONAL USE OF SUPPLEMENTS

Nutritional supplements can never take the place of a balanced diet or provide all the health benefits of a whole food, but they can provide nutritional assistance and therapeutic effects in three different ways:

1. Supplementation to correct a gross deficiency. A patient presenting with clinical signs and symptoms of a nutritional deficiency will require nutritional counselling and possibly supplementation to quickly redress the situation (e.g. vitamin C supplementation and dietary education for patients with scurvy).

2. Supplementation to address a sub-clinical deficiency. A patient may not be presenting with overt clinical signs or symptoms of deficiency, but may benefit from an increased intake of certain nutrients or food components to prevent disease or reduce the incidence of other adverse outcomes (e.g. maternal folic acid supplementation and gestational health and development).

3. Supplementation to address symptoms not associated with nutrient deficiency. A patient presents with symptoms or disease unrelated to nutritional deficiency, but evidence indicates that nutritional supplementation can provide health benefits. This describes the use of nutritional supplements in pharmacological doses to achieve a specific health-related purpose, much like a therapeutic drug (e.g. high-dose riboflavin supplementation for migraine prophylaxis or coenzyme Q10 supplementation in hypertension). Many more examples are found in the monograph section of this book.

Table 3.3 provides a general guide for healthcare professionals when considering nutritional aspects of their patients' situation and nutritional supplementation.

TABLE 3.3 THE RATIONAL USE OF NUTRITIONAL SUPPLEMENTS

- Be informed and seek out unbiased information — do not rely on label claims, product information manuals or other commercial sources of information alone.
- Know the common nutrient deficiency signs and symptoms.
- Know the RDIs and where relevant suggested dietary targets.
- Know the benefits and risks of nutrients at levels beyond RDI and upper-limit levels (ULs) that increase the risk of adverse effects.
- Be able to detect inadequate dietary intakes or refer to a healthcare professional who can do so.
- Ensure that all healthcare professionals involved in a patient's care remain informed of nutritional supplement use.
- Take care with children, the elderly and pregnant or lactating women.
- Take care when high-risk medicines are being taken.
- Take care with HIV, cancer and other serious illnesses.
- Know the manufacturer or supplier details.
- Store medicines appropriately.

REFERENCES

Acuff RV et al. Transport of deuterium-labeled tocopherols during pregnancy. Am J Clin Nutr 67.3 (1998): 459–464.

Ames BN. A role for supplements in optimizing health: the metabolic tune-up. Arch Biochem Biophys 423.1 (2004): 227–234.

Anderson JW. Whole grains protect against atherosclerotic cardiovascular disease. Proc Nutr Soc 62.1 (2003): 135–142.

Australian Institute of Health and Welfare 2012. Australia's food & nutrition 2012. Cat. no. PHE 163. Canberra: AIHW.

Australian Population Health Development Principal Committee (APHDPC). The prevalence and severity of iodine deficiency in Australia. (2007). Available at: www.foodstandards.gov.au (accessed 24/01/2013).

Barzi F et al. Mediterranean diet and all-causes mortality after myocardial infarction: results from the GISSI-Prevenzione trial. Eur J Clin Nutr 57.4 (2003): 604–611.

Burton GW et al. Human plasma and tissue alpha-tocopherol concentrations in response to supplementation with deuterated natural and synthetic vitamin E. Am J Clin Nutr 67.4 (1998): 669–684.

Calle EE et al. Overweight, obesity, and mortality from cancer in a prospectively studied cohort of U.S. adults. N Engl J Med 348.17 (2003): 1625–1638.

Camp KM, Trujillo E. Position of the Academy of Nutrition and Dietetics: Nutritional Genomics. J Acad Nutrit Dietetics 114.2 (2014): 299–312.

Cashel K. What are Australian children eating? Med J Aust 173 (Suppl) (2000): S4–S5.

CSIRO, University of South Australia 2008. 2007 Australian national children's nutrition and physical activity survey — main findings. Canberra: Commonwealth of Australia.

Fairfield KM et al. Vitamins for chronic disease prevention in adults: scientific review. JAMA 287.23 (2002): 3116–3126.

Fenech M. Genome health nutrigenomics and nutrigenetics — diagnosis and nutritional treatment of genome damage on an individual basis. Food and Chemical Toxicology 46.4 (2008): 1365–1370.

Ferguson LR. Natural and man-made mutagens and carcinogens in the human diet. Mutat Res 443.1–2 (1999): 1–110.

Ferguson LR. Natural and human-made mutagens and carcinogens in the human diet. Toxicology 181.2 (2002): 79–82.

Fletcher RH, et al. Vitamins for chronic disease prevention in adults: clinical applications. JAMA 287.23 (2002): 3127–3129.

FSANZ (Food Standards Australia New Zealand). Food Standards Code; Standard 1.5.2 Available at: http://www.foodstandards.gov.au/code/Pages/default.aspx 20/7/2014.

FSANZ (Food Standards Australia New Zealand). Labelling. Available at: http://www.foodstandards.gov.au/consumer/labelling/Pages/default.aspx 20/7/2014.

Gaboon NEA. Nutritional genomics and personalized diet. Egyptian J Med Hum Genetics 12.1 (2011): 1–7.

Gibson RS et al. Risk of suboptimal iron and zinc nutriture among adolescent girls in Australia and New Zealand: causes, consequences, and solutions. Asia Pac J Clin Nutr 11 (Suppl 3) (2002): S543–S552.

Giskes K et al. Socio-economic differences in fruit and vegetable consumption among Australian adolescents and adults. Public Health Nutr 5.5 (2002): 663–669.

Goran MI et al. Obesity and risk of type 2 diabetes and cardiovascular disease in children and adolescents. J Clin Endocrinol Metab 88.4 (2003): 1417–1427.

Guh D et al. The incidence of co-morbidities related to obesity and overweight: A systematic review and meta-analysis. BMC Public Health 9.88 (2009): 1–20.

Gunton JE et al. Iodine deficiency in ambulatory participants at a Sydney teaching hospital: is Australia truly iodine replete? Med J Aust 171.9 (1999): 467–470.

Guttikonda K et al. Recurrent iodine deficiency in Tasmania, Australia: a salutary lesson in sustainable iodine prophylaxis and its monitoring. J Clin Endocrinol Metab 87.6 (2002): 2809–2815.

Hamrosi MA et al. Iodine status in pregnant women living in Melbourne differs by ethnic group. Asia Pac J Clin Nutr 14.1 (2005): 27–31.

He K et al. Fish consumption and risk of stroke in men. JAMA 288.24 (2002): 3130–3136.

Horwath C et al. Attaining optimal bone status: lessons from the 1997 National Nutrition Survey. NZ Med J 114.1128 (2001): 138–141.

Keller KB, Lemberg L. Obesity and the metabolic syndrome. Am J Crit Care 12.2 (2003): 167–170.

Kimlin M et al. Does a high UV environment ensure adequate vitamin D status? J Photochem Photobiol B 89.2–3 (2007): 139–147.

Ley SJ et al. Attention is needed to the high prevalence of vitamin D deficiency in our older population. NZ Med J 112.1101 (1999): 471–472.

Li M et al. Re-emergence of iodine deficiency in Australia. Asia Pac J Clin Nutr 10.3 (2001): 200–203.

Milner JA. Nutrition and cancer: essential elements for a road map. Cancer Letters 269.2 (2008): 189–198.

Mozaffarian D et al. Cardiac benefits of fish consumption may depend on the type of fish meal consumed: the Cardiovascular Health Study. Circulation 107.10 (2003): 1372–1377.

NHMRC (National Health and Medical Research Council). Nutrient reference values for Australia and New Zealand, 2006. Available online: http://www.nhmrc.gov.au/PUBLICATIONS/synopses/n35syn.htm 21-07-09.

Nowson CA, Margerison C. Vitamin D intake and vitamin D status of Australians. Med J Aust 177.3 (2002): 149–152.

Pasco JA et al. Calcium intakes among Australian women: Geelong Osteoporosis Study. Aust NZ J Med 30.1 (2000): 21–27.

Peeters A et al. Obesity in adulthood and its consequences for life expectancy: a life-table analysis. Ann Intern Med 138.1 (2003): 24–32.

Renwick AG et al. Risk-benefit analysis of micronutrients. Food Chem Toxicol 42.12 (2004): 1903–1922.

Rissanen TH et al. Low intake of fruits, berries and vegetables is associated with excess mortality in men: the Kuopio Ischaemic Heart Disease Risk Factor (KIHD) Study. J Nutr 133.1 (2003): 199–204.

Russell R. Setting dietary intake levels: problems and pitfalls. in: Bock G, Goode J (eds). Dietary supplements and health, 1st edn. Chichester: Wiley, 2007, pp 29–45.

Slavin J. Why whole grains are protective: biological mechanisms. Proc Nutr Soc 62.1 (2003): 129–134.

Stover PJ, Caudill MA. Genetic and epigenetic contributions to human nutrition and health: managing genome-diet interactions. J Am Diet Ass 108.9 (2008): 1480–1487.

Sydney-Smith M. Nutritional assessment in general practice. Curr Ther 41 (2000): 12–24.

van der Mei IA et al. The high prevalence of vitamin D insufficiency across Australian populations is only partly explained by season and latitude. Environ Health Perspect 115.8 (2007): 1132–1139.

Wahlqvist M et al. Food and nutrition. Sydney: Allen & Unwin, 1997.

Wardlaw G et al. Contemporary nutrition, 3rd edn. Dubuque: Brown and Benchmark, 1997.

Yates AA. Nutrient requirements, international perspectives. In: Benjamin C (ed). Encyclopedia of human nutrition. Oxford: Elsevier, 2005, pp 282–292.

CHAPTER 4

INTRODUCTION TO AROMATHERAPY

The term 'aromatherapy' refers to the use of essential oils and is an aspect of phytotherapy (botanical medicine). Essential oils are volatile liquid substances extracted from plant material by a variety of methods. However, 'aromatherapy' is frequently associated with cosmetic products that often do not contain any essential oils, even though the term 'aromatherapy' is included on the labels and advertising material of such products. There are several definitions of aromatherapy. Hirsch, for example, defines it as 'the use of odorants as inhalants to treat underlying medical or psychiatric symptoms' (Hirsch 2001), but this definition does not mention essential oils or differentiate between essential and fragrant (synthetic) oils, which are not usually recommended for use in healthcare. In addition, for the administration method Hirsch refers only to inhalation. Thus, Hirsch's definition does not accurately define aromatherapy nor does it describe the way it is practised. For the purposes of this chapter, aromatherapy is defined as follows:

> *The controlled use of essential oils from named botanical sources using a variety of application (external) or administration (internal) methods to promote and support health and wellbeing using a patient-centred evidence based approach.*
> **Dunning 2005**

In this context 'controlled' encompasses:
- quality use of essential oils (QUEO) (Dunning 2005), which is based on the principles of the Quality Use of Medicines (Department of Health and Aged Care 1999)

- qualifications and competence of practitioners
- accurate diagnosis
- appropriate selection of essential oils based on a thorough assessment, stating the botanical name of the plant and plant part from which the oil was extracted and evidence for use where possible, and the administration/application, dose and dose frequency method
- appropriate documentation, including adverse-event reporting when relevant, and monitoring the effects according to the aims of the treatment
- appropriate storage and handling of essential oils to reduce deterioration and oxidation and meet infection control and disposal standards
- regulatory standards, including scheduling, manufacturing and advertising processes.

HISTORICAL OVERVIEW

Use of essential oils is recorded in most ancient civilisations in healthcare, religion and cosmetics, and to enhance the environment. For example, the ancient Egyptians used them to embalm the dead as well as in healthcare. Almost all cultures used odorants, including plant oils, as preventive measures and to fumigate people and environments during illnesses, such as the plague. In the Middle East, Avicenna (AD 980–1037) is credited with developing the original steam distillation process for extracting essential oils. In the late 1800s, Chamerland undertook research into the antiseptic properties of essential oils and in the 20th century Cavel, who studied the antiseptic properties of 35 essential oils in sewage cultures, extended Chamerland's work.

A great deal of modern research concerns the relationship between odours and emotional states, cognitive performance (Jellinek 1998/99, Svoboda 2002, Van Toller & Dodd 1988) and stress management. It also focuses on the management of common health problems, such as upper respiratory tract infection (URTI) and acute and chronic pain, in a range of healthcare settings that include aged care, midwifery and acute care such as coronary care units. Often the research is conducted upon isolated chemical components of the essential oil, which does not reflect usual aromatherapy practice.

René Gattéfosse is credited with coining the term 'aromatherapy'. After burning his hand in a laboratory fire, he immersed it in a vat of lavender essential oil, which reduced the pain, and his hand subsequently healed without scarring or infection. Gattéfosse went on to use essential oils in military hospitals in World War I. Essential oils also played a major role in wound care during World War II, where Dr Jean Valnet used them in military hospitals in Europe and IndoChina. Marguerite Maury is largely responsible for the popularity of essential oils in modern beauty care. She introduced aromatherapy into the UK in the 1960s, and her technique of using low doses of essential oils dispersed in a carrier oil and applied in a massage strongly influenced aromatherapy practice in the UK and Australia (Price & Price 1995). Research into the therapeutic application of essential oils is continuing in many countries on animal and human subjects.

AROMATHERAPY PRACTICE MODELS

There are three main aromatherapy practice models, which have implications for the administration/application method, dose, dose intervals and safety. Essential oils are often combined with other conventional and complementary therapies such as massage and acupressure.

MEDICAL AROMATHERAPY

This is also known as aromatic medicine or aromatology. It is used in France and increasingly in the UK, and there is growing interest in Australia. An education program encompassing the internal use of essential oils was recently approved by the Australian National Training Authority. Medical aromatherapy utilises the internal administration of essential oils via the oral, rectal and vaginal routes, as well as in dressings, ointments and fumigation. Only steam-distilled and expressed essential oils are used internally. In France prescribing for internal use is regulated and restricted to medically qualified doctors with the relevant training. A pharmacist often formulates the prescriptions. Aromatherapists may work under the direction of a doctor. In some other countries, other practitioners can prescribe essential oils if they have the relevant qualifications.

SUBTLE AROMATHERAPY OR AROMACOLOGY

This is the German model of practice, which largely uses inhalation to influence psychological and spiritual states.

POPULAR, OR TRADITIONAL, AROMATHERAPY

Largely based on the UK model, this involves inhalation and massage. Touch, an essential aspect of massage, has its own health benefits, and this model uses topical application in massage, gels, creams and lotions, as well as inhalation for physical, psychological and spiritual effects. There are two subgroups: therapeutic aromatherapy, which is used in healthcare, and cosmetic or beauty care aromatherapy. Australian aromatherapists largely follow the UK model, but some incorporate aspects of all three models.

All three models use essential oils as the main medicinal substance. Essential oils are rarely used undiluted, but rather are incorporated into various carrier substances, depending on the administration/application route. Most aromatherapists formulate blends for individual patients, but fixed-formulation blends are available: for example, massage blends for pain relief. Aromatherapy is very popular with the general public and self-prescribing by following the directions in self-care books, magazine articles and short education courses is common. In Australia some health insurance funds reimburse the costs of aromatherapy treatments, provided the aromatherapist is qualified through an approved training facility.

ESSENTIAL OILS
CHEMISTRY

Essential oils are secondary plant metabolites and are complex chemical compounds that have a different composition from the herb extract of the same plant. Essential oils are stored in specific secretory structures in leaves, twigs, seeds, petals, bark and roots, often with resins and gums in oil cells, sacs, resin canals, ducts and hairs, and are extracted from these structures by steam distillation, expression, enfleurage, solvent extraction, maceration and more recently supercritical carbon dioxide extraction, depending on the plant source (Guba 2002, Price & Price 1995). More than 3000 odour molecules have been identified.

Chemical variations are common in plants of the same genus and these are known as chemotypes. The best known chemotypes occur in the essential oils of *Thymus vulgaris* (thyme), *Rosmarinus officinalis* (rosemary), *Ocimum basilicum* (basil) and *Melaleuca alternifolia* (tea tree). Growing conditions, harvesting, storage and handling are known to affect the chemical composition of essential oils (Guba 2004, Price & Price 1995). Common phytochemicals in essential oils are terpenes, sesquiterpenes, alcohols, phenols, aldehydes, ketones, esters, acids, phenolic ethers, oxides, lactones and coumarins (Bowles 2003, Clarke 2002). It is necessary to understand the chemical composition of essential oils in order to understand their application in healthcare and the safety aspects associated with their use.

Of the many chemicals present, the alcohols, lactones, phenols and sesquiterpenes are considered to have a major impact on the odour of the oil and are of particular significance in the cosmetic and perfumery applications of aromatherapy. Of these chemicals, alcohols are considered to be among the most important for therapeutic effect and pleasant fragrance. They often have antimicrobial properties and low toxicity, and are described as warming, uplifting and good general tonics. Two examples of alcohols found in essential oils are:
- linalool, found in the essential oils of lemon, rosemary, sage, thyme and mandarin, and which has anaesthetic, antiseptic and sedative effects

- terpineol found in the essential oils of frankincense and tea tree, and which has antiseptic activity.

The sesquiterpenes consist of three isoprene units and make up the largest group of terpenes found in the plant world. They tend to have strong odours and a variety of pharmacological effects. Two examples of sesquiterpenes found in essential oils are:
- caryophyllene, found in oil of cloves, eucalyptus, ginger, lavender, marjoram, sage, thyme, ylang ylang and valerian. It has a strong spicy, woody odour and anti-inflammatory, antispasmodic, antibacterial, fungicidal and sedative effects.
- chamazulene, found in German chamomile, which gives it the characteristic blue colour. It has analgesic, anti-inflammatory, antioxidant, antiseptic and antipyretic effects.

Optical isomerism also influences the odour of a substance, so two different oils containing the same specific chemical may have different odours because the chemicals are stereoisomers. For example, *d*-limonene found in citrus oils, pine leaves and peppermint has a citrus odour, whereas its stereoisomer *l*-limonene has a turpentine-like odour and is found in citronella and lemon verbena.

Although the pharmacological effects of many of the constituents found in essential oils have not yet been fully investigated, a few that have been investigated are notable for their significant activity. For example, eugenol is a phenol found in cinnamon, oil of cloves and ylang ylang, giving the oils a spicy, pungent odour and significant antimicrobial activity. Cinnamaldehyde, chiefly found in cinnamon oil, has also been well investigated. It has antispasmodic, antimicrobial and fungicidal activities and is described as having a warm, spicy and balsamic odour.

Most of the essential oils produced are used in the food, cosmetic and, to a lesser extent, medicine industries, where strict composition standards ensure products meet relevant standards. Organisations such as the International Organisation for Standardisation (ISO), Research Institute for Fragrance Materials (RIFM), International Fragrance Association (IFRA) and Association Française de Normalisation (AFNOR) have developed composition standards for many essential oil products used in the food and perfume industries, and this is an important aspect of quality control. The ISO and AFNOR standards are often accepted as the most reliable indicators of quality.

The need to achieve compositional consistency has led some manufacturers to artificially manipulate chemical composition, using adulteration, substitution and rectification, to ensure essential oils meet the standard and to reduce the cost of expensive oils such as rose and jasmine. Plant conservation issues have also affected aromatherapy practice: for example, the sale of essential oils from some endangered species is banned in Europe. In some cases synthetic products have been developed, which may increase the potential to cause adverse events and bring aromatherapy into disrepute. The European Federation of Essential Oils was formed in 2002 to increase awareness of the need for sustainable harvesting to benefit both local communities and aromatherapy, as well as to conserve endangered plants.

Analytical techniques such as gas chromatography, mass spectrometry, infrared spectroscopy, optical rotation and refractive index are used to assess the composition and purity of essential oils. Frequently mass spectrometry and infrared spectroscopy are considered together. The analytical information, together with other safety information, is detailed in material safety data sheets, which are available from essential oil suppliers and manufacturers. More recently, the cosmetic industry has begun to examine the peroxide value (POV) of both essential and fixed vegetable oil carrier oils. POV is an indicator of the potential of an essential oil to cause skin irritation and sensitivity (Wabner 2002). In addition, the physical appearance (colour and consistency) and odour of the oil are important aspects of quality.

Currently, there is no standard for 'therapeutic-grade essential oils' (Guba 2004). However, some suppliers undertake independent quality-control tests to ensure essential oils meet aromatherapy requirements and to guarantee that their essential oils are:
- 100% pure, which means they are not adulterated in any way
- 100% natural, which means they are made from plant material and do not contain any synthetic substances

- 100% complete, which means they are single-distilled and have not had any chemical constituents removed or added.

In Australia most essential oils are listed in schedule 14 of the medicines scheduling system of the Therapeutic Goods Administration (TGA). However, TGA listing does not necessarily indicate benefit or efficacy, but does indicate that the risks associated with listed products are low. Manufacturers are not permitted to make therapeutic claims for listed products.

Aromatherapists prefer to use the entire essential oils rather than isolated compounds or synthetic oils, because the chemicals present in individual essential oils and blends have synergistic and quenching properties that enhance the beneficial effects and reduce unwanted effects. These beneficial interactions occur among the individual constituents within an oil and among the essential oils in a blend of oils (Clarke 2002, Price & Price 1995, Opdyke 1976). In most cases a blend of essential oils is used to suit the condition being treated, and the composition of the blend is modified according to the individual's response in much the same way as herbal medicines are used. Common application/administration methods and doses are shown in Table 4.2 at the end of this chapter. Recommended doses are based on a long history of traditional use and the recommendations of experts, rather than on dose-finding trials. A number of factors need to be considered when deciding on an application method, dose and dose interval, including:
- the aromatherapy model being used
- the pharmacokinetics and pharmacodynamics of the essential oils
- the mode of administration/application
- the patient's age and gender, presenting health issues and medical history, including allergies
- other conventional and herbal medicines being used
- the qualifications of the practitioner.

Most aromatherapists do not recommend using fragrant oils for therapeutic purposes, although most accept they may have a role as environmental fragrances and may have psychological effects.

CARRIER SUBSTANCES

In most cases essential oils are dispersed in another substance known as a carrier. Carrier substances for massage are usually cold-pressed or fixed vegetable oils, such as sweet almond, grapeseed and macadamia nut oil, depending on the aims of treatment. In massage, the carrier oils primarily provide lubrication for the therapist's hands to allow smooth movement over the skin and to enhance absorption of the essential oils; however, some fixed oils, such as those of calendula (*Calendula officinalis*) or St John's wort (*Hypericum perforatum*), also have therapeutic properties.

Other carriers include honey, Aloe vera, shea and cocoa butter, and waxes, which are used for capsules, ointments and suppositories intended for internal use. Purified clays such as bentonite are also used as carriers for essential oils to be applied in compresses, poultices and face and body masks/packs in beauty care. Incipients (dispersants) are usually required if essential oils are added to water to keep them in solution because essential oils are generally insoluble in water.

HYDROSOLS

A hydrosol is the condensed water co-produced with the essential oil during steam distillation (Catty 2001). Each litre of hydrosol contains low doses of essential oils, between 0.05 and 0.02 mL, depending on the solubility of the constituents in the oil being distilled, the duration of the distillation process and the hydrophilic/lipophilic nature of the constituents. Therefore, the chemical profile is different from the essential oil obtained from the same distillation. Hydrosols can be used as carrier substances or prepared as tinctures, spritzers and compresses; frequently, they can also be drunk (Catty 2001).

PHARMACOKINETICS AND PHARMACODYNAMICS

Essential oils are absorbed, metabolised and excreted in a similar way to fat-soluble medicines (Tisserand & Balacs 1995). They have a short life span in the blood, from where they are distributed to muscle and adipose tissues over a longer period. They may bind to plasma proteins for transportation, and detoxification primarily occurs in the liver. The exact pharmacokinetics and pharmacodynamics depend on many factors, including the route of administration.

Research into the pharmacodynamics and pharmacokinetics of essential oils indicates that they are metabolised and excreted between 72 and 120 hours after administration/application depending on the:

- body size of the subject
- chemical composition of the carrier substance of the essential oil/s
- carrier substance
- application/administration route
- dose, dose form and dose interval
- individual's health status.

Essential oils are absorbed through the skin, but the absorption rate of the various chemical components in a particular essential oil depends on a number of factors, including the size of the individual molecules, the percentage of essential oils in the blend, total dose applied, the area covered and the state of the circulation. Jager et al (1992) detected linalool and linalyl acetate (components of lavender) in the blood at 5 minutes after a 10-minute abdominal massage using 2% *Lavandula angustifolia* in peanut oil.

Likewise, salicylate was detected in subcutaneous tissue within 30 minutes and for up to 60 minutes after the application of 20% methyl salicylate to the forearm (Cross et al 1997). Larger molecules, such as the coumarins, take up to 1 hour to penetrate (Ford et al 2001). Covering the area after applying the essential oils enhances absorption. Absorption is usually rapid from the rectal and buccal mucosa. Gastrointestinal factors such as diarrhoea and vomiting can affect absorption of oral doses.

Research is currently underway to ascertain whether essential oils enhance the absorption of topically applied medicines. Components such as limonene, 1,8-cineole and nerolidol enhance the penetration of both hydrophilic and lipophilic substances (Cornwall et al 1996, Duke 1998). Such research suggests topical application of essential oils may be contraindicated or caution required if conventional topical medicines such as anti-anginal agents, nicotine patches or hormone replacement therapy (HRT) are used at the same time.

SAFE USE

Safe use of essential oils is a complex topic that includes similar issues to those concerning herbal medicine safety. It is largely based on the long history of safe traditional use, case reports and animal studies to determine lethal doses (e.g. LD_{50}). The lethal dose (LD) may not provide useful information about topical applications. Even less is known about effective doses (ED) or the effects of organ disease, such as liver, renal or cardiac disease, on the metabolism and elimination of essential oils, although it is reasonable to expect these would be important considerations for internal dosing, as would the state of the skin for absorption of topical applications. Safety information can be found in the essential oil material data sheets, *The complete German Commission E monographs* (Blumenthal et al 1998) and the *ESCOP monographs: The scientific foundation for herbal medicinal products* (ESCOP 2003), as well as Poisons Information Centres (see Appendix 3).

Common potential risks are:

- skin, eye and mucous membrane irritation to the person using the oils and people in the vicinity (this is also an occupational hazard for practitioners)

- phototoxicity

- local irritation

- allergy (regular use of the same essential oils increases the risk of cumulative effects and allergy)

- respiratory difficulties, asthma or migraines in susceptible individuals triggered by odours

- unwanted psychological effects (e.g. euphoria in people with dementia).

Essential oils that contain aldehydes, phenols and furocoumarins — especially citrus oils such as bergamot (*Citrus bergamia*) — are more likely to irritate the eyes, mucous membranes and skin, and cause sensitisation. Contact sensitisation related to monoterpene oxidation (Tisserand & Balacs 1995) is frequently the result of poor storage conditions (Burfield 2000). If a skin reaction occurs, the area should be blotted with tissue to remove or dilute the oils and a carrier substance applied and removed with tissue. The process may need to be repeated several times. Removing with soap and water may exacerbate the reaction (Bensouilah & Buck 2006). The reaction should be noted in the individual's health history and an adverse event notification filed depending on its severity.

Cross-sensitisation to other essential oil components and foods has also been reported: for example, between Thai food and *Cymbopogon flexuosus* (East Indian lemongrass) (Bleaser et al 2002, Clarke 2002). Perfume and fragrant products found in candles, aerosols, incense and soaps are common irritants and often contain limonene, coumarin, geraniol and cinnamaldehyde (Harris 2005). Some also contain carcinogenic substances such as styrene or naphthalene, and some contain formaldehyde in amounts many times the safe limit, which is < 2 micrograms/m^3 of air (Harris 2005).

Patch testing of susceptible individuals (e.g. those with atopy) is recommended. Allergy from inhaled essential oils is known to occur, but data about exposure levels are limited and many of the reports concern perfumes rather than essential oils (Burfield 2000). Cumulative effects can occur. Essential oils that are not commonly used in aromatherapy have been associated with cancer, neurotoxicity (ketones) and hepatoxicity in large doses in animals, and these adverse events are most likely to occur with internal use (Tisserand & Balacs 1995).

Potentially carcinogenic essential oils

There is no evidence that essential oils cause cancer in humans, although some constituents are potentially carcinogenic, particularly saffrole, iso-saffrole, oestagole, methyl chavicol, methyl eugenol, elemicin, asarone and *d*-limonene (Tisserand & Balacs 1995). High doses and prolonged use of essential oils containing these constituents should be avoided; however, most of these are not commonly used in aromatherapy.

Use in pregnancy

Essential oils are widely used in midwifery units in Australia, the UK and USA. Women use them largely to manage backache, nausea, discomfort from varicose veins, prevent or reduce stretch marks and reduce perineal discomfort. Essential oil massages are often used in the last trimester to relieve backache and to aid relaxation and mental wellbeing. In Australia there is little internal use of aromatherapy oils; however, the practice is starting to attract interest. Internal use of essential oils should be undertaken with caution in pregnancy, as there are a number of reports of adverse effects following oral ingestion or vaginal use. This may be because higher doses achieved with oral dosing are likely to reach the fetus, as the placenta is permeable to essential oils because of their small molecular size (< 500 molecular units). This does not necessarily represent a risk to the fetus, but the fetal liver may not be mature enough to detoxify the oils or their components. In contrast, there are no case reports of topically applied or inhaled essential oils causing harm, but there is also no definitive evidence confirming safety in the first 16 weeks of pregnancy. A low dose, ~2%, is therefore recommended for full body massage during pregnancy, based on expert opinion rather than definitive evidence.

Although there is good evidence that fetal organs and tissues are sensitive to different chemicals at different stages of development, no such data is available for essential oils (Tisserand & Balacs 1995). When deciding about the risks and benefits of using essential oils during pregnancy the woman's medical history, obstetric history, weeks of gestation and current health need to be considered. Table 4.1 shows essential oils that should be used with caution, those that should be avoided throughout pregnancy and those generally considered safe to use. Taking a cautious view, aromatherapy experts recommend that essential oils with the potential to cause fetal damage be avoided throughout pregnancy. Essential oils containing sabinyl acetate and apiol represent the greatest risk to the fetus. Essential oils with a high proportion of antheol have mild oestrogenic effects, therefore internal use of these oils is not recommended. Many aromatherapists recommend emmenagogue essential oils be avoided, although there is little scientific evidence to indicate they cause adverse outcomes when used topically or inhaled.

Some of the current recommendations are based on contraindications for the herb extract; however, as has already been pointed out, essential oils and herbs may contain very different chemical components, even when they are derived from the same plant. Until more is known, caution is recommended.

INTERACTIONS

It is difficult to determine whether interactions between conventional medicines, herbal medicines and essential oils occur. Most texts focus on interactions with conventional medicines, and there is little information about interactions with herbal medicines. Interactions between topically applied essential oils and medicines are most likely if they are both applied to the same local site. Only very small amounts are absorbed from topical application, so clinically significant interactions are unlikely, but the potential for interactions increases with internal use (see Table 4.2). The

TABLE 4.1 USE OF ESSENTIAL OILS DURING PREGNANCY			
GENERALLY CONSIDERED SAFE	**GENERALLY CONSIDERED SAFE TO USE EXTERNALLY**	**USE WITH CAUTION**	**AVOID. THESE CONTAIN CAMPHOR, APIOL, SABINYL ACETATE OR PINOCAMPHONE**
Cardamom Roman and German chamomile Clary sage Coriander Geranium Ginger Lavender Neroli Palmarosa Patchouli Petitgrain Rose Rosewood Sandalwood Sweet orange or mandarin	Anise Fennel Lavandin Lavender spike *Lavandula stoechas* Rosemary Star anise Yarrow Mace	Artemisia Cangerana Cotton lavender Oakmoss Perilla Rue	Camphor Ho leaf Hyssop Indian dill *Juniperus pfitzeriana* Parsley leaf Plectranthus Spanish sage Savin

TABLE 4.2 COMMON APPLICATION METHODS, RECOMMENDED DOSES AND SAFETY TIPS FOR ESSENTIAL OILS		
APPLICATION METHOD	**DOSES (USING A STANDARD ESSENTIAL OIL DROPPER TOP)**	**SAFETY TIPS**
Massage	*Adults* The recommended dose is between 3.5% and 5% of an essential oil blend in a carrier oil. However, larger doses can be used safely (e.g. 15% in an aqueous cream, 10% in a gel). The dose also depends on the presenting problem (e.g. undiluted tea tree or lavender oil might be applied to an insect bite or a small burn, whereas lower doses would be used for chronic diseases). *Children* Children > 7 years and the elderly: 1–1.5%. Children 2–7 years: 0.5%. *Babies* 0–1 year: no essential oils. Approximately 25–30 mL of a carrier substance is needed for a full adult body massage, depending on size of the individual, skin condition and amount of body hair.	To avoid cumulative effects and reduce the likelihood of sensitivity developing over time, the same essential oils should not used for long periods. Essential oils containing aldehydes, phenols and furocoumarins, especially cinnamon (or cassia) and citrus oils such as bergamot (*Citrus bergamia*), are more likely to irritate the eyes, mucous membranes and skin, and cause sensitisation. Geranium, ginger, pine and citronella should be avoided by people with sensitive skin or a history of dermatitis. Essential oils are not recommended for use on babies.
Bath	4–7 drops of essential oils added to a warm bath directly or first mixed in a carrier substance and agitated into the bath water.	Take care that bath water with oils is not ingested and does not enter eyes. The oil must be mixed into the water before the person gets into the bath, not left floating on the surface.
Vaporiser	4–7 drops applied onto the surface of the water that is to be vaporised.	Keep vaporisers out of the reach of children and confused people who might drink from them. Poisoning has been reported in children drinking from vaporisers.
On a tissue, cotton ball, pillowcase or clothing	1–2 drops applied directly and inhaled from these items.	
Steam inhalation	Fill a bowl with 2 cups of almost boiling water and add 2–4 drops of essential oils. The scented steam should be inhaled for 5–10 minutes. Low doses of essential oils should be used to reduce the risk of irritating the respiratory mucous membranes and the eyes, especially when the oils are highly volatile (i.e. top notes). Five drops of essential oil yields approximately 35 mg of essential oil from a nebuliser.	Take care with people who have asthma because some oils can exacerbate symptoms. High doses, and some essential oils such as eucalyptus, can irritate the eyes.
Unscented lotions, creams or ointments	4–5 drops/60 mL of vehicle such as aqueous cream, white soft paraffin or vitamin E cream.	
Gargle and mouth wash	2–3 drops in 30 mL of distilled or spring water; for children, 1 drop mixed in honey before adding to water. Hydrosols can be used as mouthwashes and gargles.	Not to be ingested orally.

(Continued)

TABLE 4.2 COMMON APPLICATION METHODS, RECOMMENDED DOSES AND SAFETY TIPS FOR ESSENTIAL OILS *(continued)*

APPLICATION METHOD	DOSES (USING A STANDARD ESSENTIAL OIL DROPPER TOP)	SAFETY TIPS
Room sprays and spritzers	8–10 drops in 500 mL of distilled water. Spritzers are useful when the person cannot be massaged (e.g. for herpes zoster 15–20 drops in 50 mL can be used to relieve pain and itch). Hydrosols can be used as spritzers.	Use glass bottles or stainless steel spray cans, not plastic containers. Do not spray into the eyes.
Poultice	2–3 drops in ½ cup of chopped up solid or semi-solid medium, e.g. clay, oatmeal, linseeds, chopped comfrey. Hot water can be added to the mixture to make a paste, which is then spread onto a piece of gauze and covered with a second piece of gauze. Fold over the ends to secure the contents and apply warm to the affected area.	
Compress — hot or cold Cold compresses are used when there is inflammation, swelling or headache; hot compresses for muscle aches and pains, menstrual pain or boils.	2–6 drops, depending on the size of the area to be covered by the compress: 2–3 drops for a finger; 5–6 drops for a knee. A soft piece of fabric (e.g. flannel, towelling) is sufficient for both types. Put 6–10 drops of essential oil into 0.5 L of water (ice-cold or hot) and place the fabric on top of the water. Squeeze the fabric to prevent it from dripping when lifted out; however, don't allow the fabric to become too dry. Place the compress on the area to be treated and reapply when it has warmed or cooled to body temperature.	
Undiluted on the skin (tea tree, lavender)	1–2 drops onto a cotton bud and applied directly to the affected area.	Essential oils should not be applied directly to the skin unless under the direction of an aromatherapist. Some low-irritant essential oils, such as lavender and rosewood, are generally safe.
Oral, buccal (not generally used in Australia or New Zealand)	30 mg/dose for adults in a gel, capsule or lozenge. *Acute conditions* 60 mg three times daily for 3 days. *Chronic conditions* 30–45 mg three times daily for 15 days.	Essential oils should be used orally only under the direction of an aromatherapist qualified in this method of use. Many essential oils irritate mucous membranes.
Rectal suppositories (not generally used in Australia or New Zealand)	*Adults* 150–450 mg/day three times daily for 3 days. *Chronic conditions* 150 mg/day for 15 days.	Essential oils should be used only under the direction of an aromatherapist qualified in this method of use. Many essential oils irritate mucous membranes.
Vaginal suppositories (not generally used in Australia or New Zealand)	150 mg on 1 g suppository. 1–5% with an excipient in a douche. Up to 10% in a carrier substance on tampons.	Essential oils should be used only under the direction of an aromatherapist qualified in this method of use. Many essential oils irritate mucus membranes.

exact mechanism of actual or potential interactions is difficult to define. Most are theoretical, largely based on animal studies, and most are not thoroughly researched.

SAFETY PRECAUTIONS

- Most available essential oils are considered safe and present few risks when used appropriately.
- Most essential oils should not be applied undiluted to the skin.
- Susceptible individuals, such as those with a history of allergies or eczema, can develop a sensitivity to any essential oil.
- The risk of serious adverse events is higher with internal administration methods, especially oral.
- Essential oils containing aldehydes and phenols are more likely to cause allergic reactions. Patch testing before using essential oils for the first time may be indicated, especially in at-risk individuals.
- Using the same essential oils for long periods may lead to cumulative effects and cause sensitivity after a period of time. After 3 weeks of use, cessation for at least 24 hours is recommended.
- Although there is not any quality evidence to support recommendations for the use of essential oils in certain groups of people, traditional precautions and contraindications concerning pregnancy and lactation, epilepsy, asthma, people with alcohol or other addictions, certain age groups and disease states should be considered.
- Use traditional doses and dose intervals. Most aromatherapists use low doses, although effective therapeutic doses and dose ranges for specific situations are unclear.
- Some essential oils are not used in aromatherapy because of their known toxicity: for example, wormwood, rue, camphor, bitter almond and sassafras. Oil of wintergreen is sometimes on the exclusion list, but if it is used appropriately, it is an effective analgesic in a massage blend for muscular aches and arthritic pain.
- Essential oils must be appropriately stored and kept out of the reach of children, the cognitively impaired or suicidal patients to avoid inadvertent or deliberate overdose. Vaporisers should also be placed out of reach.
- Essential oils are highly flammable. Products must be used and disposed of appropriately to reduce the fire risk.
- Educating patients who self-apply essential oils is an important aspect of safe use.

For safety and medicolegal reasons healthcare professionals and the general public are advised to buy essential oils from reputable sources that label and store their products correctly. Labels are an important source of information and should contain the following information:
- botanical name, species, and if relevant the chemotype of the plant from which the oil was extracted or, in the case of a blend, for all the oils in the blend
- part or parts of the plant from which the essential oil was extracted
- country where the plants were grown (country of origin)
- extraction method
- statement of purity (however, this is not a regulatory requirement and not all suppliers make such statements)
- batch number, so that the batch can be identified if an adverse event occurs to determine whether the reaction was idiosyncratic or occurred because of the manufacturing process
- expiry date and storage precautions
- in some cases, specific warnings: for example, phototoxicity risk in Australia
- supplier details.

STORAGE

Essential oils are volatile and readily evaporate, so they should be stored in airtight amber glass bottles to protect them from light and air. Plastic is usually avoided because there can be transference of chemicals in the oil to the plastic and vice versa, thereby changing the chemical composition of the oil. Essential oils should also be stored in a cool place, preferably away from direct sunlight. Some aromatherapists store oils in a refrigerator. The 'top notes' of the oil have the lowest boiling points and are highly volatile and evaporate first, thereby altering the aroma of the oil. In general, oils should be used within 1 year of opening; however, their shelf-life can be extended with careful use and storage.

AROMATHERAPY IN PRACTICE

The level of evidence for aromatherapy use is an important aspect given the current focus on evidence-based care. The level of evidence is judged according to the quality of the research, considering factors such as statistical power, study design, accuracy of the measurements and the outcomes. Overall, most clinical aromatherapy research is low-level evidence (Dana-Farber Cancer Institute 2008). In addition, individual practice varies considerably, which means that the management of specific health conditions varies considerably.

As with all clinical practice, it is important to be clear about the goals of treatment and decide what treatment/s and forms of administration will achieve those goals. For aromatherapy, this means choosing the correct essential oils and whether the topical and/or inhaled method of administration is suitable. Psychological, physical and practical requirements are also assessed, together with relevant safety information. When using oils topically in children, the elderly or allergenic people, it is recommended that a skin test be performed first. One drop of oil applied with a cotton ball or swab to the inside of the elbow or wrist is usually sufficient. The application area should be marked and left unwashed for 24 hours. If a reaction occurs (redness and itch) the offending oil should be avoided. See Table 4.2 (p. 50) for more information about using oils in practice.

CHOOSING AN AROMATHERAPIST

Aromatherapy may be particularly beneficial for managing stress and inducing relaxation. It can also be useful in skin care, for managing topical fungal and bacterial infections, to relieve respiratory symptoms, as topical analgesia, and to reduce muscle spasm, especially when combined with massage. A key aspect of safe, effective aromatherapy treatment is choosing a knowledgeable and competent aromatherapist.

EDUCATION AND COMPETENCE

The aromatherapist should belong to a professional association, such as the International Federation of Aromatherapists (IFA) or the Australian Aromatic Medicine Association (AAMA), that has defined membership criteria, including the expectation that the aromatherapy training curriculum was approved by the Australian National Training Authority and/or state training authorities, whose competencies are consistent with national competency standards for aromatherapy, continuing professional development requirements and a code of professional conduct. These associations maintain membership lists and can be accessed via the telephone directory or their respective websites. Aromatherapists in Australia are not regulated, but membership of such an association suggests self-regulatory processes are in place. Undertaking short courses is adequate for self-care, but not for the therapeutic application of essential oils, even by healthcare professionals such as doctors and nurses.

PROFESSIONAL COURTESY

The aromatherapist should communicate with other relevant healthcare providers, document the care provided, including monitoring outcomes and adverse events, provide advice that includes the benefits and risks of using essential oils and recommend that people with serious conditions seek medical advice.

Safety

The aromatherapist should adhere to relevant occupational health and safety standards and other relevant Acts and regulations: although aromatherapists are not regulated, regulations apply to the products they use and their premises.

Clarity of outcome

The aromatherapist should be clear about what aromatherapy can offer and their personal competencies.

REFERENCES

Bensouilah J, Buck P. Aromadermatology: Aromatherapy in the treatment and care of common skin conditions. Oxford: Radcliffe Publishing, 2006.
Bleaser N et al. Allergic contact dermatitis following exposure to essential oils. Aust J Dermatol 45 (2002): 211–213.
Blumenthal M et al. The complete German Commission E monographs: therapeutic guide to herbal medicines. Austin, TX: American Botanical Council, 1998.
Bowles J. Basic chemistry of aromatherapeutic essential oils. Sydney: Allen & Unwin, 2003.

Burfield T. Safety of essential oils. Int J Aromather 10 (2000): 16–29.

Catty S. Hydrosols: The next aromatherapy. Rochester: Healing Arts Press, 2001.

Clarke S. Essential oil chemistry for safe aromatherapy. Edinburgh: Churchill Livingstone, 2002.

Cornwall PA et al. Modes of action of terpene penetration enhancers in human skin differential scanning calorimetry, small angle X-ray diffraction and enhancer uptake studies. Int J of Pharm 127 (1996): 9–26.

Cross S et al. Is there tissue penetration after application of topical salicylate formulations? Lancet 350 (1997): 636.

Dana-Farber Cancer Institute. Website: http://www.dana-farber.org/can/complementary-and-alternative-medicine, accessed June 2008.

Department of Health and Aged Care. National strategy for the quality use of medicines. Canberra: DHAC, 1999. Available online: www.health.gov.au November 2005.

Duke J. Fragrant plant aromathematics. Int J Aromather 9 (1998): 22–35.

Dunning T. Applying a quality use of medicines framework to essential oil use in nursing practice. Complement Ther Clin Pract 11 (2005): 172–81.

ESCOP (European Scientific Cooperative on Phytotherapy). ESCOP monographs: The scientific foundation for herbal medicinal products. Exeter, UK: ESCOP, 2003.

Ford R et al. The in vivo dermal absorption and metabolism of [4-^{14}C] coumarin by rats and by human volunteers under simulated conditions of use in fragrances. Food Chem Toxicol 39 (2001): 153–162.

Guba R. The modern alchemy of carbon dioxide extraction. Int J Aromather 12.3 (2002): 120–126.

Guba R. Quality matters: 'natural variation'. Essential News 15 (2004): 3–4.

Harris R. Use of essential oils in child care. Int J Aromather 2 (2005): 26–34.

Hirsch A. Aromatherapy: art, science or myth? In: Weintraub M (ed.), Alternative and complementary treatment in neurological illness. New York: Churchill Livingstone, 2001, pp 128–150.

Jager W et al. Percutaneous absorption of lavender oil from a massage oil. J Soc Cosmetic Chem 43 (1992): 49–54.

Jellinek S. Odour and mental states. Int J Aromather 9 (1998/99): 115–120.

Opdyke D. Inhibition of sensitisation reactions induced by certain aldehydes. Food, Cosmetic Toxicol 14.3 (1976): 197–198.

Price S, Price L. Aromatherapy for health professionals. Edinburgh: Churchill Livingstone, 1995.

Svoboda K. Case study: the effects of selected essential oils on mood, concentration and sleep in a group of 10 students monitored for 5 weeks. Int J Aromather 12 (2002): 157–161.

Tisserand R, Balacs T. Essential oil safety: A guide for health professionals. Edinburgh: Churchill Livingstone, 1995.

Van Toller S, Dodd G. Fragrance: The psychology and biology of perfume. Barking, UK: Elsevier, 1988.

Wabner D. The peroxide value: a new tool for the quality control of essential oils. Int J Aromather 12 (2002): 142–144.

CHAPTER 5

INTRODUCTION TO FOOD AS MEDICINE

Let food be your medicine and medicine be your food.
(Hippocrates)

The maxim coined by Hippocrates, the father of Western medicine, around the 5th century BC, is as true today as it was then. Hippocrates observed that certain foods had the potential to both prevent and treat disease, and recognised the effects of nutritional deficiencies and excesses on health (Jensen 1993). Hippocrates' axiom went largely ignored in the evolution of Western medicine, but the pioneering work of researchers such as Linus Pauling and Victor Rocine in the early 20th century created a renewed interest in the therapeutic value of food and its influence, both positive and negative, on health.

Over the last 100 years a number of significant developments have been made in nutritional science, including:

- identifying essential nutrients and documenting their associated biochemical pathways

- defining nutrient reference values and RDIs required to prevent nutritional deficiencies

- establishing dietary guidelines that include increasing consumption of fruits, vegetables and fibre, and reducing fat

- developing food guides, such as food pyramids, that can be used for daily meal planning.

Nutritional science has also led to the recognition that diet plays a major role in the chronic diseases that cause the bulk of morbidity and mortality in modern societies, such as heart disease, diabetes, hypertension and cancer.

Together with an increasing understanding of the potential benefits and negative consequences of food choices comes an unprecedented availability of different foods. Despite this, a problem of oversupply has arisen in developed countries and many Australians are consuming vast amounts of kilojoule-laden, yet nutrient-deficient, foods resulting in nutritional depletion and suboptimal nutrition. Largely as a result of this phenomenon, nutrition research has shifted from focusing exclusively on deficiency states to investigating the association between disease prevention, healthy ageing and adequate dietary intake in order to optimise quality of life and long-term health (Kennedy 2006).

FUNCTIONAL FOODS

The foods and substances we ingest affect us even at the most basic cellular level. In recent years scientists have discovered many thousands of previously unidentified substances in food and described their therapeutic actions. Currently around 50,000 (of a likely 200,000 substances) have been identified and described, yet for the most part we know very little about their functions (Hounsome 2008). These substances are known as phytonutrients, secondary metabolites, phytochemicals or a–nutrients.

Phytonutrients are generally classified according to their chemical structures, and major classes include phenolic and polyphenolic compounds (flavonoids, phenolic acids, lignins, anthocyanidins, catechins, isoflavones), terpenoids (carotenoids, tocopherols and tocotrienols, quinines, sterols), alkaloids (including saponins) and sulfur-containing compounds (glucosinolates, indoles, allylic sulfides) (Goldberg 2003). They impart colour, taste and smell, as well as possessing therapeutic properties such as antioxidant, anticarcinogenic, antimicrobial, antihypertensive, anti–inflammatory and cholesterol lowering properties.

When plants are under stress they produce these chemicals to defend themselves against infection or predation. In the absence of synthetic pesticides and fertilisers organic farming practices encourage these endogenous plant defence mechanisms and therefore result in higher levels of many phytonutrients (Brandt et al 2011). An example is salicylic acid, a phenolic compound that acts as a signalling molecule when a plant is under attack. It is also the active compound in aspirin which exerts anti-inflammatory and anti-platelet effects (Baxter et al 2001).

A brief summary of some of the better known phytonutrients, their major actions and therapeutic uses is shown in Table 5.1. Although thousands of studies have already been conducted to identify phytonutrients in foods and understand their properties and influence on human health, much remains unknown.

In parallel with the advances in nutritional science, there has been growing consumer interest in food's potential to have a positive impact on health and wellbeing, as well as in developments in food technology that allow foods to be produced, processed, preserved and fortified so as to maximise their nutritional values. This has led to changes in food-labelling laws that permit certain foods to make claims about health benefits, and has given rise to the development of functional foods.

The concept of a 'functional' food originated in Japan and is now being further developed, mainly in Japan, the United States and Europe. Functional foods are foods or dietary components that provide a health benefit that goes beyond their nutritional value, such as improving wellbeing and/or reducing the risk of disease. These may include traditional foods that have been shown to impart a positive biological effect or foods that have been modified to impart health benefits. Other terms that

TABLE 5.1 EXAMPLES OF PHYTONUTRIENTS FOUND IN FUNCTIONAL FOODS AND THEIR MAIN ACTIONS AND USES			
CLASS/ PHYTONUTRIENT	MAIN FOOD SOURCES	MAIN ACTIONS	CLINICAL USE
Carotenoids			
Beta-carotene	Carrots, sweet potatoes, spinach, pumpkin, apricots, rockmelon (cantaloupe)	Anticarcinogenic Antioxidant	May reduce the risk of lung cancer in smokers May protect against UV radiation (Stahl & Sies 2012)
Lutein, zeaxanthin	Green leafy vegetables such as kale, chard, spinach Egg yolk	Antioxidant Antitumour (breast, colon)	May reduce the risk of macular degeneration and cataracts, cardiovascular disease and some cancers (Koushan et al 2013, Ribaya-Mercado & Blumberg 2004)
Lycopene	Tomatoes cooked with oil Watermelon, guava, pink grapefruit, papaya	Antioxidant Anticarcinogenic (bladder, breast, cervix, prostate) Anti-inflammatory Hypocholesterolaemic	May reduce the risk of some cancers (especially prostate) and atherosclerosis (Bommareddy et al 2013, Bhuvaneswari & Nagini 2005)

(Continued)

TABLE 5.1 EXAMPLES OF PHYTONUTRIENTS FOUND IN FUNCTIONAL FOODS AND THEIR MAIN ACTIONS AND USES *(continued)*

CLASS/ PHYTONUTRIENT	MAIN FOOD SOURCES	MAIN ACTIONS	CLINICAL USE
Thiols/dithiols			
Alpha-lipoic acid (dithiol)	Potato, spinach Liver	Hypoglycaemic Antioxidant (water & lipid soluble) Hypotensive	May assist in the prevention of diabetic complications and cardiovascular disease Recycles other antioxidants (Rochette et al 2013, Eddey 2005, Smith et al 2004, Wollin & Jones 2003)
Glutathione (thiol)	Garlic, fruits, vegetables Meat (found in all cells of plants and animals)	Antioxidant Chemoprotective	Important endogenous antioxidant
Phenolic compounds (including flavonoids)			
Phenolic acids	Most fruits and vegetables, especially the cruciferous family (cabbage family), tomatoes, berries	Antioxidant Anti-inflammatory Inhibits platelet activity	
Polyphenols	Fruits and vegetables Wine Green tea Extra virgin olive oil Dark chocolate and other cocoa products	Anti-allergenic Antioxidant Anti-inflammatory	
Anthocyans (anthocyanins, glycosides, and their aglycons, anthocyanidins)	Fruits and berries	Anticarcinogenic Antioxidant	May reduce the risk of cancer and cardiovascular disease (Domitrovic 2011)
Caffeic acid (phenolic acid)	Fruits (apples, pears, citrus fruits) Some grains and vegetables	Antioxidant Antihypertensive Antithrombotic Antitumour Antiviral	May contribute to maintenance of healthy vision and cardiovascular health (Jiang et al 2005)
Ellagic acid (polyphenol)	Fruits, nuts and vegetables (e.g. pomegranate, strawberries, raspberries, grape seeds, onions)	Aldose reductase inhibitor (Duke 2003) Anticarcinogenic (cervix, colon, oesophagus, mouth) Antioxidant	Counteracts synthetic and naturally occurring carcinogens (Stoner & Mukhtar 1995)
Proanthocyanidins (catechin and epicatechin)	Fruits (e.g. apples, pears, grape seeds and peaches) Vegetables, nuts, beans (e.g. cocoa) Seeds, flowers and bark (e.g. pine) Tea Cocoa, chocolate	Antioxidant	May stabilise capillary walls and enhance wound healing May assist in the treatment of pancreatitis

TABLE 5.1 EXAMPLES OF PHYTONUTRIENTS FOUND IN FUNCTIONAL FOODS AND THEIR MAIN ACTIONS AND USES *(continued)*

CLASS/ PHYTONUTRIENT	MAIN FOOD SOURCES	MAIN ACTIONS	CLINICAL USE
Quercetin	Onions, beans Red wine Green tea, black tea Apples, berries	Anti-allergic Anti-inflammatory Antioxidant Antiviral	May assist in the treatment of allergies Prevention of diabetic complications
Resveratrol	Red wine and red grape juice	Anticarcinogenic (breast, prostate, skin) (Duke 2003) Antifungal Anti-inflammatory Antioxidant Antithrombotic	May reduce risk of cardiovascular disease and cancer (Raederstorff et al 2013, Fremont 2000)
Diphenols (phyto-oestrogens)			
Isoflavones (daidzein, genistein, glycitein)	Soybeans and soy-based products	Anticarcinogenic (breast) (Duke 2003) Antioxidant Phyto-oestrogenic	May ameliorate menopausal symptoms and contribute to the maintenance of bone and cardiovascular health
Lignans	Flax/linseed Some legumes and grains	Anticarcinogenic Antioxidant Phyto-oestrogenic	May contribute to maintenance of cardiovascular and immune function May reduce risk of breast and prostate cancers
ISOTHIOCYANATES			
Sulforaphane	Broccoli (especially young), broccoli sprouts, cauliflower, cabbage, kale, horseradish	Anti-apoptotic Anticarcinogenic Antioxidant	May reduce the risk of cancer and degeneration of the nervous system (Tarozzi et al 2013, Fimognari et al 2005, Gills et al 2005)
INDOLES			
Cruciferous indoles (indole-3-carbinol)	Cabbage, broccoli, Brussels sprouts, Chinese cabbage, Chinese greens, kale	Anticarcinogenic	May induce the metabolism of a cancer-preventive form of oestrogen and reduce the risk of cancer
FATTY ACIDS			
Conjugated linoleic acid	Dairy products and cooked meats	Anticarcinogenic Anti-inflammatory	May assist with fat loss and cardiovascular disease prevention (Dilzer & Park 2012)
Mono-unsaturated fatty acids	Olives, olive oil Canola oil	Anti-atherogenic Antihypertensive Anti-inflammatory	May reduce risk of cardiovascular disease and diabetes (Schwingshackl & Hoffmann 2012, Eddey 2005)
Omega-3 PUFAs (ALA, DHA, EPA)	Fish (deep sea/cold water) Flax/linseed, walnuts	Anti-arrhythmic Anticarcinogenic Antihypertensive Anti-inflammatory Cardioprotective	May reduce risk of cardiovascular disease (Lorente-Cebrián et al 2013, Eddey 2005) May contribute to maintenance of mental and visual function

(Continued)

TABLE 5.1 EXAMPLES OF PHYTONUTRIENTS FOUND IN FUNCTIONAL FOODS AND THEIR MAIN ACTIONS AND USES *(continued)*

CLASS/ PHYTONUTRIENT	MAIN FOOD SOURCES	MAIN ACTIONS	CLINICAL USE
Dietary fibre			
Beta-glucan	Oat bran, wholegrain oats	Antihypertensive Hypocholesterolaemic	May reduce risk of cardiovascular disease Reduces GI of meal
Insoluble fibre	Wheat bran, celery, dried beans	Anticarcinogenic	May contribute to the maintenance of a healthy digestive tract May reduce the risk of colon, lung, breast, cervical cancers
Soluble fibre	Psyllium seed husk, pectin, oat bran, broccoli	Hypocholesterolaemic Modulates bowel function	May lower cholesterol and reduce risk of cardiovascular disease May improve gastrointestinal health
Prebiotics/probiotics			
Inulin, oligofructose	Globe artichoke, garlic, onions, leeks, asparagus Whole grains Some fruits Honey	Anti-inflammatory Modulates immune function Prebiotic	Stimulates colonic production of short-chain fatty acids and favours the growth of lactobacilli and/or bifidobacteria (Guarner 2005) Increases calcium and magnesium absorption Influences blood glucose levels and reduces the levels of cholesterol and serum lipids (Lopez-Molina et al 2005)
Lactobacilli/ bifidobacteria	Yoghurt; some other fermented foods	Probiotic	May reduce diarrhoea (Guandalini 2011) Improve gastrointestinal health and systemic immunity

Data adapted from International Food Information Council Foundation. Functional foods. 2011. Available at: http://www.foodinsight.org/; Dr Duke's Phytochemical and Ethnobotanical Databases. Available at: www.ars-grin.gov/duke.

See respective monographs for more detail.

are used for functional foods are super foods, designer foods, fortified foods, nutraceuticals, cosmaceuticals, medifoods, vitalfoods and Foods for Specified Health Use (FOSHU) (Ashwell 2002).

Many commonly prescribed 'herbal medicines' can also be considered as functional foods and are commonly used for both medicinal and culinary purposes. Many of these foods and food derivatives are included in the monographs in this book: for example, celery seed, chamomile, cloves, cranberry, dandelion, fenugreek, fish oils, garlic, ginger, green tea, honey, horseradish, lemon balm, licorice, linseeds, noni, oats, peppermint, probiotics, raspberry, rosemary, sage, stinging nettle, thyme and turmeric.

There is some disagreement regarding how functional foods should be defined and the standards of scientific evidence required to support health claims (Verschuren 2002). Functional foods can be foods in which a component has been enhanced through special growing conditions or foods in which a component has been added, removed, modified or had its bioavailability increased. Functional foods cannot be marketed as medicines because they cannot make therapeutic claims for treating specific diseases; rather, they are designed to be marketed to healthy consumers to enhance health and prevent disease (Ashwell 2002). As such, functional foods are distinct from dietetic foods, which are designed for treating illness and are marketed to health professionals.

Examples of functional foods include garlic, blueberries, oats, yoghurt and probiotics, vitamin- and mineral-fortified breakfast cereals, iodised salt and sports drinks (which are proven to promote rapid gastric emptying and fast intestinal absorption, to improve water retention, thermal regulation and physical performance, and to delay fatigue) (Ashwell 2002).

Although functional foods retain their identity as foods and do not include pills, the line between food and medicine is a fine one and the line between food and herbal medicine even finer. In Australia, foods (including herbal medicines) are regulated according to their intended use either by the TGA or by Food Standards Australia New Zealand (FSANZ). Recently, recognition of the therapeutic value of foods has led to a review of the extension of permissible health claims, substantiated by scientific evidence, that are allowed on food packaging. Regulations currently allow for 'nutrition-content claims' (e.g. 'high in fibre'), 'general health level claims' such as calcium is good for bones and teeth and 'high level health claims' such as phytosterols may reduce blood cholesterol (FSANZ 2013). Health claims must be based on substantiated food–health relationships.

Although the primary aim of altering foods to make them 'functional' is to promote their beneficial effects, consideration should also be given to the potentially negative implications of manipulating foods, such as altering the natural synergy of nutrients, the introduction of synthetic nutrients and the possibility of detrimental effects. In the USA, for example, mandatory fortification of cereal and grain products with folic acid has raised concerns about increasing colon cancer risk (Lucock & Yates 2009), masking the haematological abnormalities of vitamin B_{12} deficiency, thereby allowing the progression of neurological complications to continue undetected (Rothenberg 1999), as well as placing some individuals at risk of exceeding the recommended safe upper limit of 1000 micrograms synthetic folate daily (Jamison 2005), while still failing to meet the peri-conceptual requirements of others (see Monographs: *Folate*).

SUPPLEMENTS VERSUS FOOD

Food, not nutrients, is the fundamental unit in nutrition.
Jacobs & Tapsell 2007

The actions of a whole food cannot be completely understood by studying its various components in isolation, because phytonutrients often interact with one another and, when used together, can produce different outcomes from those predicted for an isolated compound. Thus supplementation with individual food components may produce different effects from those produced by the consumption of the whole food. For example, epidemiological studies supporting the use of foods containing beta–carotene for the prevention of lung cancer in smokers have not been supported by clinical trials of supplementation with synthetic beta-carotene (Ziegler et al 1996) (see Monographs: *Beta-carotene*). Similarly, there is strong evidence to suggest that eating a variety of fibre-rich foods is beneficial in the prevention and management of diabetes; however, studies using fibre supplements have produced contradictory results (Venn & Mann 2004).

The results of these and other studies substantiate the value of 'whole foods' as medicine and suggest that epidemiological studies supporting the use of certain foods cannot necessarily be extrapolated to confirm the benefits of isolated supplementary nutrients. Furthermore, the practice of refining foods and then enriching them with synthetic versions of some of the lost nutrients cannot be deemed to be the equivalent of the whole food.

Nutritional supplements may prove lifesaving in an overt deficiency state and may enhance the individual's nutritional status when dietary intake is insufficient to meet physiological requirements, such as during periods of increased biological demand. Fundamentally the body uses nutrients as building blocks to create the tissues and structures of the body, and as chemicals in reactions that drive the functions of the body. Problems may arise when the availability of these nutrients is insufficient to meet the structural and functional demands of the body.

Some of the isolated nutritional supplements discussed in this book are used at doses unattainable through dietary modification alone. In such cases they are not only used to correct a deficiency/insufficiency state, but may also have direct pharmacological activity. However, such studies often elicit contradictory results and this may be because the prime benefit of nutrients is to ensure that the biological demands are met and actual pharmacological benefits may be less common. An individual's nutritional status is dependent upon supply and demand. Supply will be affected not only by the intake of nutrients from the diet (or supplementary sources), but also on how well those nutrients are absorbed. This is dependent on a number of factors including digestive function and the structural form of the nutrient. Demands may vary between individuals and during times of increased physiological need, such as infection or stress, and may also be compounded by losses that occur as a result of factors, including medication use, bleeding, etc. As such individuals will vary in their nutritional requirements, so studies that do not assess baseline nutritional status may fail to recognise that participants who commence a study with depleted stores of the nutrient/s in question may respond while others who may be depleted in other nutrients may not respond. Just as with building materials or chemicals in a laboratory, having excess stockpiles of select individual nutrients doesn't make up for a lack of others.

A further issue is that nutrients do not generally work in isolation and require cofactors. Some nutritional supplements may not produce the desired or anticipated effect because of the absence of significant but as yet unidentified cofactors that are important for bioavailability, pharmacological activity or safety of the individual constituent. While a nutritional supplement will contain a limited number of nutrients at specific doses it may not contain, or the individual taking it may not be replete in, other nutrients required as cofactors. An individual food will contain many different nutrients and phytonutrients, those that science has identified and others that science has yet to identify. These individual foods will generally also be consumed in combination with other foods as part of a whole meal and a whole diet. As a result, the likelihood that an individual will attain the specific nutrients they require is increased with the intake of a varied whole food diet.

INDIVIDUALISING FOOD

An old Chinese proverb states 'Whatsoever was the father of disease, an ill diet was the mother'. Traditional medicine systems such as traditional Chinese medicine (TCM) and Ayurvedic medicine continue to understand and practise using food as medicine, and view food within a conceptual framework that includes the energetic value of food in addition to its physical qualities. An assessment of different foods may be based on the food's 'vitality' or 'life force', otherwise known as 'chi' in TCM and 'prana' in Ayurvedic medicine. The type of food and its biological, nutritional and sensual properties, together with the many agricultural practices, production processes and preparation methods, make a contribution to this force. Every step in the process of producing a food may potentially affect the energetic value, net nutritional content and overall therapeutic benefits.

In traditional medicine systems, foods may be classified as having properties such as 'heating', 'cooling', 'drying' or 'moistening', and may be considered to be energetically aligned with one or more of five phases of transformation, or 'elements', that correspond to the different organ systems and tissues within the body, as well as to the different emotions, seasons, colours and so on. These properties, as well as constitutional typing of the patient, may be used to make a sophisticated assessment of an individual and to design dietary prescriptions based on an individual's constitution, propensities for disease development and/or responses to different foods. Thus traditional medicine systems can be seen to practise 'nutriphenomics', whereby a food is used as a medicine based on a person's phenotype.

Biomedical science has not matched the same degree of sophistication in individualising diet as traditional medicines; however, it is moving in this direction. Just as in pharmaceutical medicine the emerging science of pharmacogenomics promises to provide drugs best suited to a person's genetic makeup, the emerging science of nutrigenomics promises to deliver an understanding of how different nutrients affect genes to cause specific conditions, and the ability to design foods and dietary recommendations based on an assessment of an individual's genotype (see also Chapter 3). The success of such developments and their impact in human health, however, are yet to be determined.

FOOD QUALITY ISSUES

The health benefits of different foods must be considered in relation to the many agricultural farming practices and production processes that are involved. As soon as produce is picked or an animal is killed, it starts to decompose and lose nutritional value. When a ripe organic apple is picked in season directly from the tree and eaten immediately its nutritional value is at its maximum. How does this compare to the apple grown in nutritionally depleted soil, using pesticides and synthetic fertilisers, out of season, picked before ripening and kept in cold storage to extend its shelf life, potentially for months, even years?

Every step in the process, from paddock to plate and beyond, may potentially affect the nutrients, as well as the 'energetic' quality and therapeutic benefits of the food. Thus food quality can be affected by multiple factors:

- farming conditions, which include genetic variety (seed/animal species), chemical exposure (e.g. pesticides, fertilisers), maturity at harvest, location, water availability, soil composition, animal care and feeding practices, climate, seasons, aspect and sunlight exposure
- transport and handling conditions
- processing, such as milling, refining and enriching
- preservation methods, which may include chemical additives, cold storage, drying, salting, irradiation
- packaging methods and the conditions and length of storage
- meal preparation methods, such as cutting, crushing or tossing
- cooking methods, such as no cooking (i.e. food is raw), steaming, frying, microwaving
- how food is consumed, which includes duration of mastication, food combinations and the biochemical individuality of the person consuming the food (Gliszczynska-Swiglo et al 2005, Jeffery et al 2003, Podsedek 2005).

PESTICIDE RESIDUES

The creation of a global food industry and the emergence of agribusiness have led to the increasing use of pesticides in food production. At the same time there is growing worldwide public concern about the impact of these pesticides on human health. Currently, it is reasonable to expect that most animals on the planet have accumulated pesticide residues through water, air or the food chain and, although acute effects of pesticides are well documented, the chronic effects of pesticide exposure are more difficult to assess.

Given that the intended purpose of pesticides is to damage or kill living organisms, it is not surprising that there are many published studies attesting to a link between pesticide exposure and health risks. In a systematic review conducted for the Ontario College of General Physicians in 2004 (Sanborn et al 2004) a positive relationship was identified between exposure to pesticides and the development of many cancers (Bassil et al 2007); as well as the risk of genotoxic, immunotoxic, neurotoxic and reproductive effects; and an increased incidence of psychiatric and dermatological conditions (Sanborn 2007). The review was updated in 2012 with a focus on reproductive, neurodevelopmental, behavioural and respiratory health outcomes (Sanborn et al 2012). It highlighted specific concerns for elevated risk of preterm birth as well as birth defects, including hypospadias, neural tube defects and diaphragmatic hernia; and called for measures to reduce exposure of pregnant women to pesticides. It also found that prenatal pesticide exposure is consistently associated with measurable deficits in child neurodevelopment from impaired mental development in newborns, to attention deficit hyperactivity disorder (ADHD) and reduced IQ in older children. The review further highlighted multiple studies reporting associations between pesticide exposure and asthma, chronic obstructive lung diseases and reduced lung function. An earlier review, which focused on the effects of pesticides on children, indicated that pesticide residues have been implicated in causing reproductive problems, including miscarriages and spontaneous abortion, birth defects, childhood cancer and neurological, neurobehavioural and endocrine effects (Garry 2004).

Children appear to be particularly vulnerable to the effects of pesticides because they eat and drink more per kilogram of body weight than adults, and their diets are often rich in foods that contain higher levels of pesticides, such as fresh fruits, vegetables and juices. It should be noted that such contaminants are often bio-accumulated in the fatty tissue of animals, and that concerns over pesticide exposure should not lead to the removal of nutrient-rich foods from the diet, but rather to minimising exposure by choosing organic foods whenever possible.

Children's exposure to pesticides may also be increased through breast milk. This provides many immunological, physiological, nutritional and psychological advantages, but is nevertheless commonly contaminated with high levels of pesticides. For example, it has been found that serum concentrations of organochloride compounds are significantly higher ($P < 0.0001$) in breastfed infants than in bottle-fed infants (Lackmann et al 2004), and that an infant's measured intake of organochlorines from breast milk may greatly exceed the adult acceptable daily intake (ADI) (Quinsey et al 1995, 1996). The fact that children born today have a longer life expectancy in which to develop diseases with long latency periods places them at further risk (Sanborn et al 2004). In addition, children have less developed detoxification pathways; for example, newborn infants have low levels of the enzymes carboxylesterase and paraoxonase-1 (PON-1), which detoxify certain pesticides (Chen et al 2003, Yang et al 2009) and in childhood there can be reduced activity of PON-1, although the extent of this effect appears to vary depending on the genotype (Huen et al 2009). Serum PON-1 levels and activity also vary widely between different ethnic populations due to polymorphisms (Mohamed Ali & Chia 2008).

The dietary exposure of the Australian population to pesticides and other food contaminants was previously monitored every 2 years via the Australia Total Diet Survey (ATDS) conducted by Food Standards Australia New Zealand (FSANZ). The 23rd ATDS was released in November 2011. Pesticides were tested for the first time since the 20th ATDS, which was conducted in 2001 and published in early 2003. The survey examined dietary exposure to 214 agricultural and veterinary chemicals in 92 foods and beverages. This represented a wider range than the 88 pesticides and 65 foods previously surveyed. A total of 46 agricultural chemicals were detected in this study. Seven had dietary exposures exceeding 10% of the Acceptable Daily Intake (ADI) and estimated dietary exposures tended to be highest in 2–5-year-olds (FSANZ 2011, 2014). Other residue testing is also conducted on fresh produce in Australia (e.g. FreshTest and the National Residue Survey), but this is largely funded and directed by industry bodies.

Although safety assessments are conducted on pesticides and guidelines are set for maximum residue levels (MRLs), this does not necessarily guarantee food safety as numerous other factors need to be considered. Safety assessments usually examine only single chemicals at high doses and often only in animals, which may lead to a significant underestimation of the potential risk associated with the numerous mixtures of compounds that consumers are typically exposed to. The actual pesticide formulations used may be several hundred times more toxic than the active principle that has been tested (Mesnage et al 2014). The combined toxic effect of multiple chemicals is not necessarily predictable by adding up the toxic potential of each chemical; mixtures of chemicals can also interact to produce synergistic toxic effects (Laetz et al 2009). Thus it is possible that there may be greatly enhanced toxicity of these compounds when they are combined, and this is supported by research documenting reproductive, immune and nervous system effects not expected from the individual compounds acting alone (Boyd et al 1990, Porter et al 1993, 1999, Thiruchelvam et al 2000). Pregnant and lactating women require specific consideration to minimise exposure of the fetus or infant during critical periods of development and consistent research on the risks to children have led to calls to limit children's exposures to pesticides as much as possible (Roberts & Karr 2012). A report for the American Academy of Pediatrics expressed concern about the subclinical effects of long-term, low-dose exposure and recommended ongoing research describing toxicological vulnerabilities and exposure factors across the life span to inform regulation and allow for appropriate interventions (AAP 2012).

GENETIC MODIFICATION (TRANSGENIC FOODS)

Conventional methods of selective breeding and cross-breeding have been used for centuries to alter the genetic makeup of the foods we consume; for example, the wheat that we consume today is significantly different from the wheat consumed by our ancestors. However, these methods allow only for the selective enhancement of characteristics that already exist within a species or compatible species. In recent years transgenic technology, commonly (if not entirely accurately) known as 'genetic engineering', has been developed. This allows for the introduction of genetic material from unrelated species, which would not be possible using conventional methods. Transgenic crops have been grown commercially since the mid-1990s, but at present no livestock or fish have been commercially released for food or agricultural purposes.

While advocates maintain that there is the potential for biotechnology to have a positive impact on the nutritional properties of transgenic foods and to allow for their cultivation in areas where farming is difficult, it has been argued that most transgenic foods have so far produced greater benefits for producers than consumers. The Food and Agriculture Organisation of the United Nations has expressed concerns that developments in biotechnology 'have not sufficiently benefited smallholder farmers and producers and consumers' (FAO 2014a).

As yet, the long-term safety implications of genetically modified organisms (GMOs) are unclear and most of the published studies have been conducted by biotechnology companies responsible for commercialising these products (Domingo & Gine Bordonaba 2011). In 2013 the FAO established the GM Foods Platform to share information on safety assessment of foods derived from recombinant-DNA plants (FAO 2014b). The long-term safety implications of genetic engineering, a self-regulated industry, are being hotly debated by activists and the public alike. Some of the issues under discussion focus on:

- the consequences of introducing into the food chain questionable genetic material that may produce unpredictable results

- the introduction of lectins, causing immunological effects, such as allergic reactions

- the use of bacteria and viruses to introduce foreign material into cells

- the use and potential spread of antibiotic-resistant genes

- the greater use of pesticides and herbicides with transgenic crops

- the contamination of non-transgenic crops with modified genes

- the use of terminator genes and prevention of seed-saving.

Consequently, many communities are divided as to whether transgenic foods should be allowed in their country. The prospect that transgenic crops could be used for mass medication and vaccination programs also raises concern in some circles. In reality, the ultimate benefits and detriments of genetic engineering are unlikely to be known for several generations.

A number of GM crops have been approved for sale in Australia and New Zealand: canola corn, cotton/cottonseed oil, lucerne, potatoes, rice, soybeans and sugar beet. In Australia, to enable consumer choice, food producers are required to label foods that contain a GM-derived component or a GM protein introduced through genetic engineering; however, there are numerous exceptions and the genetic material that has been used is not specified (FSANZ 2014).

ANTIBIOTIC RESISTANCE

The use of antibiotics in conventional agriculture has led to the fear that widespread antibiotic-resistant bacteria have emerged that can cause disease in humans and animals that will be difficult to treat (Forman & Silverstein 2012). There are also concerns about the impact of chronic cumulative exposure to antibiotics, the risk of allergic reactions to antibiotics and the disruption of gut microbiota (Dolliver & Gupta 2008).

Although the widespread use of antibiotics in animal production ceased in Europe in 2006, it remains commonplace in countries such as Australia. On last count, approximately two-thirds of the antibiotics used in Australia were used in intensive animal production (JETACAR 1999).

Sub-therapeutic doses of antibiotics are utilised on conventional farms for the control of infection, which is a particular concern in large-scale animal confinement operations, but they are also used as growth promotants (Dolliver & Gupta 2008). Antibiotics are routinely added to the food and water of healthy livestock and may be retained in animal products and therefore consumed by humans. Alternatively they may be excreted unaltered and then contaminate groundwater (Blackwell et al 2009) or soil used for growing human (or livestock) food, and accumulate up the food chain (Rosenblatt-Farrell 2009); and affect soil quality by inhibiting microbial and enzyme activities (Liu et al 2009). Furthermore, antibiotic-resistant genes are sometimes added as marker genes to GM food.

As such practices are largely restricted in organic agriculture (AQIS 2009) the presence of antibiotic-resistant bacteria is significantly lower in organic produce (Smith-Spangler et al 2012). Antibiotic residues have been reported in animal tissue samples collected as part of the National Residue Survey (NRS) as have ractopamine (a beta-agonist used as a growth promotant) and antiparasitics (anthelmintics, anticoccidials) (DAFF 2012).

FOOD ADDITIVES AND IRRADIATION

Additives are listed as either numbers, known as additive codes, or by name; 'de-coders' are readily available in many bookshops and online. Up-to-date lists of the food additives used in Australian and New Zealand food products are available from the FSANZ website (FSANZ 2012). Food additives include preservatives, artificial sweeteners, colourings, flavourings and hydrogenated fats. The prevalence of food additive intolerance in school-aged children is estimated to be around 1–2% (Fuglsang et al 1993). Reactions may occur to preservatives (atopic dermatitis, asthma, rhinitis), colouring agents (atopic dermatitis, asthma, urticaria, gastrointestinal symptoms) or other substances (Fuglsang et al 1994). Artificial colourings and preservatives have been associated with hyperactivity in some children, and a UK study reported that the proportion of hyperactive children halved when additives were removed from their diets (Bateman et al 2004).

A further concern is the long-term safety of consuming irradiated foods. Currently irradiation is used for the purpose of food preservation, to control microbes and to protect against critical quarantine pests. Irradiated food is exposed to gamma rays from a radioactive source, which kill insects, eggs, larvae and pathogenic microorganisms.

The Food Standards Code in Australia allows for the irradiation of a select number of products including spices, herbs, herbal teas, tomatoes, capsicum and some tropical fruits (FSANZ 2013) as a disinfestation measure for pests such as the fruit fly. However, the practice is not common in Australia because it is expensive and the dose required to inactivate pathogens is often too high to be tolerated by the fresh produce without undesirable changes in nutrients and quality (Gomes et al 2011). The safety data from toxicological analysis of irradiated food and animal feeding experiments is relatively strong, but the issue remains controversial due to concerns about nutrient impairment, effects on beneficial gut microbiota and the use of nuclear technology (Shea 2000).

PROCESSING AND PREPARATION

While production and preservation methods may affect food quality, processing techniques may also significantly affect the therapeutic value of a food, and both benefits and detrimental effects are possible. For example, as both fibre and other nutrients are concentrated in the outer part of the grain, significant losses of not only fibre, but also of B vitamins, fat-soluble vitamins and other nutrients occur when grain is refined (Jamison 2006). Similarly, food preparation methods can significantly affect a food's therapeutic qualities. Consider the potentially different nutritional and energetic effects of the same food consumed raw, juiced, steamed, boiled, fried, barbecued or microwaved. For example, steaming and drying may actually increase the sulforaphane content and antioxidant activity of broccoli, while freezing and boiling diminishes the polyphenol concentration (Mahn & Reyes 2012). The microwaving of broccoli has been found to destroy 97% of the flavonoids; conventional boiling destroys 66% and high-pressure boiling causes considerable leaching into the cooking water, whereas steaming produces minimal loss (Vallejo et al 2003).

Cooking does not always have detrimental effects and can sometimes increase the bioavailability of bioactive compounds; for example, the lycopene in tomatoes is more bioavailable when tomatoes are cooked in oil. The concentration of phenolic compounds in a food may also be increased by thermal processing, resulting in a significant increase in overall antioxidant status, despite some loss of heat-sensitive antioxidant nutrients such as vitamin C (Jamison 2006).

Food combination is another factor that influences the therapeutic value of a meal; for example, consuming red meat with leafy greens and a citrus salad dressing synergistically improves iron absorption. The consumption of antioxidants in the diet, such as the tocopherols, coenzyme Q10, carotenoids, vitamin A, ascorbic acid, reduced glutathione, selenomethionine, flavonoids and other polyphenolic compounds, together with spices and synthetic antioxidants added to food, may counteract the effects of pro-oxidants found in food and the environment. Applying this concept, it could be suggested that foods containing high levels of pro-oxidants (e.g. meat) should be served with plenty of antioxidant-containing vegetables, together with sauces, juices, fruits and teas high in antioxidants (Surai et al 2004). This is supported by a study of 2814 male smokers who participated in the Belgian Interuniversity Research on Nutrition and Health study. This found that men with the highest oxidative balance score had a higher relative risk of all-cause mortality (RR = 1.44, 95% confidence interval [CI]: 1.13–1.82) and of total cancer mortality (RR = 1.62, 95% CI: 1.07–2.45), compared with men in the lowest-score group (Van Hoydonck et al 2002).

Glycaemic index

The glycaemic index (GI) ranks carbohydrates based on their immediate effects on blood glucose levels. Carbohydrate-containing foods that cause a rapid rise in blood glucose are said to have a high GI (> 70), whereas those that cause a slow, steady rise in blood glucose, a more ideal situation, have a low GI (< 55). As insulin is released in response to circulating glucose levels, foods with a high GI will cause a rapid rise in insulin levels. In the presence of chronically-elevated levels of circulating glucose and insulin, cells begin to shut down receptor sites, resulting in insulin resistance. Foods that have a low GI rating cause a much slower rise in blood glucose levels and therefore less insulin is secreted in response.

Observational studies indicate that a low-GI diet reduces elevated low-density lipoprotein (LDL) and triglyceride levels, raises high-density lipoprotein (HDL) levels (Dushay & Abrahamson 2005) and improves fasting glucose and glycated protein values (Anderson et al 2004). Recent reviews also reveal beneficial effects on fasting insulin and pro-inflammatory markers such as C-reactive protein (Schwingshackl et al 2013). In addition to beneficial effects in diabetes and obesity, low-glycaemic-load diets have also demonstrated benefits in conditions such as acne (Smith et al 2007).

As some foods have a low GI because of their fat content, the GI rating should not be used in isolation, but as part of a sensible approach that limits the amount of saturated and *trans*-fatty acids in the diet. Additionally, other foods that have a high GI, such as potatoes, may also contain substances such as lipoic acid, which is beneficial for the prevention of the long-term complications of diabetes. As such, it is more important to consider the GI or glycaemic load (GL) of the *entire* meal than to eliminate all foods with a high GI. The GL is calculated by multiplying the number of grams of carbohydrate in a serving of food by the GI value, and is expressed as a percentage: GL = GI (%) × grams of carbohydrate per serving.

Social, cultural and environmental aspects

In addition to being influenced by physico-chemical properties, the therapeutic qualities of food may further be affected by a person's psychological state and/or intention while preparing and eating food, as well as by the social, cultural, economic, ethical, religious and environmental impact of the food. It has been said that 'eating is essentially an act of communion with the living forces of nature' (Robbins 1992). Indeed, most cultures and traditions have developed mealtime rituals that acknowledge the source of their food and attempt to align mind and body with the greater forces of nature. Food also features prominently in many spiritual traditions and practices. Thus, the idea of saying grace before meals and then eating 'gracefully' and mindfully, without rushing, may make significant contributions to psychological and spiritual health.

The effects of 'un-mindful' eating have been demonstrated in a study that revealed that television viewing increases energy intake by delaying normal mealtime satiation and reducing satiety signals from previously consumed foods (Bellissimo et al 2007). The boys in the study consumed on average an extra 228 kcal (approximately one and a half pieces of pizza) over a 30-minute period while watching an episode of *The Simpsons*. When we are not eating mindfully we are not able to recognise when we have had enough. In contrast, studies have shown that an eating-focused mindfulness-based intervention can result in statistically significant decreases in weight, eating disinhibition, binge eating and psychological distress in obese individuals (Dalen et al 2010). Benefits have also been noted in people with eating disorders (Hepworth 2011).

Food and health are both multidimensional and interrelated. Food choices not only influence physiological functioning, but have much broader social, economic, ethical and environmental ramifications, which may in turn affect personal health and wellbeing. Some of these aspects are becoming acknowledged in wider food-related social movements, such as the Fair Trade Federation, International Slow Food Movement and Food Miles.

Food is not just a means of providing nutrition and sustaining health, it is also a global industry that affects everyone. In the new global economy, there is a fear that the production, trade and retailing of most goods and services are being increasingly concentrated under the control of a small number of corporations that have enormous influence. It is questionable whether all corporations take sufficiently seriously the responsibility of providing quality foods while protecting workers and their environment, and whether free-trade agreements do any more than just offer global protection for a company's intellectual and property rights. For example, global trade in coffee and cocoa has led to social disruption, environmental damage and the mistreatment of workers, including children, who earn meagre wages while corporations make huge profits (Cavanagh 2006).

To counter this trend, the Fair Trade Federation (2014) sets standards for commodities, such as coffee, tea, sugar, cocoa and fruits, that will support living wages and safe, healthy conditions for workers in the developing world. Fair Trade standards stipulate that traders must pay a price to cover the costs of sustainable production and living, and the organisation attempts to support food-producing communities by paying a premium that producers can invest in development, making partial advance payments when requested by producers and signing contracts that allow for long-term planning and sustainable production practices.

The environmental, economic, social and health consequences of the global trade in food are not only influenced by how food is produced, but also by its transportation. Nutrients have their best chance to develop under certain climatic conditions; this means that foods grown and harvested seasonally have an advantage and are also more appropriate for eating at those times of year. The ability to transport food around the world allows seasonal food to be eaten year round and creates an enormous economic, social and environmental burden. The environmental and social implications of the rapid escalation in 'food miles', which is the distance that food travels before being consumed, have been reviewed by Sustain (2011), which also considers the effects of food on behaviour and mental health.

The interests of the food industry and agribusiness are not always aligned with the interests and needs of consumers; for example, the widespread availability of fast foods and their enormous popularity threatens gastronomic traditions, traditional cultivation and processing techniques, while standardising taste. The Slow Food Movement is an international movement that originated in Italy; it attempts to address these concerns by:

- promoting regional food and wine cultures, while defending food and agricultural biodiversity worldwide
- opposing the standardisation of taste
- defending the need for consumer information
- protecting cultural identities tied to food and gastronomic traditions
- safeguarding traditional foods (Slow Foods Movement 2014).

Unfortunately the exploitation of natural and human resources comes at a cost. For too long, the external costs of agribusiness have been delayed, resulting in the availability of artificially 'cheap' but nutritionally depleted food. The food production industry is now faced with new challenges: the results of years of hyperintensive farming practices (soil erosion, contamination of water sources, superbugs), the effects of climate change, water shortages; rising oil prices (required for transportation, food processing and the production of pesticides and fertilisers); the diversion of food grain for ethanol production; and the loss of arable land to urbanisation. All these challenges must be met with nutritionally, socially and environmentally responsible solutions.

PRINCIPLES OF USING FOOD AS MEDICINE

It is often said that 'you are what you eat'; however, it may be more accurate to say that 'you are what you absorb in relation to your individual demands'. Differences in flavonoid bioavailability may result from variations in gut physiology and flora (Grinder-Pedersen et al 2003). Demand for nutrients may also vary both between and within individuals depending on their circumstances. Additional nutrients may be required to support the body during times of stress, infection, blood loss, etc. Demand may also be increased to support the metabolism of environmental toxins.

Food choices can exert a profound positive or negative influence on individual health, as well as on the health of communities and the environment. While the research community establishes the mechanisms by which foods exert their biological effects, there are some general recommendations that can enhance the positive impact of food, summarised by the mnemonic SLOW: consume food that is:

S **S**easonal
L **L**ocally produced with Lots of colour and variety
O **O**rganic
W **W**hole, fresh and with minimal processing.

THERAPEUTIC POTENTIAL OF COMMON FOODS

When consuming or prescribing functional foods, consideration should be given not only to the selection of foods for their potential therapeutic benefits, but also to the quality of the food consumed (as discussed earlier), and to the digestive function and health status of the individual. It should be noted that no single food should be eaten to the exclusion of others,

and the inclusion of functional foods should form part of an otherwise balanced diet. Several examples of foods that may be incorporated into the diet for physiological benefit are discussed here, but a range of foods are covered in greater depth in the monographs.

Blueberries (and other berries)

A growing body of research suggests that the dietary intake of berry fruits has a 'positive and profound impact on human health, performance, and disease' (Seeram 2008). Berry cousins – blueberry (*Vaccinium corymbosum*), cranberry (*Vaccinium macrocarpon*) and bilberry (*Vaccinium myrtillus*) — have demonstrated significant benefits in the past, and there has recently been increased interest in other berry-type fruits, such as pomegranate (*Punica granatum*), goji berry (*Lycium barbarum*), mangosteen (*Garcinia mangostana*) and the Brazilian acai berry (*Euterpe oleraceae*).

Blueberries, native to East Asia and the United States (Natoli 2005), are readily available fresh during the warmer months and frozen or juiced year round. They were traditionally used by the North American Indians for the treatment of diarrhoea and labour pains (Pratt & Matthews 2004a) and are an excellent source of antioxidant nutrients and phenolic compounds that work synergistically within the body (including vitamin C, beta-carotene, flavonoids, anthocyanins and resveratrol) (Natoli 2005, Pratt & Matthews 2004a). The anthocyanins are powerful antioxidant and anti-inflammatory agents, responsible for the deep blue-purple colour of blueberries; the deeper the colour, the greater the anthocyanin content (Pratt & Matthews 2004a).

The majority of studies to date rely on in vitro, animal and epidemiological evidence. Blueberry and its cousins appear to 'limit the development and severity of certain cancers and vascular diseases, including atherosclerosis, ischaemic stroke and neurodegenerative diseases of ageing' (Neto 2007). Anticarcinogenic properties have been demonstrated in prostate cell lines, and blueberry extracts have been shown to suppress tumour growth, protect the integrity of DNA (Natoli 2005), reduce angiogenesis (Atalay et al 2003), inhibit the proliferation of androgen-dependent prostate cancer cells (Schmidt et al 2006), prevent oestrogen-induced mammary tumours (Jeyabalan et al

2013, Aiyer 2008) and reduce the risk of metastasis (Matchett et al 2006). Studies have demonstrated improved insulin sensitivity (Stull et al 2010), a reduction in fat cell production and proliferation (Moghe et al 2012), a reduction in total and LDL cholesterol (Kalt 2008), reduction in blood pressure in hypertensive rats (Wiseman et al 2011) and reduced risk of cardiovascular disease (Ahmet et al 2009, Kalea et al 2006, Youdim et al 2002). Blueberries are thought to improve memory (Krikorian et al 2010, Carey et al 2014), and the antioxidant and anti-inflammatory effects of blueberries have been associated with an improvement in age-related cognitive and motor deficits, spatial working memory tasks and neurodegenerative disorders such as Alzheimer's disease, and improved growth capacity in neural transplants (Bickford et al 1999, 2000, de Rivera et al 2005, Galli et al 2006, Lau et al 2005, Ramirez et al 2005, Wang et al 2005, Williams 2008, Willis 2008). Animal studies suggest blueberry may also assist with prevention of bone loss (Devareddy et al 2008) and may act synergistically with cranberry to inhibit *Helicobacter pylori* (Vattem et al 2005). Human clinical trials have demonstrated improved exercise capacity in hot environments (McAnulty et al 2004) and accelerated recovery of muscle peak isometric strength after exercise (McLeay et al 2012).

Choose dark blue-purple berries that move freely in the container. Damaged berries will inhibit movement and be prone to mould and should be discarded before storage. Organic fruit is preferable because it has higher concentrations of malic acid, phenolics, anthocyanins and overall higher antioxidant activity (Wang et al 2008). Although the vitamin C content degrades rapidly during heating and storage, many of the phenolic compounds may actually become more bioavailable, improving the overall antioxidant capacity (Wehrmeister et al 2005). Frozen berries maintain the phenolic compounds and provide an excellent source for year-round availability (Srivastava 2007). As blueberries contain salicylates, those with a known sensitivity should be cautious about consuming them (Natoli 2005).

Broccoli (and cruciferous vegetables)
Broccoli, originally grown in the Mediterranean region and cultivated by the ancient Romans, belongs to the cruciferous family of vegetables (Brassicaceae), so-called because of the cross-shaped structure of the leaves and flowers (Pratt & Matthews 2004b). The family also includes cauliflower, Brussels sprouts, cabbage and kale, which have also demonstrated significant therapeutic potential. Broccoli is low in kilojoules and an excellent source of fibre; calcium; folate; vitamins C, E and K; coenzyme Q10; iron; sulforophane; indoles; phenolic compounds (quercetin, kaempferol, hydroxycinnamoyl acids); and the carotenoids beta-carotene, cryptozanthin, lutein and zeaxanthin (Damon et al 2005, Lucarini et al 1999, Podsedek 2005, Pratt & Matthews 2004b). The antioxidant nutrients in broccoli work in synergy to reduce reactive oxygen species and recycle each other (Podsedek 2005); however, significant variations occur in nutrient levels because of differences in variety, maturity at harvest, soil quality, sunlight exposure, growing environment, processing and storage conditions (Jeffery et al 2003, Gliszczynska-Swiglo et al 2005, Podsedek 2005).

Numerous epidemiological studies have established an inverse association between the consumption of cruciferous vegetables and the incidence of cancer (especially lung, colon, stomach, rectal, bladder and premenopausal breast cancers) (Brennan et al 2005, Cortizo & Vitetta 2004, Kim et al 2003, Pratt & Matthews 2004b, Tang 2008). A possible explanation for this is the effect of glucoraphanin (a glucosinolate) on mitochondrial function (Armah et al 2013). When broccoli is crushed or chewed, glucoraphanin is converted by the action of myrosinase into isothiocyanates, the most studied of which is the powerful anticarcinogenic compound known as sulforophane (Matusheski et al 2004). Young broccoli shoots are the best source of the chemoprotective glucosinolates, containing 20–50-fold the content of the more mature vegetable (Cortizo & Vitetta 2004). In animal and in vitro studies, isothiocyanates have demonstrated chemoprotective activity against different types of tumours, enhancing detoxification of carcinogens, blocking the initiation of chemically-induced carcinogens, inducing apoptosis and modulating cell-cycle progression in highly proliferative cancer cells (Cortizo & Vitetta 2004, Fimognari et al 2005, Gills et al 2005, Hintze et al 2003, Jadhav et al 2007, Rose et al 2005). Indoles, such as indole-3-carbinol, have also been shown to exert chemopreventive effects in liver, colon and mammary tissue (Kang et al 2001) and to arrest human tumour cells in the G1 phase of the cell cycle (Matsuzaki et al 2004). They may also block oestrogen receptors in breast cancer cells (Pratt & Matthews 2004b).

Although the anticarcinogenic, antioxidant and anti-inflammatory benefits of broccoli compounds help to explain their therapeutic effects, the exact mechanisms are still unclear and contradictory evidence exists for a role in inhibiting phase I and inducing phase II enzymes (Cortizo & Vitetta 2004, Knize et al 2002, Myzak & Dashwood 2005, Perocco et al 2006, Steinkellner et al 2001, Vang et al 2001). Furthermore, several authors warn of potential risks resulting from uncontrolled use of isolated compounds from broccoli (Fimognari et al 2005, Perocco et al 2006, Wiseman 2005); therefore, consumption of the plant itself is currently more advisable than isolated extracts.

Human clinical trials have demonstrated improvements in HDL-cholesterol in overweight subjects (Jeon et al 2013) and a reduction in LDL-cholesterol in hypercholesterolaemic patients (Takai et al 2003). The consumption of broccoli sprouts has also been shown to improve insulin resistance in people with type 2 diabetes (Bahadoran et al 2012). Additional benefits for cardiovascular health are suggested by in vitro evidence indicating that broccoli compounds may bind to bile acids (Kahlon et al 2007) and have an ACE inhibitor activity (Lee et al 2005). Broccoli contains high amounts of selenium and glucosinolates, which can exert a cardioprotective effect (Mukherjee et al 2008). Because of its known nutrient content, broccoli may support the immune system; it may also reduce the risk of cataracts, osteoporosis and neural tube birth defects (Podsedek 2005, Pratt & Matthews 2004b).

Choose young plants or shoots with a dark-green–purplish colour. As broccoli is prone to infestation and has a large surface area, agricultural chemical residue can be an issue, and ideally organic broccoli should be purchased and inspected for pests. Broccoli will store at 5°C (non-packaged) for 1–3 weeks without significant nutrient loss (Favell 1998, Leja et al 2001), although processing methods may affect nutrient quality (Podsedek 2005). The bioavailability of sulforaphane is around ten times higher in soups made from fresh compared to frozen broccoli (Saha et al 2012). Although cooking degrades the vitamin C and isothiocyanate content, the carotenoids may become more bioavailable, increasing the potential overall antioxidant activity (Bernhardt & Schlich 2005, Pratt & Matthews 2004b, Turkmen et al 2005, Tang et al 2008). Light steaming (approximately 1 minute) of raw broccoli is likely to maintain the best nutritional profile. Despite concerns that goitrogenic compounds in broccoli may increase the risk of thyroid cancer, a meta-analysis found no correlation (Cortizo & Vitetta 2004); nevertheless, broccoli should not be consumed in excess by those with known thyroid disease. A serving size of half to 1 cup per day is associated with a significant reduction in cancer risk (Pratt & Matthews 2004b).

Single-cell foods

Microalgae are both single cells and whole plants that are at the bottom of the food chain and are the most productive organisms on the planet, using light approximately three times more efficiently than higher plants (Pirt 1980). Gram for gram, microalgae may also be the most nutrient-dense food on earth (Passwater & Solomon 1997), with minimal indigestible structures in contrast to higher plants or animals, in which less than half their dry weight is typically nutritionally useful (Bruno 2001).

Microalgae, which include *Spirulina* and *Chlorella* species, and the 'red-orange' algae *Dunaliella salina*, contain a range of macro- and micronutrients, such as chlorophyll, carotenoids, phytonutrients, amino acids, polysaccharides, essential fatty acids, carbohydrates and vitamins and bioavailable minerals (Cases et al 1999, Chamorro et al 2002, Kay 1991). They may also promote the growth of lactic acid bacteria in the gastrointestinal tract (Parada et al 1998).

These organisms can be considered to be a mix of food, supplement and medicine. As single-cell plants, they represent 'whole' foods; however, they are often marketed in capsules and can be taken as supplements and/or medicines. In contrast to the reductionist approach to nutrition, which leads to supplementation with only a few specific nutrients, microalgae provide a complex mix of nutrients developed over millions of years of evolution. Although accumulating research suggests that microalgae have many health benefits, further research is required to determine their clinical applications.

The cyanobacteria *Spirulina* spp (usually *Spirulina platensis* or *S. maxima*) contains pigments, called phycobilins or phycobiliproteins (including phycocyanin and allophycocyanin), that are similar in structure to bile pigments (Pinero Estrada et al 2001). *Spirulina* spp are said to possess antiviral, hypocholesterolaemic, antioxidant, anti-inflammatory, hepatoprotective, anti-allergic and immunomodulatory activities and have been used to treat certain allergies, anaemia, cancer, viruses, cardiovascular diseases, hyperlipidaemia, immune deficiency and inflammatory processes (Chamorro et al 2002, Hirahashi et al 2002).

In vitro studies of spirulina suggest antiviral and antiretroviral activity by inhibiting the penetration of viruses into host cells and also the replication of several enveloped viruses, including human cytomegalovirus, measles virus, mumps virus, influenza A virus and HIV-1 (Ayehunie et al 1998, Hayashi & Hayashi 1996, Hernandez-Corona et al 2002).

Spirulina extracts enhance macrophage activity (Quereshi & Ali 1996), and humoral and cell-mediated immune functions in animal studies (Quereshi et al 1996), and may also act as anticlastogenic (Ruiz Flores et al 2003) and antitumour agents (Li et al 2005). They inhibit mast-cell-mediated immediate-type allergic reactions in vivo and in vitro (Kim et al 1998), possibly by inhibiting mast-cell degranulation.

Animal studies have demonstrated that spirulina reduces vascular reactivity (Mascher et al 2006), possesses hypocholesterolaemic (Devi & Venkataraman 1983), anti-atherogenic (Kaji et al 2002, 2004) and antioxidant activity (Pinero Estrada et al 2001), reduces chromosomal damage and lipid peroxidation and increases liver enzymes and non-enzymatic antioxidants (Premkumar et al 2004). The hepatoprotective effects are likely to be caused by the antioxidant activity. Although some green foods are touted as being a good source of vitamin B_{12} for vegetarians, and this is true of chlorella, the B_{12} in spirulina appears to be in a largely inactive form (Watanabe et al 2002). Spirulina extract is an excellent selenium carrier and therefore enriched sources can provide a

highly bioavailable source of selenium (Cases et al 1999).

Chlorella (usually *Chlorella vulgaris* or *C. pyrenoidosa*) has been promoted as an anticarcinogenic, immunomodulatory, hypolipidaemic and gastric mucosa-protective agent. As with other green foods, the antitumour activity is thought to be mediated by an immunopotentiation mechanism (Noda et al 1996), and extracts of chlorella have demonstrated antitumour activity against both spontaneous and experimentally-induced metastasis in the lymphoid organs of mice (Tanaka et al 1998). Based on animal studies, chlorella may also ameliorate some of the side effects of 5-fluorouracil chemotherapy treatment (Konishi et al 1996).

Chlorella vulgaris extract enhances resistance to *Listeria monocytogenes* through augmentation of Th1 responses, producing gamma-interferon (Hasegawa et al 1999). It may be useful for the prevention of allergic diseases (Kralovec et al 2005), especially in those people with a predominantly Th2 response (Hasegawa et al 1999).

In some animal experiments, chlorella appears to possess hypolipidaemic (Sano et al 1988) and anti-atherogenic effects (Sano & Tanaka 1987). It may prevent dyslipidaemia in animals chronically fed a high-fat diet by preventing intestinal absorption of redundant lipids and thus reducing triglyceride, and total and LDL-cholesterol levels (Cherng & Shih 2005). In addition, inhibition of advanced glycation end products in vitro suggests a possible role for reducing atherogenesis, diabetic microangiopathy and Alzheimer's dementia (Yamagishi et al 2005).

Chlorella may also exhibit hypoglycaemic activity (Cherng & Shih 2006), improve insulin sensitivity (Jong-Yuh & Mei-Fen 2005) and prevent stress-induced ulcers (Tanaka et al 1997), according to animal studies.

Although it has been suggested that a diet high in spirulina may be a risk for kidney stones, this may be the case only with a high or excessive intake of oxalic acid (e.g. beetroot leaves or rhubarb) (Farooq et al 2005), as the antioxidant activity of phycocyanin appears to aid in the prevention of calcium oxalate stones (Farooq et al 2004). Occasional gastrointestinal symptoms and allergic reactions have been reported for spirulina and chlorella, and those taking warfarin should avoid chlorella, which can be high in vitamin K.

Doses of spirulina range from 250 mg to 5 g daily (PDRHealth 2014). High doses of chlorella (10 g/day) have been used successfully in clinical trials for fibromyalgia (Holdcraft et al 2003, Merchant & Andre 2001), but the standard dose is usually 200–500 mg/day (PDRHealth 2014).

Dunaliella salina is a soft-celled microalga found in many coastal waters and saltwater lakes (see Monographs: *Dunaliella*). It is one of the most salt-tolerant life forms known, and is adapted to extremely high UV radiation. To cope with these extreme environments, *Dunaliella* produces very high levels of antioxidant molecules. On a per-gram basis, *Dunaliella* has more than twice the chlorophyll, five times the mineral content and more than 6000 times the carotenoid antioxidants content of spirulina (Table 5.2), with the carotenoids giving it an orange rather than a green colour. Furthermore, *Dunaliella*'s soft-cell membrane makes it easily digestible, compared with other microalgae that have hard cell walls (Ben-Amotz & Avron 1983). To date, most of the clinical research on *Dunaliella* has been on beta-carotene-containing extracts rather than on the whole organism, but recent advances in production technology have allowed the whole, dried *Dunaliella* biomass with its full range of nutrients and minerals to become commercially available (Table 5.3) (Tracton & Bobrov 2005 and more studies).

Medicinal mushrooms (reishi, shiitake)

Mushrooms such as shiitake (*Lentinus edodes*), reishi (*Ganoderma lucidum*), oyster (*Pleurotus ostreatus*) and maitake (*Grifola frondosa*), to name just a few, have also been used as medicinal agents in Asia for thousands of years (Chang 1996, Sliva 2004). More recently the benefits of the common button mushroom (*Agaricus bisporus*), widely cultivated in the West, have also begun to be elucidated (Beelman et al 2004). Although the nutritional and medicinal potential of mushrooms may differ because of variations in species, cultivation techniques, maturity at harvest and other factors, numerous common features arise. (See also Monographs: *Coriolus versicolor*).

In general, mushrooms contain significant amounts of water (>90%), and, as a result, nutrients measured on the fresh-weight values may appear to be quite low. Nevertheless, they are low in kilojoules and a good source of fibre (including glucans and chitin), amino acids, B vitamins, copper, selenium, potassium, germanium, ergosterol (Beelman et al 2004) and lipids, especially linoleic acid (Yilmaz et al 2005).

TABLE 5.2 NUTRIENT CONTENT OF DUNALIELLA vs SPIRULINA AND CARROTS (per 100 g)			
NUTRIENT	**DUNALIELLA**	**SPIRULINA**	**CARROTS**
Protein	7.4 g	57 g	1 g
Fat (total)	7 g	8 g	0
Carbohydrates	29.7 g	24 g	10 g
Energy	893 kJ	1214 kJ	180 kJ
Fibre	0.4 g	4 g	3 g
Chlorophyll	2210 mg	1000 mg	NA
Minerals	49 g	6.2 g	1 g
Beta-carotene	2100 mg	0.34 mg	8.3 mg
Alpha-carotene	53 mg	0.0 mg	3.5 mg
Lutein/zeaxanthin	97.6 mg	0.0 mg	0.26 mg
Cryptoxanthin	46.5 mg	0.0 mg	0.1 mg

Data obtained from: US Department of Agriculture. National nutrient database for standard references (release 18) 2005 (www.nal.usda.gov), National Measurement Institute (Australia) (www.measurement.gov.au), Craft Technologies Inc. (USA) (www.crafttechnologies.com).

TABLE 5.3 COMPARISON OF THE NUTRIENT AND TRACE MINERALS IN 'SUPER' FOODS (mg/100 g)							
FOOD	Ca	Mg	Na	K	Cu	Zn	Fe
Dunaliella salina	178	5394	7513	5	0.4	4	23.5
Spirulina	547	330	>999	5	1.1	2	50.5
Chlorella	201	211	106	5	0.1	1	214
Kelp powder	1443	796	>999	7	0.2	3	27
Wheat grass	937	83	315	6	0.4	2	13.7
Green barley	384	186	818	6	0.6	2	8.4
FOOD	Mn	Cr	Se	B	Co	Mo	S	Li	Rb
Dunaliella salina	1.8	0.2	1.02	25.4	0.022	0.041	3105	0.9	0.66
Spirulina	2.6	0.53	0.03	0.25	0.13	0.11	<2000	0.093	0.13
Chlorella	4	0.06	0.01	0.03	0.038	0.042	<2000	0.01	0.066
Kelp powder	3.8	0.23	0.69	11.1	0.045	0.094	2426	0.068	0.85
Wheat grass	5.1	0.09	0.04	0.33	0.005	0.05	<2000	0.008	1.0
Green barley	3.9	0.11	0.15	1.05	0.004	0.066	<2000	0.023	0.51

Data obtained from: Trace Elements Inc. (USA) (www.traceelements.com).

The immunostimulatory properties of a variety of polysaccharides found in mushrooms are thought to contribute to their anticancer effects, and other biologically active substances, including triterpenes, cerebrosides and phenols, have been identified and characterised in the medicinal mushrooms in particular (Sliva 2004). Mushrooms may also protect against oxidative damage to DNA (Beelman et al 2004).

Shiitake mushrooms (*Lentinus edodes*) possess immunomodulating, antitumour, hypolipidaemic, antibacterial (Hirasawa et al 1999) and antioxidant properties (Cheung et al 2003), and may help to reduce dental caries, according to in vitro and animal studies (Shouji et al 2000). They have been traditionally used for exhaustion, colds, intestinal parasites, poor circulation and liver problems (PDRHealth 2014).

Lentinan, which is a biologically active beta-glucan in shiitake mushrooms, modulates the immune system (including T-lymphocytes and cytokines); suppresses hepatic expression of cytochrome P1A (Okamoto et al 2004); and has demonstrated antitumour and antimetastatic activity against chemical and viral carcinogens (Mitamura et al 2000, Ng & Yap 2002, Zheng et al 2005). However, clinical trials using shiitake extract in men with prostate cancer were not successful in reducing levels of prostate-specific antigen (White et al 2002), although other compounds may also contribute to the antitumour effects (Sia & Candlish 1999). The consumption of shiitake in patients undergoing chemotherapy is thought to be safe and may improve quality of life and immune function (Yamaguchi et al 2011).

Lentinus edodes mycelia inhibit atherosclerotic development in rabbits (van Nevel et al 2003) and contains eritadenine, a hypocholesterolaemic compound that also acts as an immunomodulator and tumour-inhibitor in animal models (Beelman et al 2004, Yamada et al 2002). Extracts from shiitake mushrooms have been shown to elevate plasma insulin and reduce plasma glucose, total cholesterol and triglyceride levels in rats (Yang et al 2002). Lentinan is antifungal and may also exert an inhibitory effect on HIV-1 reverse transcriptase and proliferation of leukaemia cells (Ngai & Ng 2003).

Ganoderma lucidum (reishi) has been used in TCM for thousands of years for the treatment of asthma, cough, fatigue, insomnia and weakness, and was popular as a cancer chemotherapy agent in ancient China (Sliva 2003). There is some confusion about the taxonomical classification of reishi mushrooms and, as a result, a variety of different medicinally active compounds with significantly different pharmacological effects may be attributed to different strains, adding confusion to the body of evidence available (Szedlay 2002).

A small clinical trial has reported mild antidiabetic effects and improved lipid profiles in subjects with elevated blood glucose levels (Chu et al 2012). The anticancer activity may be due to direct cytotoxic effects against tumour cells, inhibition of angiogenesis (Lin & Zhang 2004), and the effects of immunomodulatory polysaccharides (Chen et al 2004), which act by stimulating the expression of cytokines (especially IL-1, IL-2 and IFN-gamma) (Wang et al 2002) and modulating humoral and cellular immunity (Lin 2005).

Dietary intake of *Agaricus bisporus* (white button mushrooms) may improve mucosal immunity by accelerating salivary IgA secretion (Jeong et al 2012). Studies have also suggested that it may modulate aromatase activity and function, resulting in chemoprevention of the deleterious effects of in situ oestrogen in breast cancer (Grube et al 2001), and may be a potential agent for preventing scarring and promoting healthy wound-healing (Batterbury et al 2002, Kent et al 2003). The brown strains (Swiss browns, portabellas) harvested when fully mature, with open caps, appear to be the most useful (Beelman et al 2004).

High doses of shiitake mushrooms may cause rash, diarrhoea and bloating, and consumption of 4 g shiitake powder has been associated with marked eosinophilia (Levy et al 1998). Reishi mushrooms should not be consumed daily in the long term (> 3–6 months), as they may cause dizziness, dry mouth, nose bleeds and gastrointestinal upset, and may potentially produce additive effects with anticoagulant medications (PDRHealth 2014).

Agaricus bisporus contains agaratine, a hydrazine compound with suspected carcinogenic potential (Hashida et al 1990). To date, animal studies have demonstrated different outcomes between species and no conclusive evidence exists for a cause–effect relationship between mushroom intake and cancer prevalence in humans. In addition, the potential anticarcinogenic properties of other compounds in mushrooms may provide protection (Beelman et al 2004). Although there are concerns about heavy metal toxicity in wild *Agaricus* mushrooms, levels of mercury and cadmium in commercially cultivated mushrooms have been found to be very low (Kalac & Svoboda 2000, Vetter & Berta 2005).

Agaricus mushrooms (including Swiss browns and portabellas) and shiitake mushrooms are readily available fresh or dried, and dried reishi mushrooms can sometimes be found in Asian grocery stores. Dried mushrooms can be reconstituted in warm water for use in cooking. Cooking mushrooms may increase free polyphenolic compounds (Choi et al 2006) but can make them tough and result in losses of manganese, zinc and iron (Coskuner & Ozdemir 1997).

FUTURE DIRECTIONS

Despite advancements in medicine and pharmaceutical drug development, dietary choices remain the cornerstone of preventive medicine and enhance the health of individuals and societies. Emerging research indicates exceptional potential for the benefits of using 'food as medicine'. Recognising the inherent therapeutic value of foods or their potential to induce harmful health consequences means that we can tailor the diet to produce better health outcomes.

REFERENCES

Ahmet I et al. Survival and cardioprotective benefits of long-term blueberry enriched diet in dilated cardiomyopathy following myocardial infarction in rats. PLoS One. 4.11 (2009).

Aiyer HS, Srinivasan C, Gupta RC. Dietary berries and ellagic acid diminish estrogen-mediated mammary tumorigenesis in ACI rats. Nutr Cancer 60.2 (2008): 227–34.

American Academy of Pediatrics (AAP). Pesticide exposure in children. Pediatrics 130.6 (2012): e1757–1763.

Anderson JW et al. Carbohydrate and fiber recommendations for individuals with diabetes: a quantitative assessment and meta-analysis of the evidence. J Am Coll Nutr 23.1 (2004): 5–17.

AQIS. National Standard for Organic and Bio-Dynamic Produce. (2009). Australian Quarantine & Inspection Service. Available: http://www.tasorganicdynamic.com.au/national-standard-1-July-2009.pdf 13 June 2014.

Armah CN et al. 'A Diet Rich in High-Glucoraphanin Broccoli Interacts with Genotype to Reduce Discordance in Plasma Metabolite Profiles by Modulating Mitochondrial Function.' Am J Clin Nutr 98.3 (2013): 712–722.

Ashwell M. Concepts of functional foods. International Life Sciences Institute Europe, Brussels (2002).

Atalay M et al. Anti-angiogenic property of edible berry in a model of hemangioma. FEBS Lett 544.1–3 (2003): 252–257.

Ayehunie S et al. Inhibition of HIV-1 replication by an aqueous extract of Spirulina platensis (Arthrospira platensis). J Acquir Immune Defic Synd Hum Retrovirol 18 (1998): 7–12.

Bahadoran Z et al. Effect of broccoli sprouts on insulin resistance in type 2 diabetic patients: A randomized double-blind clinical trial. Int J Food Sci Nutr, 63.7 (2012): 767–771.

Bassil K et al. Cancer health effects of pesticides: Systematic review. Can Fam Physician, 53.10 (2007): 1704–1711.

Bateman B et al. The effects of a double blind, placebo controlled, artificial food colourings and benzoate preservative challenge on hyperactivity in a general population sample of preschool children. Arch Dis Child 89.6 (2004): 506–511.

Batterbury M et al. Agaricus bisporus (edible mushroom lectin) inhibits ocular fibroblast proliferation and collagen lattice contraction. Exp Eye Res 74.3 (2002): 361–370.

Baxter GJ et al. Salicylic acid in soups prepared from organically and non-organically grown vegetables. Eur J Nutr 40 (2001): 289–292.

Beelman R et al. Bioactive components in Agaricus bisporus (J. Lge) Imbach of nutritional, medicinal, or biological importance (Review). In: Proceedings of the XVI International Congress on the Science and Cultivation of Edible and Medicinal Fungi. March 14–17, 2004, Miami FL, USA. Available at: Pennsylvania State University (online) www.foodscience.psu.edu.

Bellissimo N et al. Effect of television viewing at mealtime on food intake after a glucose preload in boys. Pediatr Res 61 (2007):745–749.

Ben-Amotz A, Avron M. Accumulation of metabolites by halotolerant algae and its industrial potential. Annu Rev Microbiol 37 (1983): 95–119.

Bernhardt S, Schlich E. Impact of different cooking methods on food quality: Retention of lipophilic vitamins in fresh and frozen vegetables. J Food Eng 77 (2005): 327–333.

Bhuvaneswari V, Nagini S. Lycopene: a review of its potential as an anticancer agent. Curr Med Chem Anticancer Agents 5.6 (2005): 627–635.

Bickford PC et al. Effects of aging on cerebellar noradrenergic function and motor learning: nutritional interventions. Mech Ageing Dev 111.2–3 (1999): 141–54.

Bickford PC et al. Antioxidant-rich diets improve cerebellar physiology and motor learning in aged rats. Brain Res 866.1–2 (2000): 211–217.

Blackwell PA et al. Effects of agricultural conditions on the leaching behaviour of veterinary antibiotics in soils. Chemosphere, 75(1) (2009), 13–19.

Bommareddy, A., Eggleston, W., Prelewicz, S., Antal, A., Witczak, Z., McCune, D.F., & Vanwert, A.L. (2013). Chemoprevention of prostate cancer by major dietary phytochemicals. Anticancer Res, 33(10), 4163–4174.

Boyd CA et al. Behavioural and neurochemical changes associated with chronic exposure to low-level concentrations of pesticide mixtures. J Toxicol Environ Health 30 (1990): 209–21.

Brandt K et al. Agroecosystem Management and Nutritional Quality of Plant Foods: The Case of Organic Fruits and Vegetables. Critical Reviews in Plant Sciences, 30.1–2 (2011): 177–197.

Brennan P et al. Effect of cruciferous vegetables on lung cancer in patients stratified by genetic status: a mendelian randomisation approach. Lancet 366.9496 (2005): 1558–1560.

Bruno JJ. Edible microalgae: a review of the health research. Center of Nutritional Psychol Press, 2001. Available: www.ediblemicroalgae.com 13 June 2014.

Carey AN, Gomes SM, Shukitt-Hale B. Blueberry supplementation improves memory in middle-aged mice fed a high-fat diet. J Agric Food Chem. January (2014).

Cases J et al. Glutathione-related enzymic activities in rats receiving high cholesterol or standard diets supplemented with two forms of selenium. Food Chem 65.2 (1999): 207–211.

Cavanagh J. Why fair trade? A brief look at free trade in the global economy. Fair Trade Federation (2006). Available: www.fairtradefederation.org.

Chamorro G et al. [Update on the pharmacology of Spirulina (Arthospira), an unconventional food]. Arch Latinoam Nutr 52.3 (2002): 232–240.

Chang R. Functional properties of edible mushrooms. Nutr Rev 54 (1996): S91–93.

Chen H et al. Studies on the immuno-modulating and anti-tumor activities of Ganoderma lucidum (Reishi) polysaccharides. Bioorg Med Chem 12.21 (2004): 5595–5601.

Chen J et al. Increased influence of genetic variation on PON1 activity in neonates. Environ Health Perspect 111.11 (2003): 1403–1410.

Cherng JY, Shih MF. Preventing dyslipidemia by Chlorella pyrenoidosa in rats and hamsters after chronic high fat diet treatment. Life Sci 76.26 (2005): 3001–3013.

Cherng JY, Shih MF. Improving glycogenesis in Streptozocin (STZ) diabetic mice after administration of green algae Chlorella. Life Sci 78.11 (2006): 1181–1186.

Cheung LM et al. Antioxidant activity and total phenolics of edible mushroom extracts. Food Chem 81.2 (2003): 249–255.

Choi Y et al. Influence of heat treatment on the antioxidant activities and polyphenolic compounds of Shiitake (Lentinus edodes) mushroom. Food Chem 99.2 (2006): 381–387.

Chu TT et al. Study of potential cardioprotective effects of ganoderma lucidum (lingzhi): Results of a controlled human intervention trial. Br J Nutr 107.7 (2012): 1017–1027.

Cortizo F, Vitetta L. Broccoli and cranberry. J Complement Med 3.4 (2004): 65.

Coskuner Y, Ozdemir Y. Effects of canning processes on the elements content of cultivated mushrooms (Agaricus bisporus). Food Chem 60.4 (1997): 559–562.

Dalen J et al. Pilot study: Mindful Eating and Living (MEAL): weight, eating behavior, and psychological outcomes associated with a mindfulness-based intervention for people with obesity. Complement Ther Med 18.6 (2010): 260–264.

Damon M et al. Phylloquinone (vitamin K1) content of vegetables. J Food Comp Anal 18.8 (2005): 751–8.

Department of Agriculture, Fisheries and Forestery (DAFF). National Residue Survey 2010–2011. (2012) Available: http://www.daff.gov.au/agriculture-food/nrs/nrs-results-publications/annual-reports.

De Rivera C et al. The effects of antioxidants in the senescent auditory cortex. Neurobiol Aging 27 (2005): 1035–44.

Devareddy L et al. Blueberry prevents bone loss in ovariectomized rat model of postmenopausal osteoporosis. J Nutr Biochem 19.10 (2008): 694–9.

Devi M, Venkataraman L. Hypocholesterolemic effect of blue-green algae Spirulina platensis in albino rats. Ann Nutr Rep Int 28 (1983): 519–30.

Dilzer A, Park Y. Implication of conjugated linoleic acid (cla) in human health. Crit Rev Food Sci Nutr 52.6 (2012): 488–513.

Dolliver H, Gupta S. Antibiotic losses in leaching and surface runoff from manure-amended agricultural land. J Environ Qual 37.3 (2008): 1227–1237.

Domingo JL, Gine Bordonaba J. A literature review on the safety assessment of genetically modified plants. Environ Int, 37.4 (2011): 734–742.

Domitrovic R. The molecular basis for the pharmacological activity of anthocyans. Curr Med Chem 18.29 (2011): 4454–4469.

Duke JA. Dr Duke's phytochemical and ethnobotanical databases. US Department of Agriculture, Agricultural Research Service, National Germplasm Resources Laboratory. Beltsville Agricultural Research Center, Beltsville, MD, 2003. Available: www.ars-grin.gov/duke 16 June 2014.

Dushay J, Abrahamson MJ. Insulin resistance and type 2 diabetes: a comprehensive review, (2005).

Eddey S. Fatty acid facts. J Complement Med 4.2 (2005): 50–4.

Fair Trade Federation website. (2014) Available: www.fairtradefederation.org. 14 June 2014.

Farooq SM et al. Prophylactic role of phycocyanin: a study of oxalate mediated renal cell injury. Chemico-Biol Interact 149.1 (2004): 1–7.

Farooq SM et al. Credentials of Spirulina diet on stability and flux related properties on the biomineralization process during oxalate mediated renal calcification in rats. Clin Nutr 24.6 (2005): 932–42.

Favell DJ. A comparison of the vitamin C content of fresh and frozen vegetables. Food Chem 62.1 (1998): 59–64.

Fimognari C et al. Micronucleus formation and induction of apoptosis by different isothiocyanates and a mixture of isothiocyanates in human lymphocyte cultures. Mutat Res Genet Toxicol Environ Mutagen 582.1–2 (2005): 1–10.

Food and Agriculture Organisation of the United Nations (FAO). (2014). Biotechnology. Available: http://www.fao.org/biotechnology/en/ 16 June 2014

Food and Agriculture Organisation of the United Nations (FAO). (2014b). FAO GM Foods Platform. Available: http://www.fao.org/food/food-safety-quality/gm-foods-platform/en/. 16 June 2014

Food Standards Australia New Zealand (FSANZ). Australian total diet study. (2011) Available: http://www.foodstandards.gov.au/science/monitoring/Pages/australiantotaldiets1914.aspx 16 June 2014.

Food Standards Australia New Zealand (FSANZ). Additives. (2012) Available: http://www.foodstandards.gov.au/consumer/additives/additiveoverview/Pages/default.aspx 16 June 2014.

Food Standards Australia New Zealand (FSANZ). Food irradiation (2013). Available: http://www.foodstandards.gov.au/consumer/foodtech/irradiation/Pages/default.aspx 16 June 2014.

Food Standards Australia New Zealand (FSANZ). Nutrition, health and related claims. (2013). Available: http://www.foodstandards.gov.au/industry/labelling/Pages/Nutrition-health-and-related-claims.aspx 16 June 2014.

FSANZ (Food Standards of Australia and New Zealand) 2013. website. Available: http://www.foodstandards.gov.au/consumer/additives/additiveoverview 13 June 2014.

Food Standards Australia New Zealand (FSANZ). 'Current GM applications and approvals.' (2014). Available: http://www.foodstandards.gov.au/consumer/gmfood/applications/Pages/default.aspx 16 June 2014.

Forman J, Silverstein, J. American College of Pediatrics Committee on Nutrition and Council on Environmental Health. Organic foods: Health and environmental advantages and disadvantages. Pediatrics 130 (2012): e1406–e1416.

Fremont L. Biological effects of resveratrol. Life Sci 66 (2000): 663–73.

Fuglsang G et al. Prevalence of intolerance to food additives among Danish school children. Pediatr Allergy Immunol 4.3 (1993): 123–129.

Fuglsang G et al. Adverse reactions to food additives in children with atopic symptoms. Allergy 49.1 (1994): 31–37.

Galli RL et al. Blueberry supplemented diet reverses age-related decline in hippocampal HSP70 neuroprotection. Neurobiol Aging 27.2 (2006): 344–50.

Garry VF. Pesticides and children. Toxicol Appl Pharmacol 198.2 (2004): 152–63.

Gills JJ et al. Sulforaphane prevents mouse skin tumorigenesis during the stage of promotion, 2005. Cancer Lett 236.1 (2006): 72–9.

Gliszczynska-Swiglo A et al. The effect of solar radiation on the flavonol content in broccoli inflorescence. Food Chem 100 (2005): 241–245.

Goldberg G. Plants: diet and health. The report of a British nutrition foundation task force. Blackwell, Oxford (2003).

Gomes C, Moreira RG, Castell-Perez E. Microencapsulated antimicrobial compounds as a means to enhance electron beam irradiation treatment for inactivation of pathogens on fresh spinach leaves. J Food Sci, 76.6 (2011): E479–488.

Grinder-Pedersen L et al. Effect of diets based on foods from conventional versus organic production on intake and excretion of flavonoids and markers of antioxidative defense in humans. J Agric Food Chem 51(19) (2003): 5671–5676.

Grube BJ et al. White button mushroom phytochemicals inhibit aromatase activity and breast cancer cell proliferation. J Nutr 131.12 (2001): 3288–93.

Guandalini S. Probiotics for prevention and treatment of diarrhea. J Clin Gastroenterol, 45 Suppl (2011): S149–153.

Guarner F. Inulin and oligofructose: impact on intestinal diseases and disorders. Br J Nutr 93 (Suppl 1) (2005): S61–5.

Hasegawa T et al. Oral administration of hot water extracts of Chlorella vulgaris reduces IgE production against milk casein in mice. Int J Immunopharmacol 21.5 (1999): 311–323.

Hashida C et al. [Quantities of agaritine in mushrooms (Agaricus bisporus) and the carcinogenicity of mushroom methanol extracts on the mouse bladder epithelium]. Nippon Koshu Eisei Zasshi 37.6 (1990): 400–5.

Hayashi T, Hayashi K. Calcium spirulan, an inhibitor of enveloped virus replication, from a blue-green alga Spirulina platensis. J Nat Prod 59 (1996): 83–7.

Hepworth NS. A mindful eating group as an adjunct to individual treatment for eating disorders: a pilot study. Eat Disord 19.1 (2011): 6–16.

Hernandez-Corona A et al. Antiviral activity of Spirulina maxima against herpes simplex virus type 2. Antiviral Res 56.3 (2002): 279–285.

Hintze KJ et al. Induction of hepatic thioredoxin reductase activity by sulforaphane, both in Hepa1c1c7 cells and in male Fisher 344 rats. J Nutr Biochem 14.3 (2003): 173–179.

Hirahashi T et al. Activation of the human innate immune system by Spirulina: augmentation of interferon production and NK cytotoxicity by oral administration of hot water extract of Spirulina platensis. Int Immunopharmacol 2.4 (2002): 423–434.

Hirasawa M et al. Three kinds of antibacterial substances from Lentinus edodes (Berk.) Sing. (Shiitake, an edible mushroom). Int J Antimicrob Agents 11.2 (1999): 151–7.

Holdcraft LC et al. Complementary and alternative medicine in fibromyalgia and related syndromes. Best Pract Res Clin Rheumatol 17.4 (2003): 667–83.

Hounsome N et al. Plant metabolites and nutritional quality of vegetables. J Food Sci 73.4 (2008): R48–65.

Huen K et al. Developmental changes in pon1 enzyme activity in young children and effects of pon1 polymorphisms. Environ Health Perspect 117 (2009): 1632–1638.

Jacobs DR, Tapsell LC. Food, not nutrients, is the fundamental unit in nutrition. Nutrition Reviews 65.10 (2007): 439–450.

Jadhav U et al. Dietary isothiocyanate iberin inhibits growth and induces apoptosis in human glioblastoma cells. J Pharmacol Sci 103.2 (2007): 247–251.

Jamison J. Folate. J Complement Med 4.1 (2005): 46–49.

Jamison J. Whole foods and processing. J Complement Med 5.1 (2006): 66–8.

Jeffery EH et al. Variation in content of bioactive components in broccoli. J Food Comp Anal 16.3 (2003): 323–30.

Jensen B. Foods that heal. Avery, New York (1993).

Jeon SM et al. 'Randomized double-blind placebo-controlled trial of powdered brassica rapa ethanol extract on alteration of body composition and plasma lipid and adipocytokine profiles in overweight subjects.' [In eng]. J Med Food 16.2 (2013): 133–138.

Jeong SC, Koyyalamudi SR, Pang G. Dietary intake of agaricus bisporus white button mushroom accelerates salivary immunoglobulin a secretion in healthy volunteers. Nutrition 28.5 (2012): 527–531.

JETACAR. The use of antibiotics in food producing animals: antibiotic resistant bacteria in animals and humans. Report of the Joint Expert Technical Advisory Committee on Antibiotic Resistance. (1999). Available: http://www.health.gov.au/internet/main/publishing.nsf/Content/health-pubhlth-strateg-jetacar-reports.htm 16 June 2014.

Jeyabalan J et al. Chemopreventive and therapeutic activity of dietary blueberry against estrogen-mediated breast cancer. J Agric Food Chem (2013).

Jiang RW et al. Chemistry and biological activities of caffeic acid derivatives from Salvia miltiorrhiza. Curr Med Chem 12.2 (2005): 237–246.

Jong-Yuh C, Mei-Fen S. Potential hypoglycemic effects of Chlorella in streptozotocin-induced diabetic mice. Life Sci 77.9 (2005): 980–990.

Kahlon TS et al. In vitro binding of bile acids by spinach, kale, brussels sprouts, broccoli, mustard greens, green bell pepper, cabbage and collards. Food Chem 100.4 (2007): 1531–1536.

Kaji T et al. Repair of wounded monolayers of cultured bovine aortic endothelial cells is inhibited by calcium spirulan, a novel sulfated polysaccharide isolated from Spirulina platensis. Life Sci 70.16 (2002): 1841–1848.

Kaji T et al. Sodium spirulan as a potent inhibitor of arterial smooth muscle cell proliferation in vitro. Life Sci 74.19 (2004): 2431–2439.

Kalac P, Svoboda L. A review of trace element concentrations in edible mushrooms. Food Chem 69.3 (2000): 273–281.

Kalea AZ et al. Wild blueberry (Vaccinium angustifolium) consumption affects the composition and structure of glycosaminoglycans in Sprague-Dawley rat aorta. J Nutr Biochem 17.2 (2006): 109–116.

Kalt W et al. Effect of blueberry feeding on plasma lipids in pigs. Br J Nutr 100.1 (2008): 70–78.

Kang JS et al. Post-initiation treatment of Indole-3-carbinol did not suppress N-methyl-N-nitrosourea induced mammary carcinogenesis in rats. Cancer Lett 169.2 (2001): 147–154.

Kay RA. Microalgae as food and supplement. Crit Rev Food Sci Nutr 30.6 (1991): 555–573.

Kennedy ET. Evidence for nutritional benefits in prolonging wellness. Am J Clin Nutr 83.2 (2006): 410–414S.

Kent D et al. Edible mushroom (Agaricus bisporus) lectin modulates human retinal pigment epithelial cell behaviour in vitro. Exp Eye Res 76.2 (2003): 213–219.

Kim DJ et al. Chemoprevention of colon cancer by Korean food plant components. Mutat Res Genet Toxicol Environ Mutagen 523/524 (2003): 99–107.

Kim HM et al. Inhibitory effect of mast cell-mediated immediate-type allergic reactions in rats by Spirulina. Biochem Pharmacol 55.7 (1998): 1071–1076.

Knize MG et al. Factors affecting human heterocyclic amine intake and the metabolism of PhIP. Mutat Res Genet Toxicol Environ Mutagen 506/507 (2002): 153–162.

Konishi F et al. Protective effect of an acidic glycoprotein obtained from culture of Chlorella vulgaris against myelosuppression by 5-fluorouracil. Cancer Immunol Immunother 42 (1996): 268–274.

Koushan K et al. The role of lutein in eye-related disease. Nutrients 5.5 (2013): 1823–1839.

Kralovec JA et al. An aqueous Chlorella extract inhibits IL-5 production by mast cells in vitro and reduces ovalbumin-induced eosinophil infiltration in the airway in mice in vivo. Int Immunopharmacol 5.4 (2005): 689–698.

Krikorian R et al. Blueberry supplementation improves memory in older adults. J Agric Food Chem 58.7 (2010): 3996–4000.

Lackmann M et al. Organochlorine compounds in breast-fed vs. bottle-fed infants: preliminary results at six weeks of age. Sci Total Environ 329.1–3 (2004): 289–293.

Laetz CA et al. The synergistic toxicity of pesticide mixtures: Implications for risk assessment and the conservation of endangered pacific salmon. Environ Health Perspect, 117.3 (2009): 348–353.

Lau FC et al. The beneficial effects of fruit polyphenols on brain aging. Neurobiol Aging 26.1, Suppl 1 (2005): 128–132.

Lee JE et al. Tyr-Pro-Lys, an angiotensin I-converting enzyme inhibitory peptide derived from broccoli (Brassica oleracea Italica). Food Chem 99 (2005): 143–148.

Leja M et al. Antioxidant ability of broccoli flower buds during short-term storage. Food Chem 72.2 (2001): 219–222.

Levy AM et al. Eosinophilia and gastrointestinal symptoms after ingestion of shiitake mushrooms. J Allergy Clin Immunol 101.5 (1998): 613–620.

Li B et al. Effects of CD59 on antitumoral activities of phycocyanin from Spirulina platensis. Biomed Pharmacother 59.10 (2005): 551–560.

Lin ZB. Cellular and molecular mechanisms of immuno-modulation by Ganoderma lucidum. J Pharmacol Sci 99.2 (2005): 144–153.

Lin ZB, Zhang HN. Anti-tumor and immunoregulatory activities of Ganoderma lucidum and its possible mechanisms. Acta Pharmacol Sin 25.11 (2004): 1387–1395.

Liu F et al. Effects of six selected antibiotics on plant growth and soil microbial and enzymatic activities. Environ Pollut, 157.5 (2009): 1636–1642.

Lopez-Molina D et al. Molecular properties and prebiotic effect of inulin obtained from artichoke (Cynara scolymus L.). Phytochemistry 66 (2005): 1476–1478.

Lorente-Cebrián S et al. Role of omega-3 fatty acids in obesity, metabolic syndrome, and cardiovascular diseases: A review of the evidence. J Physiol Biochem, 69.3 (2013): 633–651.

Lucarini M et al. In vitro calcium availability from brassica vegetables (Brassica oleracea L.) and as consumed in composite dishes. Food Chem 64.4 (1999): 519–523.

Lucock M, Yates Z. Folic acid fortification: A double-edged sword. Curr Opin Clin Nutr Metab Care 12.6 (2009): 555–564.

Mahn A, Reyes A. An overview of health-promoting compounds of broccoli (brassica oleracea var. Italica) and the effect of processing. Food Sci Technol Int 18.6 (2012): 503–514.

Mascher DM et al. Ethanolic extract of Spirulina maxima alters the vasomotor reactivity of aortic rings from obese rats. Arch Med Res 37.1 (2006): 50–57.

Matchett MD et al. Inhibition of matrix metalloproteinase activity in DU145 human prostate cancer cells by flavonoids from lowbush blueberry (Vaccinium angustifolium): possible roles for protein kinase C and mitogen-activated protein-kinase-mediated events. J Nutr Biochem 17.2 (2006): 117–125.

Matsuzaki Y et al. Indole-3-carbinol activates the cyclin-dependent kinase inhibitor p15INK4b gene. FEBS Lett 576.1–2 (2004): 137–140.

Matusheski NV et al. Heating decreases epithiospecifier protein activity and increases sulforaphane formation in broccoli. Phytochemistry 65.9 (2004): 1273–1281.

McAnulty SR et al. Consumption of blueberry polyphenols reduces exercise-induced oxidative stress compared to vitamin C. Nutr Res 24.3 (2004): 2092–221.

McLeay Y et al. Effect of New Zealand blueberry consumption on recovery from eccentric exercise-induced muscle damage. J Int Soc Sports Nutr 9.1 (2012): 19.

Merchant RE, Andre CA. A review of recent clinical trials of the nutritional supplement Chlorella pyrenoidosa in the treatment of fibromyalgia, hypertension, and ulcerative colitis. Altern Ther Health Med 7.3 (2001): 79–91.

Mesnage R et al. Major pesticides are more toxic to human cells than their declared active principles. BioMed Research International 2014 (2014).

Mitamura T et al. Effects of lentinan on colorectal carcinogenesis in mice with ulcerative colitis. Oncol Rep 7.3 (2000): 599–601.

Moghe SS, et al. Effect of blueberry polyphenols on 3T3-F442A preadipocyte differentiation. J Med Food 15.5 (2012): 448–452.

Mohamed M S et al. Administration of lycopene and betacarotene decreased risks of pneumonia among children. Pak J Nutr 7.2 (2008): 273–217.

Mukherjee S et al. Broccoli: a unique vegetable that protects mammalian hearts through the redox cycling of the thioredoxin superfamily. J Agric Food Chem 56.2 (2008): 609–617.

Myzak MC, Dashwood RH. Chemoprotection by sulforaphane: Keep one eye beyond Keap1. Cancer Lett 233 (2005): 208–218.

Natoli S. Berries. J Complement Med 4.4 (2005): 52–6.

Neto C. Cranberry and blueberry: Evidence for protective effects against cancer and vascular diseases. Mol Nutr Food Res 51.6 (2007): 652–664.

Ng ML, Yap AT. Inhibition of human colon carcinoma development by lentinan from shiitake mushrooms (Lentinus edodes). J Altern Complement Med 8.5 (2002): 581–589.

Ngai PH, Ng TB. Lentin, a novel and potent antifungal protein from shiitake mushroom with inhibitory effects on activity of human immunodeficiency virus-1 reverse transcriptase and proliferation of leukemia cells. Life Sci 73.26 (2003): 3363–3374.

Noda K et al. A water-soluble antitumor glycoprotein from Chlorella vulgaris. Planta Med 62 (1996): 423–426.

Okamoto T et al. Lentinan from shiitake mushroom (Lentinus edodes) suppresses expression of cytochrome P450 1A subfamily in the mouse liver. Biofactors 21.1–4 (2004): 407–409.

Parada JL et al. Lactic acid bacteria growth promoters from Spirulina platensis. Int J Food Microbiol 45.3 (1998): 225–228.

Passwater R, Solomon N. Algae: The next generation of superfoods. Exp Optimal Health J 1 (1997): 2.

PDRHealth. Chlorella/Shiitake/Spirulina. Available: http://www.pdrhealth.com 16 June 2014.

Perocco P et al. Glucoraphanin, the bioprecursor of the widely extolled chemopreventive agent sulforaphane found in broccoli, induces Phase-I xenobiotic metabolizing enzymes and increases free radical generation in rat liver. Mutat Res Genet Toxicol Environ Mutagen 595.1–2 (2006): 125–136.

Pinero Estrada JE et al. Antioxidant activity of different fractions of Spirulina platensis protean extract. Farmaco 56.5–7 (2001): 497–500.

Pirt SJ. The effects of oxygen and carbon dioxide partial pressures on the rate and efficiency of algal (Chlorella) photosynthesis. Biochem Soc Trans 4 (1980): 479–481.

Podsedek A. Natural antioxidants and antioxidant capacity of Brassica vegetables. A review. Food Sci Technol 40 (2005): 1–11.

Porter WP et al. Endocrine, immune, and behavioural effects of alicarb (carbamate), atrazine (triazine) and nitrate (fertiliser) mixtures at ground water concentrations. Toxicol Ind Health 15 (1999): 133–150.

Porter WP et al. Groundwater pesticides: interactive effects of low concentrations of carbamates aldicarb and methomyl and the triazine

metribuzin on thyroxine and somatotrophin levels in white rats. J Toxicol Environ Health 40 (1993): 15–34.

Pratt S, Matthews K. Blueberries. In: Superfoods. London: Bantam Books, 2004a: 74–86.

Pratt S, Matthews K. Broccoli. In: Superfoods. London: Bantam Books, 2004b: 87–96.

Premkumar K et al. Protective effect of Spirulina fusiformis on chemical-induced genotoxicity in mice. Fitoterapia 75.1 (2004): 24–31.

Quereshi M et al. Dietary Spirulina platensis enhances humoral and cell-mediated functions in chickens. Immunopharmacol Immunotoxicol 18 (1996): 465–476.

Quereshi M, Ali R. Spirulina platensis exposure enhances macrophage phagocytic function in cats. Immunopharmacol Immunotoxicol 18 (1996): 457–463.

Quinsey PM et al. Persistence of organochlorines in breast milk of women in Victoria. Australia. Food Chem Toxicol 33.1 (1995): 49–56.

Quinsey PM et al. The importance of measured intake in assessing exposure of breast-fed infants to organochlorines. Eur J Clin Nutr 50.7 (1996): 438–442.

Raederstorff D, Kunz I, Schwager J. Resveratrol, from experimental data to nutritional evidence: The emergence of a new food ingredient. Ann N Y Acad Sci, 1290 (2013): 136–141.

Ramirez MR et al. Effect of lyophilised Vaccinium berries on memory, anxiety and locomotion in adult rats. Pharmacol Res 52.6 (2005): 457–62.

Ribaya-Mercado JD, Blumberg JB. Lutein and zeaxanthin and their potential roles in disease prevention. J Am Coll Nutr 23.6 (Suppl) (2004): 567–87S.

Robbins J. Diet for a new world. Avon, New York (1992).

Roberts JR, Karr CJ Pesticide exposure in children. Pediatrics 130.6 (2012): e1765–1788.

Rochette L et al. Direct and indirect antioxidant properties of alpha-lipoic acid and therapeutic potential. Mol Nutr Food Res, 57.1 (2013): 114–125.

Rose P et al. Broccoli and watercress suppress matrix metalloproteinase-9 activity and invasiveness of human MDA-MB-231 breast cancer cells. Toxicol Appl Pharmacol 209.2 (2005): 105–113.

Rosenblatt-Farrell N. The landscape of antibiotic resistance. Environ Health Perspect, 11.6 (2009): A244–250.

Rothenberg SP. Increasing the dietary intake of folate: pros and cons. Semin Hematol 36.1 (1999): 65–74.

Ruiz Flores L et al. Anticlastogenic effect of Spirulina maxima extract on the micronuclei induced by maleic hydrazide in Tradescantia. Life Sci 72.12 (2003): 1345–1351.

Saha S et al. Isothiocyanate concentrations and interconversion of sulforaphane to erucin in human subjects after consumption of commercial frozen broccoli compared to fresh broccoli. Mol Nutr Food Res 56.12 (2012): 1906–1916.

Sanborn M. Non-cancer health effects of pesticides. Systematic review and implications for family doctors. Canadian Family Physician, 53.10 (2007): 1712–1720.

Sanborn, M., Bassil, K., Vakil, C., Kerr, K., & Ragan, K. (2012). 2012 systematic review of pesticide human health effects. Retrieved 25 January, 2014, from http://www.ocfp.on.ca/docs/pesticides-paper/2012-systematic-review-of-pesticide.pdf

Sanborn M et al. Systematic review of pesticide human health effects: Pesticides literature review. Ontario College of Family Physicians. (2004) Available: http://www.ocfp.on.ca/local/files/Communications/Current%20Issues/Pesticides/Final%20Paper%2023APR2004.pdf 16 June 2014.

Sano T et al. Effect of lipophilic extract of Chlorella vulgaris on alimentary hyperlipidemia in cholesterol-fed rats. Artery 15 (1988): 217–224.

Sano T, Tanaka Y. Effect of dried, powdered Chlorella vulgaris on experimental atherosclerosis and alimentary hypercholesterolemia in cholesterol-fed rabbits. Artery 15 (1987): 76–84.

Schmidt BM et al. Differential effects of blueberry proanthocyanidins on androgen sensitive and insensitive human prostate cancer cell lines. Cancer Lett 231.2 (2006): 240–246.

Schwingshackl L, Hoffmann G. Monounsaturated fatty acids and risk of cardiovascular disease: Synopsis of the evidence available from systematic reviews and meta-analyses. Nutrients, 4.12 (2012): 1989–2007.

Schwingshackl L et al. Long-term effects of low glycemic index/load vs. high glycemic index/load diets on parameters of obesity and obesity-associated risks: a systematic review and meta-analysis. Nutr Metab Cardiovasc Dis 23.8 (2013): 699–706.

Seeram NP. Berry fruits: compositional elements, biochemical activities, and the impact of their intake on human health, performance, and disease. J Agric Food Chem 56.3 (2008): 627–629.

Shea KM. Technical report: irradiation of food. Committee on Environmental Health. Pediatrics 106.6 (2000): 1505–1510.

Shouji N et al. Anticaries effect of a component from shiitake (an edible mushroom). Caries Res 34.1 (2000): 94–98.

Sia GM, Candlish JK. Effects of shiitake (Lentinus edodes) extract on human neutrophils and the U937 monocytic cell line. Phytother Res 13.2 (1999): 133–137.

Sliva D. Ganoderma lucidum (Reishi) in cancer treatment. Integr Cancer Ther 2.4 (2003): 358–364.

Sliva D. Cellular and physiological effects of Ganoderma lucidum (Reishi). Mini Rev Med Chem 4.8 (2004): 873–879.

Slow Foods Movement. website. Available: http://www.slowfood.com/ 13 June 2014.

Smith AR et al. Lipoic acid as a potential therapy for chronic diseases associated with oxidative stress. Curr Med Chem 11.9 (2004): 1135–1146.

Smith-Spangler C et al. Are organic foods safer or healthier than conventional alternatives?: a systematic review. Ann Intern Med 157.5 (2012): 348–366.

Smith RN et al. A low-glycemic-load diet improves symptoms in acne vulgaris patients: a randomized controlled trial. Am J Clin Nutr 86.1 (2007): 107–115.

Srivastava A et al. Effect of storage conditions on the biological activity of phenolic compounds of blueberry extract packed in glass bottles. J Agric Food Chem 55.7 (2007): 2705–2713.

Stahl W, Sies H. 'beta-Carotene and other carotenoids in protection from sunlight.' Am J Clin Nutr 96.5 (2012): 1179S–1184S.

Steinkellner H et al. Effects of cruciferous vegetables and their constituents on drug metabolizing enzymes involved in the bioactivation of DNA-reactive dietary carcinogens. Mutat Res Genet Toxicol Environ Mutagen 480/481 (2001): 285–297.

Stoner GD, Mukhtar H. Polyphenols as cancer chemopreventive agents. J Cell Biochem Suppl 22 (1995): 169–180.

Stull AJ et al. Bioactives in blueberries improve insulin sensitivity in obese, insulin-resistant men and women. J Nutr 140.10 (2010): 1764–1768.

Surai KP et al. Antioxidant-prooxidant balance in the intestine: Food for thought. 2. Antioxidants. Curr Top Nutraceut Res 2.1 (2004): 27–46.

Sustain. The Food Miles Report — the dangers of long-distance food transport (2011) Available: http://www.sustainweb.org/ 13 June 2014.

Szedlay G. Is the widely used medicinal fungus the Ganoderma lucidum (Fr.) Karst. sensu stricto? (A short review). Acta Microbiol Immunol Hung 49.2–3 (2002): 235–243.

Takai M et al. 3P-0811 LDL-cholesterol-lowering effects of a mixed green vegetable and fruit beverage containing broccoli and cabbage in hypercholesterolemic subjects. Atheroscler Suppl 4.2 (2003): 239.

Tanaka K et al. Oral administration of a unicellular green algae, Chlorella vulgaris, prevents stress-induced ulcer. Planta Med 63 (1997): 465–466.

Tanaka K et al. A novel glycoprotein obtained from Chlorella vulgaris strain CK22 shows antimetastatic immunopotentiation. Cancer Immunol Immunother 45 (1998): 313–320.

Tang L et al. Consumption of raw cruciferous vegetables is inversely associated with bladder cancer risk. Cancer Epidemiology Biomarkers & Prevention 17 (2008): 938–944.

Tarozzi A et al. Sulforaphane as a potential protective phytochemical against neurodegenerative diseases. Oxid Med Cell Longev (2013). 415078.

Thiruchelvam M et al. The nigrostriatal dopaminergic system as a preferential target of repeated exposures to combined paraquat and maneb: implications for Parkinson's disease. J Neurosci 20.24 (2000): 9207–9214.

Tracton I, Bobrov Z. World's first organic, super-antioxidant, wholefood to be released. Sydney: NutriMed Group (media release), June 2005: 23.

Turkmen N et al. The effect of cooking methods on total phenolics and antioxidant activity of selected green vegetables. Food Chem 93.4 (2005): 713–718.

Vallejo F et al. Phenolic compound contents in edible parts of broccoli inflorescences after domestic cooking. J Sci Food Agric 83.14 (2003): 1511–1516.

Van Hoydonck PGA et al. A dietary oxidative balance score of vitamin C, β-carotene and iron intakes and mortality risk in male smoking Belgians. J Nutr 132.4 (2002): 756–761.

Van Nevel CJ et al. The influence of Lentinus edodes (Shiitake mushroom) preparations on bacteriological and morphological aspects of the small intestine in piglets. Arch Tierernahr 57.6 (2003): 399–412.

Vang O et al. Biochemical effects of dietary intakes of different broccoli samples. I. Differential modulation of cytochrome P-450 activities in rat liver, kidney, and colon. Metabolism 50.10 (2001): 1123–1129.

Vattem DA et al. Cranberry synergies for dietary management of Helicobacter pylori infections. Process Biochem 40.5 (2005): 1583–1592.

Venn BJ, Mann JI. Cereal grains, legumes and diabetes. Eur J Clin Nutr 58.11 (2004): 1443–1461.

Verschuren PM. Functional foods: Scientific and global perspectives. British Journal of Nutrition, 88 (2002): 125–131.

Vetter J, Berta E. Mercury content of the cultivated mushroom Agaricus bisporus. Food Control 16.2 (2005): 113–116.

Wang SY et al. Fruit quality, antioxidant capacity, and flavonoid content of organically and conventionally grown blueberries. J Agric Food Chem 56.14 (2008): 5788–5794.

Wang Y et al. Studies on the immuno-modulating and antitumor activities of Ganoderma lucidum (Reishi) polysaccharides: functional and proteomic analyses of a fucose-containing glycoprotein fraction responsible for the activities. Bioorg Med Chem 10.4 (2002): 1057–1062.

Wang Y et al. Dietary supplementation with blueberries, spinach, or spirulina reduces ischemic brain damage. Exp Neurol 193.1 (2005): 75–84.

Watanabe F et al. Characterization and bioavailability of vitamin B12-compounds from edible algae. Tokyo: J Nutr Sci Vitaminol 48 (2002): 5325–5331.

Wehrmeister AA et al. Antioxidant content of fresh, frozen, canned, and dehydrated blueberries. J Am Dietetic Assoc 105 Suppl 1 (2005): 38.

White RW et al. Effects of a mushroom mycelium extract on the treatment of prostate cancer. Urology 60.4 (2002): 640–644.

Williams CM et al. Blueberry-induced changes in spatial working memory correlate with changes in hippocampal CREB phosphorylation and brain-derived neurotrophic factor (BDNF) levels. Free Radic Biol Med 45.3 (2008): 295–305.

Willis LM et al. Dietary blueberry supplementation affects growth but not vascularization of neural transplants. J Cereb Blood Flow Metab 28.6 (2008): 1150–64.

Wiseman A. Dietary anticancer isothiocyanates (ITC) in Brassica raise the reduced-glutathione barrier to DNA-damage in the colon? Trends Food Sci Technol 16.5 (2005): 215–216.

Wiseman W et al. Feeding blueberry diets inhibits angiotensin ii-converting enzyme (ace) activity in spontaneously hypertensive stroke-prone rats. Can J Physiol Pharmacol, 89.1 (2011): 6771.

Wollin SD, Jones PJ. Alpha-lipoic acid and cardiovascular disease. J Nutr 133.11 (2003): 3327–3330.

Yamada T et al. Effects of Lentinus edodes mycelia on dietary-induced atherosclerotic involvement in rabbit aorta. J Atheroscler Thromb 9.3 (2002): 149–156.

Yamagishi S et al. Therapeutic potentials of unicellular green alga Chlorella in advanced glycation end product (AGE)-related disorders. Med Hypotheses 65.5 (2005): 953–955.

Yamaguchi Y, Miyahara E, Hihara J. Efficacy and safety of orally administered lentinula edodes mycelia extract for patients undergoing cancer chemotherapy: A pilot study. Am J Chin Med 39.3 (2011): 451–459.

Yang BK et al. Hypoglycemic effect of a Lentinus edodes exo-polymer produced from a submerged mycelial culture. Biosci Biotechnol Biochem 66.5 (2002): 937–942.

Yang, D et al. Human carboxylesterases hce1 and hce2: Ontogenic expression, inter-individual variability and differential hydrolysis of oseltamivir, aspirin, deltamethrin and permethrin. Biochem Pharmacol 77.2 (2009): 238–247.

Yilmaz N et al. Fatty acid composition in some wild edible mushrooms growing in the middle Black Sea region of Turkey. Food Chem 99 (2005): 168–174.

Youdim KA et al. Potential role of dietary flavonoids in reducing microvascular endothelium vulnerability to oxidative and inflammatory insults. J Nutr Biochem 13.5 (2002): 282–288.

Zheng R et al. Characterization and immunomodulating activities of polysaccharide from Lentinus edodes. Int Immunopharmacol 5.5 (2005): 811–820.

Ziegler RG et al. Nutrition and lung cancer. Cancer Causes Control 7.1 (1996): 157–177.

CHAPTER 6

INTRODUCTION TO THE PRACTICE OF INTEGRATIVE MEDICINE

Throughout history, every civilisation and culture has developed its own form of medicine. The rise of modern technology and scientific enquiry have added new therapeutic techniques, products and services to the range of traditional therapies. Thus, within today's pluralistic, multicultural and increasingly globalised societies, the wisdom and therapeutic interventions of many different traditions are becoming available. While it is impossible for any practitioner to have access to, or even know something about, the many hundreds of therapeutic interventions available, it is possible to incorporate some of the key principles into today's conventional healthcare practice. This leads to the practice of integrative medicine (IM), which attempts to define and embrace these principles.

The practice of IM is more than simply an expansion of conventional medical practice to include 'complementary therapies', such as mind–body techniques, acupuncture, herbs, nutrients and body work (for example, massage and manipulation). It involves:

- a focus on the whole person: the interplay between the physical, emotional, spiritual and psychological states

- individualised treatment plans tailored to meet the needs of the person

- the development of a therapeutic partnership between the patient and practitioner as a fundamental part of the healing process

- a primary focus on prevention, health enhancement and addressing predisposing, exacerbating and sustaining causes of disease

- integration of the best available, evidence-based, safe and ethical therapies from different traditions.

As such, IM forms the basis for clinical decision making and improving patient outcomes, by providing each patient with effective and compassionate care and healing on many levels. IM is increasingly being acknowledged as 'best practice'; however, it requires some fundamental shifts in the way healthcare is delivered, and has not yet become widely implemented (Cohen 2005a). For example, the use of complementary medicines is an integral part of IM practice, yet this use raises many issues for medical practitioners, particularly those who have not received training in how to use them. Some of the questions are:

- What can reasonably be expected by providing integrative care?

- What are the safety issues?

- Which therapies are cost-effective?

- What advice should be given to patients in the absence of definitive evidence?

- Which therapies or products are useful for which conditions and which patients?

- Where can high-quality complementary and alternative medicine (CAM) products be obtained?
- Which practitioners or modalities should patients be referred to use, and when, how and for what reasons should referrals be made?
- Where can reliable information about CAM be found, and what pathways are there for further study?

These are core issues in any healthcare practice and are not specific to the use of complementary medicines or even to the practice of IM. The practice of IM, however, poses additional challenges to medical practitioners, both professionally and personally. It requires being prepared to learn about new and different treatment systems, traditions and ways of thinking, and recognising the advantages and limitations of both complementary and conventional medicine and the potential benefits of combining them. It also requires adopting a collaborative approach with patients and a variety of different healthcare professionals, while allowing old beliefs to be challenged and re-evaluated. Furthermore, the practice of IM challenges medical practitioners to develop their intuition, empathy and compassion, address their own health and personal growth, and become role models for their patients and the wider community.

From a practical perspective, IM takes extra time. Time is needed to keep up to date with the changing evidence base, as well as to establish a rapport with and holistic understanding of patients and then apply the principles of IM to address their needs.

HOLISM AND THE INDIVIDUAL

In their professional training, medical practitioners study the biological, psychological and social aspects of health, as well as the signs, symptoms and pathophysiology of specific illnesses, to achieve an understanding of health and disease in a clinical context. This knowledge base must be updated and modified with new knowledge provided by new scientific evidence and cumulative clinical experience. Although consideration of the best available evidence is an important dimension of clinical practice, scientific data are often based on a group of observations that give statistical information about research populations, but which may not provide definitive information about what will happen to any individual patient in certain circumstances.

Each human being is unique and presents in a specific clinical context in which the outcome will be determined by personal attributes, such as attitudes, education and understanding, as well as by genetics, physiology, past experiences, socioeconomic and cultural circumstances, available resources and lifestyle. Accounting for individual differences is an essential aspect of the art of medicine and a cornerstone of many ancient systems of medicine.

Chinese medicine, Ayurvedic medicine and Western herbal medicine all have sophisticated systems of categorising people according to their different physiological and psychological characteristics in order to guide treatment selection. In comparison, modern Western medicine has been slow to accept and use this individualistic approach, preferring to standardise treatment approaches through clinical guidelines and protocols. The fields of pharmacogenomics and nutrigenomics, which have emerged out of the Human Genome Project, are beginning to provide a scientific rationale for individualising treatments. These new fields emphasise two factors: individualised response to medicines and nutrients, and the roles of dietary and genetic interactions in patient health.

The practice of IM combines both ancient and modern knowledge, and takes a holistic perspective that recognises health involves physical, psychological, social, spiritual and environmental dimensions. This is in line with increasing patient expectations to have the accompanying social and psychological aspects of their illness addressed, not just their presenting symptoms (Jonas 2001). Thus the practice of IM requires careful history-taking and physical examination, which may include obtaining information from different philosophical perspectives, together with astute and appropriate investigations, and obtaining other information from relatives or carers.

Accounting for individual factors takes considerable time, yet this time is well spent because there is mounting evidence to suggest a direct relationship between consultation length and the quality of care. Longer consultations are likely to result in better health outcomes and better handling of psychosocial problems, fewer prescriptions, more lifestyle advice and lower costs, less litigation and more patient and doctor satisfaction (Cohen et al 2002).

THERAPEUTIC RELATIONSHIPS

Although amassing personal information about a patient is a time-consuming process, it is an extremely valuable one, not only for the information gleaned but also because it facilitates the development of rapport, respect and trust, thus laying the foundation for the therapeutic relationship. The development of close and meaningful relationships with people in a clinical context is one of the great challenges of holistic or integrative practice. It is also one of the most powerful therapeutic tools clinicians have and may be more important than any specific treatment modality.

The therapeutic relationship is a profound and sacred one, acknowledged since ancient times and codified in the Hippocratic oath, which has specific phrases that dictate the principle of doctor–patient confidentiality, as well as the responsibility of clinicians to exercise a duty of care.

A therapeutic relationship is established with the specific intention of healing, and the act of establishing such a relationship, in which intuition and empathy are valued alongside information and evidence, may be therapeutic in itself. Simply articulating one's personal story and expressing traumatic experiences to a sympathetic listener can help people make connections and better understand the causes and implications of their disease, as well as providing much needed psychosocial support.

Healthcare professionals commonly see people at their worst: when they are in pain and/or feeling sick, scared, sleep deprived and fearful of the possible implications of an illness. The constant stream of 'sick people' can make it easy to start differentiating patients by their illnesses; however, thinking of people in terms of their highest level of functioning may be more productive. To this end, some of the most important questions a practitioner can ask are: 'What makes you happy?' or 'What makes you feel alive?' The answers to these questions can provide valuable insight into an individual and form the basis for a more meaningful relationship than the answer to the question: 'What is the problem?'

Developing rapport, trust and a holistic understanding of patients' lives is one of the most important elements in IM, because it places practitioners in a better position to allay their patients' fears, adequately address the issues of most concern and help to reduce the burden of stress that accompanies virtually all illness. A holistic understanding of a person also enables clinicians to recommend treatments that are more likely to be successfully integrated into a patient's social and cultural environment, thus improving efficacy and compliance. Furthermore, a sound therapeutic relationship provides the camaraderie and sense of therapeutic adventure necessary to underpin a partnership model of health and provides a solid foundation for clinical decision making.

PRACTITIONER WELLBEING

Healthcare professionals experience significant mental, physical and spiritual demands during the course of everyday practice. In addition, personal stress can influence the ability to deliver effective care, establish therapeutic relationships and maintain good health. Over time, exposure to multiple stressors can lead to physical and emotional exhaustion, or burnout, with its accompanying physical and psychological burden (Dunning 2005).

For some practitioners, there is a perceived pressure to symbolise perfect health and be invulnerable to disease. As a result, there is the temptation to avoid indications of ill health in themselves and their colleagues and a failure to see the need for self-care. The practice of IM compels clinicians to address their own health and lifestyle, explore their emotional life and develop self-care routines to maintain wellbeing and prevent disease. In addition, the therapeutic relationship developed with patients can be nurturing for the practitioner, with rewards that flow in both directions (Cohen 2005b).

In advocating a holistic view of health, the practice of IM can also motivate practitioners to become more involved in broader community, public health and global issues, such as social justice, fair trade, environmental preservation, regeneration and sustainability, as well as spiritual, ethical and philosophical debates and pursuits.

INTUITION, BEDSIDE MANNER AND PLACEBO

Medicine is an art informed by science, yet with so much recent attention being given to scientific evidence, it is easy to forget the importance of intuition and clinical experience. A holistic understanding of a patient, together with empathy and compassion for a patient's circumstances, adds important information to any clinical encounter. It is likely that the best and most inspired practice occurs when the practitioner's academic knowledge, clinical experience and intuitive understanding of the individual merge to provide a picture of the clinical situation as a coherent whole, known as the 'Gestalt' approach.

Developing an intimate therapeutic relationship and integrating rational and intuitive knowledge enlists the full capacity of the practitioner. It may also be the best way to tap into patients' unconscious healing processes and elicit the 'placebo response'. The placebo effect is often considered a source of bias and a scientific distraction that research methodology must minimise; however, the placebo response is ubiquitous and cannot be avoided in the clinical setting.

All interventions have a non-specific therapeutic action, in addition to their purported activity, and the best clinicians will always use their 'bedside manner' to harness the 'placebo response' and enhance the therapeutic benefits of any specific intervention. Herbert Benson suggested that the placebo response is based on a good therapeutic relationship, as well as positive beliefs and expectations on the part of the patient and practitioner, and, furthermore, can yield beneficial clinical results and be a powerful adjunct to therapy. Benson, who coined the term 'the relaxation response' in reference to meditation, further suggested that the placebo response should be renamed 'remembered wellness', and that it may be one of medicine's most potent assets because it is safe, inexpensive and accessible to many people (Benson & Friedman 1996).

In addition to the use of rapport, empathy, compassion, trust, confidence and intimacy, an integral part of a good bedside manner is the appropriate and thoughtful use of touch. Touch pulls together psychological and bodily experiences and is important in relationships between people in general, and the therapeutic relationship in particular. It is a basic human need that enhances communication and builds trust. A simple handshake to acknowledge each other's presence or hand-holding when bad news is delivered can provide important and reassuring support that goes beyond words. The therapeutic power of touch has been recognised and practised throughout history: for example, through the art of massage, which, when provided by a trained practitioner, can produce substantial therapeutic effects, enhance a person's sense of wellbeing and promote a sense of calm and peace.

BIAS IN MEDICAL DECISION MAKING

How do people make decisions and how do they choose between different treatment options? Decisions are made using 'heuristics', or general rules of thumb, which reduce the time and effort required. Normally this method yields fairly good results; however, there are times when they lead to systematic biases (Plous 1993). In these situations, assumptions are made and information is neglected, downplayed or overplayed, or based on what is easily recalled. In healthcare, unrecognised bias of this nature can have dire repercussions, affecting a clinician's ability to diagnose and treat effectively and a patient's ability to make good choices.

It is both normal and human to have a range of biases that influence the types of treatments that are considered appropriate, based on the individual's personal, ideological, religious, ethical, cultural, educational and philosophical ideals and experiences. Good clinicians are aware of their personal biases and will openly disclose those that may influence a patient's care. In some cases, this is easier said than done. Stating known or potential bias can be particularly sensitive when the practitioner has strongly held religious beliefs that may limit their practice or determine their attitudes to different therapies, as well as when it comes to declaring commercial interests.

Healing is a human vocation that arises from the desire to do the best for humanity. The patient–practitioner relationship, however, is not only a therapeutic one, it is commonly a commercial one. Healing is a business that sustains the personal lives of individual practitioners and drives the healthcare and pharmaceutical industries, which are among the biggest industries in the world. In 2002 the combined profits for the top 10 drug companies in the Fortune 500 list were greater than those of all the other 490 companies combined (Angell 2004).

One important source of bias that is becoming increasingly recognised concerns the millions of dollars spent by the pharmaceutical industry in a bid to influence doctors' decision making. The seemingly unlimited marketing budgets and provision of gifts, luxuries and educational events has forced the medical profession to attempt to limit these sorts of inducements (Studdert et al 2004). The extent of the industry's influence is vast and has not always been obvious. In her book on the pharmaceutical industry, Marcia Angell, a former editor-in-chief of the *New England Journal of Medicine*, states:

> *Over the past two decades the pharmaceutical industry has moved very far from its original high purpose of discovering and producing useful new drugs. Now primarily a marketing machine to sell drugs of dubious benefit, this industry uses its wealth and power to co-opt every institution that might stand in its way, including the US Congress, the FDA, academic medical centers, and the medical profession itself.*
>
> **Angell 2004**

Not only are doctors subject to the influence of the pharmaceutical industry, they may also have other pecuniary interests that could bias their clinical decision making, such as commercial interests in pathology companies and their own clinical dispensaries.

COMPLEMENTARY MEDICINE PRODUCTS

Several thousand complementary medicine products are now available on the market, the vast majority of which are available without prescription. Choosing the best product, correct dose and time-frame for use and having realistic expectations of the treatment are just some of the factors that healthcare practitioners must consider before recommending a specific product (Table 6.1). These factors, which are addressed in further detail in the monographs and chapters of this book, must be considered in the light of each individual patient's circumstances, including their condition and comorbidities, renal and hepatic function, personal preferences, financial resources and their ability to self-monitor their condition.

Complementary medicines in Australia are regulated in the same way as pharmaceutical medicines, and are evaluated for quality and safety; however, seemingly similar products will vary with respect to their efficacy and supporting scientific evidence. Most complementary medicines are available over the counter (OTC) through pharmacies, health food stores and supermarkets; however, there are also certain complementary medicines that are available as practitioner-only products. These are prescribed and dispensed only by a CAM practitioner; they can have different potencies and formulations from those available OTC and include extemporaneously compounded herbs that require time, specific knowledge and expertise to dispense. Clearly, making product choices can be confusing, and clinicians should be encouraged to become familiar with the products available and eventually identify a group of favoured products they feel confident in prescribing.

There are many good reasons for including complementary medicines into routine practice (Table 6.2). Medicines that are supported by good evidence of efficacy and safety, or which offer advantages over conventional medicines in terms of cost-effectiveness, should be considered an essential part of routine clinical practice. Indeed, there could be seen to be an ethical imperative for considering the use of such complementary medicines, as not to do so would deprive patients of potentially safe and effective treatments (see Table 6.3 and specific monographs for further details).

COST EFFECTIVENESS OF CAM

In October 2005 a report titled *The role of CAM in the NHS* examined whether treatment approaches not normally funded by the National Health Service (UK) could provide

TABLE 6.1 FACTORS TO CONSIDER WHEN RECOMMENDING A COMPLEMENTARY MEDICINE	
PRODUCT FACTORS	**COMMENTS**
Mechanism/s of action	How well established are these? Do they seem plausible?
Evidence and expectations	Is it likely to achieve treatment goals? In what time-frame? Do not rely on label claims alone. Consider the type of evidence available for this particular indication. For herbs also consider: extract and plant part/s tested. For nutrients: consider chemical form and bioavailability.
Dose and administration route	Ensure these are correct for the specific indication.
Frequency, timing and ease of use	Reduced frequency improves compliance. Consider timing, such as before, during or after meals.
Quality control standards	Not all countries impose high quality control standards on the manufacture of complementary medicines; e.g. the USA. In Australia, only use products with AUST L or AUST R numbers on the label.
Combination products or single entities	For combination products, consider dosage and potential synergy of individual ingredients.
Potential to induce adverse reactions	Consider potential likelihood of adverse reaction and consequence (see Chapter 7 for more information).
Potential to induce interactions	Are harmful, beneficial or neutral interactions possible? Should the product be avoided, used only under professional supervision, or actively prescribed? (Use METOPIA algorithm in Chapter 8.)
Contraindications	Take special care with high risk groups (see Chapters 7 and 10 for more information).
Storage	Consider sensitivity to light and heat, need for refrigeration and shelf-life.
Cost	Compare cost with that of other treatments — medicinal and non-medicinal.
Availability	Is it available OTC or only from a practitioner?

TABLE 6.2 REASONS FOR USING COMPLEMENTARY MEDICINES
Efficacy — will alleviate symptoms of disease, reduce exacerbation or present a cure. **S**afety — present a safer treatment option than other therapies. **C**ost — when they provide lower cost treatment options. **A**djunct — if the efficacy and/or safety of other interventions can be improved with adjunctive use. **P**revention — when they provide safe prevention strategies in at-risk populations. **E**nhance health — increase sense of wellbeing and quality of life. **E**nlists patients' involvement in their own healthcare.

some financial relief, while retaining good quality patient care (Smallwood 2005). The report, commissioned by HRH Prince Charles, involved an assessment of the scientific evidence, interviews with experts, such as researchers, policymakers and healthcare professionals, and case studies to draw together published and experiential information, financial data and economic forecasting.

The report suggested that acupuncture may provide cost benefits in general practice when used for musculoskeletal conditions or as an adjunct to conventional treatment for lower back pain, migraine and stroke rehabilitation. With regard to herbal medicine, the enquiry identified several OTC herbal medicines such as St John's wort, phytodolor, Echinacea, *Ginkgo biloba*, devil's claw, hawthorn, horse chestnut and saw palmetto that provide potential cost savings to the government, while offering similar or greater benefits than pharmaceutical treatments. More recently, a report on the cost effectiveness of complementary medicines produced by the National Institute of Complementary Medicine (NICM) in Australia suggested that 'millions in healthcare costs could be saved without compromising patient outcomes if complementary medicines were

TABLE 6.3 EXAMPLES OF HERBS AND NATURAL SUPPLEMENTS WITH PROVEN EFFICACY

HERB/NATURAL SUPPLEMENT	PROVEN EFFICACY
Chaste tree	Premenstrual syndrome
Cranberry	Urinary tract infection prophylaxis
Fish oils	Cardiovascular disease prevention; lipid-lowering
St John's wort	Depression
Ginkgo biloba	Dementia
Glucosamine sulphate	Osteoarthritis: symptoms and disease progression
Hawthorn	Chronic heart failure (New York Heart Association classes I–II)
Honey	Infection control/wound healing
Horse chestnut	Chronic venous insufficiency
Kava kava	Anxiety
Peppermint	Irritable bowel syndrome
Probiotics	Preventing antibiotic-induced diarrhoea
Pygeum	Benign prostatic hypertrophy (BPH)
Saw palmetto	BPH
Tea tree oil	Topical infections

more widely used' (Access Economics 2010). This report, which examined the direct costs associated with the use of selected therapies, supports the conclusions of the UK study by suggesting that acupuncture, St John's wort, fish oils and phytodolor all offer potential cost savings when used for selected conditions (see NICM 2014).

DISPENSING PRODUCTS

The choice whether or not to stock and dispense products is a complex one, with ethical, commercial and practical issues to be considered. Many medical practitioners may feel it is unethical to profit from the sale of products they prescribe (Cohen et al 2005), but the direct dispensing and selling of complementary medicines by doctors is in line with the sale of products by other registered healthcare professionals such as veterinary surgeons, pharmacists, podiatrists, physiotherapists and optometrists.

These healthcare professionals dispense advice and sell products in the same consultation, as do CAM practitioners, such as naturopaths, herbalists and traditional Chinese medicine (TCM) practitioners.

The direct dispensing of products provides practitioners with some assurance of patient compliance and promotes the use of correct dosage, administration forms and extracts. This may be particularly important for herbal products. Direct dispensing is also convenient for patients and gives them the confidence that a practitioner who is aware of their history and current needs has directed them to the best treatment. If a decision to dispense products is made, this should obviously be done in an ethical manner, and treatment plans must always be dictated by the best interests of the patient.

ETHICAL CONDUCT

The issues of ethical practitioner conduct have their basis in the Hippocratic oath, which acknowledges the inherent inequality of the practitioner–patient relationship and the responsibility of the doctor to use this to improve the health of their patients, who may be vulnerable and who entrust themselves to medical care.

The ethical conduct of doctors has since been explored by various professional associations and colleges such as the Australian Medical Association and Royal Australian College of General Practitioners. The standards of ethical conduct (AMA 2004) include:

- always acting in the best interests of patients
- not exploiting patients for any reason
- respecting the patient's right to make their own decisions and to accept or reject advice about treatment or procedures
- ensuring patients are aware of fees, and that healthcare costs are openly discussed and direct financial interests disclosed.

These standards also apply to IM, and the sale of complementary medicines must conform with these principles, insofar as the interests of the patient are the foremost consideration and patients are fully informed about the nature, benefits, risks and costs of any proposed treatment, as well as any financial interests of the practitioner. Patients also need to be aware that they have the right to accept or reject any advice (AMA 2004).

INFORMED CONSENT

The ethical precepts of informed consent and the respect for patient autonomy compel healthcare practitioners to inform their patients about the range of appropriate treatments available, their associated costs and risks, and to respect the right of patients to make their own decisions. In practice, this can be problematic, as it remains unclear how much information practitioners are expected to know themselves and how much patients require.

This issue is addressed by the joint position statement on complementary medicine made by the Royal Australian College of General Practitioners (RACGP) and the Australasian Integrative Medicine Association (AIMA):

> General practitioners require a basic understanding of natural and complementary medicine and should receive sufficient training in their undergraduate, vocational and further education to enable them to include natural/complementary medicines with proven safety and efficacy in their practice, and to discuss issues with their patients on an informed basis.
> The key principle of evidence-based medicine should be the basis of evaluating natural and complementary medicines and their use by the medical profession. It should also be the basis of any collaborative relationships between general practitioners and complementary therapists.
>
> **RACGP/AIMA 2004**

Based on this statement it would seem reasonable that all general practitioners need to know enough about widely available complementary therapies to use safe and effective, evidence-based therapies where appropriate, and to avoid predictable adverse events and interactions induced by commonly used complementary therapies. It has further been argued that doctors have an ethical and even a legal obligation to become familiar with this area and open a dialogue with their patients about complementary treatments to provide quality care and address safety concerns (Brophy 2003).

Unfortunately this is a difficult task, as most medical schools give little or no time to teaching about evidence-based complementary therapies, and the opportunities for vocational and postgraduate medical education about CAM remain limited. As a result, having ready access to quality, evidence-based, independent information sources is essential to guide clinicians when making healthcare decisions or faced with patient enquiries about CAM.

EVIDENCE-BASED MEDICINE

The idea that practitioners need to refer to evidence is the basis of evidence-based medicine (EBM), which has been described by Sackett et al (1996) as: 'the conscientious, explicit, and judicious use of current best evidence in making decisions about the care of individual patients'. These authors go on to state:

> The practice of evidence-based medicine means integrating individual clinical expertise with the best available external clinical evidence from systematic research. By individual clinical expertise we mean the proficiency and judgment that individual clinicians acquire through clinical experience and clinical practice. Increased expertise is reflected in many ways, but especially in more effective and efficient diagnosis and in the more thoughtful identification and compassionate use of individual patients' predicaments, rights, and preferences in making clinical decisions about their care.

This statement acknowledges that, in practice, for most treatment decisions the conclusive evidence simply does not yet exist, and the best available evidence may simply be clinical experience or anecdotal reports. It is also clear that each practitioner and patient must seek out the necessary information they require, and interpret this evidence in the light of each individual situation.

EVIDENCE IN PRACTICE

EBM adds another dimension to the art of medicine and requires clinicians to review the evidence of safety and efficacy for the therapy under consideration, as well as to understand the inherent limitations of the available evidence and its relevance to a specific situation. It also involves weighing up the evidence for a number of different therapies, which includes an assessment of their costs and risks versus their potential benefits (see PEACE mnemonic in Chapter 1).

In the specific case of CAM, a growing number of treatments have been subject to scientific investigation, with over 6000 RCTs identified and made available through the central Cochrane Library. Although this is encouraging, many therapies do not yet have established evidence and some remain difficult to assess under controlled conditions (e.g. massage). In practice, this should not preclude them from being viable treatment options, but it can place some limitations on use. Ultimately, clinical decision making should be guided by the evidence available (Fig. 6.1).

• When there is evidence of efficacy and safety for CAM, it should be recommended to patients where appropriate and included as part of standard care.

• When the efficacy of a treatment is unknown, due to insufficient investigation or inconclusive results, and there are no apparent safety concerns, patients deciding to use these therapies should be supported and supervised. It is prudent to set specific therapeutic objectives and time-frames, and to monitor for potential adverse outcomes.

• When there is evidence for a lack of effect, use should be discouraged, especially if there is the potential to induce adverse effects.

This approach is summarised by the four Ps: **P**rotect, **P**ermit, **P**romote and **P**artner (Jonas et al 1999). Thus, practitioners need to protect their patients by ensuring the safety and cost effectiveness of treatments, permit therapies that are safe and inexpensive, even if their efficacy has not been conclusively proven, promote proven practices and partner with patients and other complementary therapists (Jonas 2001) (Table 6.4).

Complementary therapies with rigorous evidence for efficacy and safety that do not require specialised skills or expertise to implement should be considered part of mainstream practice and used by all healthcare practitioners, whereas other therapies/medicines with less rigorous evidence or requiring specific expertise may be more appropriately used by those with a special interest and/or appropriate training. Therapies that have evidence for a lack of efficacy and safety should be abandoned along with the long list of useless and harmful therapies that have been discontinued throughout medical history.

FIGURE 6.1 Paradigm of clinical decision making (Based on Renella & Fanconi 2006, adapted from Cohen & Eisenberg 2002)

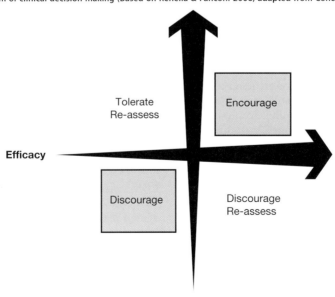

TABLE 6.4 PRINCIPLES FOR ADVISING THE USE OF COMPLEMENTARY THERAPIES		
STATUS OF EVIDENCE	SPECIAL SKILL/TRAINING REQUIRED	SPECIAL SKILL/TRAINING NOT REQUIRED
Strong evidence for quality, safety and cost-effectiveness	*Promote and partner with therapist* Encourage/recommend/implement therapy. *OR* Refer to appropriate practitioner and/or consider obtaining required skills (e.g. acupuncture).	*Promote and partner with patient* Encourage/recommend/ implement therapy. Consider as part of standard practice (e.g. dietary modification).
Insufficient or inconclusive evidence for quality, safety and cost-effectiveness	*Permit and partner with therapist* Continue therapy with caution and monitor patient in collaboration with other practitioner if necessary. *OR* Consider more appropriate therapies.	*Permit and partner with patient* Continue therapy with caution and monitor patient. *OR* Consider more appropriate therapies.
Strong evidence against quality, safety and cost-effectiveness	*Protect and partner with patient* Discourage use. Discuss reasons and desired outcomes and consider more appropriate therapies.	

A MULTIDISCIPLINARY, COLLABORATIVE APPROACH

It remains unclear which therapies should be considered within the domain of every doctor and which should be considered areas of special interest or the exclusive domain of CAM practitioners. It is clear however, that the practice of IM requires a multidisciplinary approach with collaboration and communication between the different practitioners who are aware of their own limitations and who have declared interests and expertise. It is also clear that whether or not doctors are prepared to personally use CAM, all doctors need to be prepared to discuss their use and inform patients of viable evidence-based options, as well as assess the likelihood of safety issues or interactions.

OPEN COMMUNICATION

Effective communication and teamwork is essential for the delivery of high-quality, safe patient care: communication failure is an extremely common cause of inadvertent patient harm.

Numerous surveys have shown that patients commonly combine CAM with conventional medical treatments, outside the knowledge of their various healthcare providers. This may be particularly true in hospitals, where it has been found that while almost 50% of surgical patients take complementary medicines in the perioperative period, 80% are not asked about

this use (Braun et al 2006). It is also estimated that more than 50% of users of CAM do not disclose this use to either their hospital doctors (Braun et al 2006) or their GPs (MacLennan et al 2002). In addition, many treatments are patient-initiated without professional advice.

According to a review of 12 studies, patients do not disclose use of CAM to their medical practitioner for reasons that can be grouped into three main themes (Robinson & McGrail 2004).

1. Concerns about eliciting a negative response, disapproval and rejection. Patients fear they will be persuaded to cease use and the practitioner will not continue to provide patient care.
2. Patients believe that the practitioner does not need to know about CAM use because it is irrelevant to the biomedical model of treatment; their practitioner is ignorant about CAM and would not be able to understand why it is being used or be able to contribute useful information about it.
3. Not being asked about CAM use or perceiving practitioner disinterest in the topic. (This has proved to be more significant in preventing discussion than previously thought [Braun et al 2006].)

It is therefore not unusual for there to be little coordination between patient-initiated and clinician-initiated treatments, which can result in suboptimal 'integrative care' and potentially unsafe outcomes.

As the popularity of CAM continues to grow, medical practitioners in the community and hospital settings will keep coming into contact with patients who are using, or considering using, these treatments, making the issue of communication and competence in dealing with CAM-related issues more urgent. Asking patients about possible use of complementary medicines may seem daunting; however, it is a necessary measure to promote patient safety. It also provides an opportunity to gain insight into a patient's beliefs and attitudes, as well as their willingness to be involved in their own healthcare.

Although discussions about complementary therapies may enhance the therapeutic relationship, non-disclosure can indicate a serious deficiency in this relationship, for if patients are unwilling to discuss their use, it is also possible that they will not discuss other personal information that may have an impact on their health and medical treatment. Non-disclosure also refers to a lack of interdisciplinary communication. Although many patients would like to benefit from treatment and advice from both doctors and natural therapists, effective collaboration between these groups appears to be limited and it has been estimated that of the 44% of Australians who visit natural therapists, only 13% do so on the advice of their doctors.

INTERDISCIPLINARY COLLABORATION

True collaboration can only occur in an environment of shared respect and trust, and knowledge of what can be offered. In reality, both medical and CAM practitioners have several concerns about each other's practice, which must be addressed in order to achieve a good working partnership.

For medical doctors, there are concerns that CAM practitioners may put patients at risk of delayed or missed diagnosis and/or delay the use of more effective therapies (Cohen et al 2005). There is also concern that CAM practitioners might encourage patients to refuse use of 'proven' treatments in preference for 'unproven' ones, particularly in serious diseases such as cancer or HIV-AIDS. The promotion of implausible or untrue claims or unsafe complementary therapies that waste patients' time and money, or induce adverse events, is another source of apprehension.

Complementary therapists, on the other hand, may be concerned that medical doctors too readily prescribe symptom-suppressing drugs, yet do little to address underlying causes and support natural homeostasis through diet, lifestyle and preventive approaches. There is concern that patients may waste their time and money on treatments that exert significant side effects while providing limited benefits, and that medical practitioners may advise against the use of natural therapies because of fear, ignorance or arrogance. Furthermore, natural therapists may be concerned that their positions are being usurped by doctors who take on the use of natural and complementary therapies with little specific training and little consideration for their underlying philosophies and holistic considerations (Cohen 2001).

Many of these concerns are based on ignorance and misunderstanding between the practitioner groups and can be addressed through open and honest communication and formalised communication strategies, one of the most important of which is through the provision of formal correspondence in referral letters.

REFERRAL LETTERS

Referral letters are a standardised method of professional communication between practitioners. They involve both outgoing and incoming correspondence that sets out what has been done to date and any specific requests. Referral letters may request a second opinion, ask for help in patient management through a collaborative approach or transfer patient care (Table 6.5). Upon receiving a referral letter, professional courtesy and good patient care dictates that a practitioner sends a return correspondence, thanking the referring practitioner for the referral and stating the details of any procedures undertaken, new findings, clinical impressions or recommendations, as well as their rationale, and arrangements for follow-up. Such correspondence forms an essential part of professional collaboration and may also have legal status as part of the medical record and/or eligibility for funding or patient reimbursement. It also ensures that practitioners understand each other's expectations and goes far towards fostering goodwill and mutual respect.

TABLE 6.5 ELEMENTS OF A REFERRAL LETTER	
ELEMENT	**DETAILS**
Professional letterhead	Referring practitioner's name Qualifications Practice address Phone number/fax/email Provider number if appropriate Date of referral
Practitioner and patient identification	Details of practitioner to whom referral is being made Patient identifying details: full name, date of birth, address, hospital UR (patient) number etc
Patient's history	Brief patient history including background, any special considerations, past history and present complaints Investigations, treatment to date, including current and/or proposed treatments pharmaceutical or complementary, rationale and expected outcomes including involvement of other practitioners Any psychosocial concerns
Reasons for referral	Detailed reasons for referral, including expected actions of other practitioner (e.g. second opinion, further investigation, specific intervention, help in case management, transfer of care etc)
Conclusion	Arrangements for follow up Referring practitioner's signature

Although effective communication is vital, there are still many issues that need to be resolved before interdisciplinary collaboration between complementary and conventional practitioners becomes the norm. These include the credentialling and regulation of CAM practitioners, differences in nomenclature between disciplines, equity of access in different healthcare settings, the requirements for evidence-based practice, appropriate funding models and medico-legal issues, including referrals and vicarious liability (Cohen 2004). Despite these obstacles the fruits of interdisciplinary collaboration are becoming evident, with the emergence of clinics in which doctors and natural therapists share premises and work together for the benefit of their patients. Currently this collaboration and drive towards IM seems to be in response to patient demand rather than driven by professional associations, government policy or the accumulation of supportive scientific evidence.

PATIENTS' RESPONSIBILITY

Patients now have unprecedented access to healthcare information, as well as unprecedented power to choose the type of services they receive. This power is further supported by the ethical principle of informed consent and respect for patient autonomy. With power, however, comes responsibility. Patients must therefore begin to accept the responsibility to become more informed and to be active participants in the decision-making process and the implementation of their healthcare. This responsibility also extends to implementing lifestyle interventions, as summarised by the SENSE approach (see Chapter 1). Thus in every encounter, whether patients are currently well, at risk of disease or have an established disease, practitioners should take the opportunity to enlist the patient's cooperation in implementing their own healthcare and discussing interventions that can be used to enhance health, prevent disease and complement the use of any disease-specific interventions.

PERSONAL AND PROFESSIONAL SATISFACTION

The role of the IM practitioner is particularly challenging and rewarding. It compels practitioners to develop multiple skills, be informed about many therapies, navigate between different information sources and practitioners and keep an open mind. It also broadens the capacity of practitioners to deal with a great variety of patient issues from a number of perspectives, thus providing continuous intellectual stimulation and both professional and personal satisfaction. To have people's confidence as a practitioner and to participate in their most emotionally charged moments, which may include both the beginning and the end of their life, is a great privilege, and sharing the triumphs and tragedies of individuals from different walks of life provides rewards that enrich both the professional and the personal lives of practitioners.

Our knowledge of health and disease is far from complete, and healthcare practitioners regularly deal with uncertainty. The implementation of IM, however, recognises that compassion is always helpful and healing is always possible, even when curing is not (Rakel & Weil 2003). It also recognises that practitioners must endeavour always to do their best with what they have at any point in time and to be comfortable in the knowledge that their best will continually get better.

> *By fostering interaction, cross-disciplinary research, and collaborative care, redefined standards of care will emerge that are scientifically based and interdisciplinary in nature. The outgrowth of such a paradigm shift will change the legal and practice environment from one of fear to freedom.*
>
> **Engler et al 2009**

SUMMARY POINTS

- Taking time to develop a good therapeutic relationship may be therapeutic in itself and provides the best foundation for any other therapy.
- The integrative approach compels practitioners to develop an intimate understanding of their patients' lives, and to provide social support, understanding and compassion.
- The widespread use of complementary therapies compels doctors to discuss their use with patients and to do so on an informed basis and in a non-judgemntal manner.
- All healthcare practitioners should have access to appropriate and independent information, so that they can provide sound advice and detect predictable interactions and safety issues.

- Healthcare practitioners need to be aware of their particular biases, limitations and financial interests, and to clearly state these to patients when patient care may be affected.
- Healthcare practitioners should attempt to make patients active participants in the decision-making process and the implementation of their own healthcare.
- Healthcare practitioners need to liaise with different practitioners in order to advise on and implement the most appropriate interventions.
- Complementary therapies/medicines with rigorous evidence for efficacy and safety that do not require specialised skill or expertise to implement should be considered as part of mainstream practice.
- When efficacy of treatment is unknown and there are no apparent safety concerns, patients deciding to use these therapies should be supported and supervised.
- Therapies/medicines with less rigorous evidence or requiring specific expertise may be more appropriately used by healthcare practitioners with a special interest and/or appropriate training.
- When there are differences in the supporting evidence and quality of different herbal extracts and other CAM, the recommendation of specific brands of CAM products may be appropriate.
- Compassion is always helpful and healing is always possible, even when curing is not.

REFERENCES

Access Economics. Cost effectiveness of complementary medicines, National Institute of Integrative Medicine (NICM), 2010. Available at: http://www.nicm.edu.au/research/health-economics/cost-effectiveness-of-cm-report/cost-effective-applications-of-cam.

AMA (Australian Medical Association). AMA Code of Ethics, 2004. Available at: http://www.ama.com.au/web.nsf/tag/amacodeofethics 21/7/14.

Angell M. The truth about drug companies. New York: Random House, 2004.

Benson H, Friedman R. Harnessing the power of the placebo effect and renaming it 'Remembered wellness'. Annu Rev Med 47 (1996): 193–199.

Braun L et al. Use of complementary medicines by surgical patients: undetected and unsupervised. In: Proceedings of the 4th Australasian Conference on Safety and Quality in Health Care, Melbourne. Canberra: National Medicines Symposium, National Prescribing Service, 2006.

Brophy E. Does a doctor have a duty to provide information and advice about complementary and alternative medicine? J Law Med 10.3 (2003): 271–284.

Cohen M. Interdisciplinary collaboration: obstacles and opportunities. J Aust Integr Med Assoc 17 (2001): 24–25.

Cohen M. CAM practitioners and regular doctors: is integration possible? Med J Aust 180.12 (2004): 645–646.

Cohen M. The challenges and future direction for integrative medicine in clinical practice. Evidence Based Integr Med 2.3 (2005a): 117–122.

Cohen M. Exploring emotions. In: Spa Asia [conference handbook], March/April 2005. 2005b: 100–101.

Cohen MH, Eisenberg DM. Potential physician malpractice liability associated with complementary and integrative medical therapies. Ann Int Med 136.8 (2002): 596–603.

Cohen M et al. Long consultations and quality of care. J Aust Integr Med Assoc 19 (2002): 19–22.

Cohen M et al. The integration of complementary therapies in Australian general practice: results of a national survey. J Altern Complement Med 11.6 (2005): 995–1004.

Dunning T. Caring for the wounded healer: nurturing the self. J Bodywork Movement Ther 10.4 (2005): 251–260.

Engler RJM et al. Complementary and alternative medicine for the allergist-immunologist: Where do I start? J Allergy Clin Immunol 123.2 (2009): 309–316.

Jonas WB. Advising patients on the use of complementary and alternative medicine. Appl Psychophysiol Biofeedback 26.3 (2001): 205–214.

Jonas WB et al. How to practice evidence-based complementary and alternative medicine: essentials of complementary and alternative medicine. Philadelphia: Lippincott, Williams & Wilkins, 1999: pp 72–87.

MacLennan AH et al. The escalating cost and prevalence of alternative medicine. Prev Med 35.2 (2002): 166–173.

NICM, Cost Effectiveness of Complementary Medicine (Report). 2014. Available at: http://www.nicm.edu.au/health_information/health _economics/cost_effectiveness_of_complementary_medicines_report. 14 June 2014.

Plous S. The psychology of judgement and decision making. Sydney: McGraw-Hill, 1993.

RACGP/AIMA. Joint Position Statement of the RACGP and AIMA. Complementary Medicine (2004).

Rakel D, Weil A. Philosophy of integrative medicine. In: Integrative medicine. Philadelphia: Saunders, 2003.

Renella R, Fanconi S. Decision-making in pediatrics: a practical algorithm to evaluate complementary and alternative medicine for children. European Journal of Pediatrics 165.7 (2006): 437–441.

Robinson A, McGrail MR. Disclosure of CAM use to medical practitioners: a review of qualitative and quantitative studies. Complement Ther Med 12.2–3 (2004): 90–98.

Sackett DLR et al. Evidence based medicine: what it is and what it isn't. BMJ 312.7023 (1996): 71–72.

Smallwood C. The role of complementary and alternative medicine in the NHS. London: FreshMinds, 2005.

Studdert D et al. Financial conflicts of interest in physicians' relationships with the pharmaceutical industry: self-regulation in the shadow of Federal prosecution. N Engl J Med 351.18 (2004): 1891–1900.

CHAPTER 7

SAFETY OF COMPLEMENTARY MEDICINES

Complementary medicines (CMs) are widely used by the public as a non-pharmaceutical option that can be used to prevent, treat and manage disease (MacLennan et al 2002, Braun et al 2010b). They are used by people with a range of diseases and comorbidities such as low back pain, cancer, diabetes and cardiovascular disease (Broom et al 2012, Davis et al 2010, Grant et al 2012, Manya et al 2012). They are also used by people with no diagnosed disease but wanting to prevent disease, improve quality of life and general wellbeing, or for symptom relief. While MacLennan et al (2002) reported that people assumed if a medicine was 'natural' it must therefore be safe, times have changed and more people recognise that safety is relative and some CMs have the ability to cause drug interactions or even side effects (Braun 2007).

Finding information about CM safety is not straightforward for consumers as CM products are not accompanied by comprehensive consumer product information (CPI) in the same way that many pharmaceutical medicines are; many CMs are self-selected without professional advice, which means that much-needed information is not delivered with the product (Jamison 2003, MacLennan et al 2002).

Importantly, people who use CMs do not tend to use them as true alternatives to conventional treatment and it's not uncommon for care to be received from multiple healthcare providers over a similar time period. This situation is not necessarily dangerous and can produce significant benefits when well coordinated; however, if communication is poor, and complementary and conventional practitioners remain unaware of what the other has recommended, a potentially unsafe situation can arise. The prospect of interactions or adverse drug reactions leading to misdiagnosis, induction of withdrawal effects and misleading pathology test results are examples of unwanted outcomes when combined care is not coordinated.

In the real world, people are exposed to risk whenever they actively choose to undertake a treatment or choose to do without. Some risks are identifiable, while others are unknown. In practice, in order for patients to make an informed decision, these risks must be classified into those that are acceptable and those that are unacceptable, and then considered against the potential benefit, Over-the-counter (OTC) CMs that are produced under good manufacturing practice (GMP) conditions and meet government regulations offer a lower risk and potentially more cost-effective option than other treatments for some indications, and are generally considered safe when used appropriately under 'normal' circumstances; however, they are not entirely devoid of risk.

A BRIEF HISTORY OF MEDICATION SAFETY

The potential for medical care to cause harm has been appreciated throughout history. In ancient times, knowledge of medicine, pharmacology and the healing arts developed through trial and error, with many adverse outcomes and deaths along the way. Although both practitioners and patients were aware that health could be compromised by the 'cures' used to alleviate disease, it was in ancient Greece that patient safety was formally acknowledged as the highest priority. The maxim *primum non nocere* (First, do no harm) is attributed by some historians to Galen (AD 131–201) and is still a basic tenet of modern medical practice (Ilan & Fowler 2005).

As societies developed over the centuries, so too did their systems of medicine and healing — particularly the Vedic system of medicine, which originated more than 3000 years ago in India, and Chinese medicine, which has an appreciation of the importance of dosage. Persian medicine had a major influence on the development of medicine in the Middle East and Europe, most notably with *The canon of medicine*, written by the Persian scientist Avicenna (AD 980–1037) in the 11th century. This major work documented 760 medicines, made comments about their use and effectiveness, and remained a standard medical text in western Europe for seven centuries. Avicenna recommended the testing of new medicines on animals and humans before general use, no doubt in recognition of their potential to have both beneficial and harmful effects.

In medieval Europe, there was a mixture of scientific and spiritual influences on the practice of medicine, so factors such as destiny, sin and astrology played a role in perceptions of health and disease. Two major trends appeared during this period, as the practice of medicine developed among both physicians of the upper classes and folk healers who lived in the villages. From the 14th to 17th centuries monasteries played a major role in the provision of medicine and developed great expertise in pharmacognosy. At the same time, the Christian church was instrumental in eliminating much of the practice of folk medicine through its witch hunts, which many believe retarded the development of medicine.

In the 16th century, Paracelsus (1493–1541) was one of the first physicians to believe that chemicals could cure and cause certain illnesses. He determined that specific chemicals were responsible for the toxicity of a plant or animal poison, and documented the body's responses to those chemicals. Paracelsus then concluded that the body's response was influenced by the dose received. He further discovered that a small dose of a substance may be harmless, or even beneficial, whereas a larger dose can be toxic. In essence, he started expounding the concept of a dose–response relationship. Paracelsus made an enormous contribution to medicine when he stated plainly, 'What is there that is not poison? All things are poison and nothing (is) without poison. Solely the dose determines that a thing is not a poison' (Watson 2005). As a result, he is sometimes referred to as the 'Father of Toxicology'.

In practice, this refers to the biological effect of chemicals that can be either beneficial or deleterious. Which of these effects occurs depends on the amount of active material present at the site of action (internal dose), and the concentration of the amount present relates to the amount of substance administered (external dose).

During the 18th and 19th centuries deliberate clinical testing of medicines began, and the study of dose–response relationships led to the safer use of medicines. From the 19th century onwards, developments in pharmacology, physiology and chemistry meant that drugs could be artificially synthesised and produced by large-scale manufacturing. During this time, animal- and plant-based medicines began to be replaced in clinical use by mass-produced pharmaceutical medicines which were being newly created in laboratories or synthesised from traditional medicines (e.g. morphine from *Papaver somniferum*).

Up to this point, Western herbalism had been intrinsically linked to the practice of medicine, and herbal products were an important source of treatment. Empirical knowledge accumulated and formed a body of evidence, now referred to as 'traditional evidence', a knowledge base built on the basic tenets of good clinical practice (i.e. careful observation of the patient, the environment and the diseases). This huge and diverse store of learning includes not only prescriptions for health, but also safety information. The traditional evidence base is still expanding and becoming more accessible as researchers investigate and document various healing practices worldwide. Although traditional evidence provides a valuable starting point, it has many limitations, especially with regard to issues of safety. Careful patient observation is likely to detect immediate or serious adverse effects, but is less likely to identify slow-onset responses or mild-to-moderate side effects that could be considered symptoms of a new disease. Additionally, many medicinal preparations contained multiple ingredients, making it difficult to identify which one might be responsible for inducing an adverse reaction.

More recently, the traditional evidence base has been joined by a scientific evidence base, which provides additional information about pharmacological actions, clinical effects and safety; however, much still remains unknown.

This is particularly true regarding the safety of CMs in children and in women who are pregnant or lactating, and concerning drug interactions, which is a relatively new

phenomenon. Just as Galen pronounced hundreds of years ago, 'First, do no harm' should remain the practitioner's guide.

WHAT IS SAFETY?

Safety is a complex issue that is determined by considering the interaction between 'likelihood' and 'consequence'. These two variables will differ for each medicine and individual. The likelihood can be graded from 'near impossible' to 'certainly likely', and the severity of consequence can be graded from 'negligible' to 'serious and life-threatening', with many outcomes lying somewhere between these extremes (Fig 7.1).

With regard to medication safety, avoidance of an adverse drug reaction (ADR) is paramount. Several factors are associated with an

---

CLINICAL NOTE — HISTORY OF POISONS

The history of poisons dates back to the earliest times, when humans observed toxic effects in nature, most likely by chance. By 1500 BC, written records indicate that the poisons hemlock, opium and certain metals were used in warfare and in facilitating executions. Over time, poisons were used with greater sophistication; notable poisoning victims include Socrates, Cleopatra and Claudius. Today, the 'science of poisons' is known as toxicology. This field of learning investigates the chemical and physical properties of poisons and their physiological or behavioural effects on living organisms, and uses qualitative and quantitative methods for analysis and for the development of procedures to treat poisoning (Langman & Kapur 2006). The 20th century was marked by an advanced understanding of toxicology; DNA and various biochemicals that maintain cellular functions were discovered, so that today we are discovering the toxic effects on organs and cells at the molecular level.

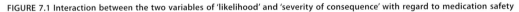

FIGURE 7.1 Interaction between the two variables of 'likelihood' and 'severity of consequence' with regard to medication safety

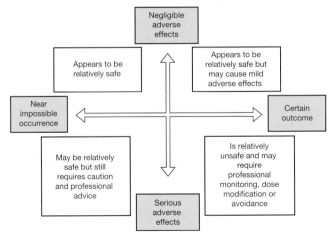

increased likelihood of developing an ADR, such as advanced age and polypharmacy, but most ADRs occur in people who are pre-scribed treatment within the limits of accepted clinical practice (Burgess et al 2005).

BENEFITS, RISK AND HARM

Many different sources of risk are associated with therapeutic products:

- **The product itself** — side effects and tox-icity of ingredients, administration form, potential harm through excessive dosage and length of time used.
- **Manufacturing factors** — poor manufac-turing process, which introduces contami-nants, uses unsafe excipients or incorrect ingredients, incorrect labelling etc.
- **Prescribing faults** — incorrect product prescribed, based on insufficient information about it, the patient or the disease, or simply negligence.
- **Patient factors** — incorrect use of a product when information for appropriate use is poorly understood, or insufficient or inappropriate self-diagnosis and treatment.

Whenever a treatment is chosen, it is done so in the belief that its potential benefit will out-weigh its potential to cause harm. Practice guidelines and traditions provide guidance when making risk–benefit evaluations and are based on common treatment decisions made many times before by many clinicians, together with the available evidence. Table 7.1 lists the potential risks associated with the use of com-plementary medicines. The safety information tends to come from a variety of sources, such as post-marketing surveillance and spontaneous reporting schemes, laboratory and animal studies, anecdotal reports, theoretical reasoning and, increasingly, formal studies.

The amount of safety literature published on pharmaceutical medicines is overwhelming. It has been estimated that 30% of the primary published literature about ADR appears in anecdotal reports and 35% as formal studies or randomised controlled trials (Aronson et al 2002). Regarding the safety of complementary medicines, traditional evidence and theoretical reasoning are heavily relied upon to provide guidance together with post-market surveil-lance studies and information from adverse event databases. Some clinical studies have looked at safety of the test intervention; however, this tends to be a secondary aim and often studies are not sufficiently powered to identify side effects. This poses a challenge for practitioners when making a rational decision about the relative risks of treatment and is one of the great difficulties of CM practice. For the public who are interested in using OTC

TABLE 7.1 POTENTIAL RISKS ASSOCIATED WITH THE USE OF COMPLEMENTARY MEDICINES	
TYPE OF HARM	**CIRCUMSTANCES**
Delay in diagnosis	When a patient has avoided or delayed seeking medical advice because they are self-treating with CMs. When a complementary medicine practitioner has not referred a patient to a medical practitioner for early diagnosis.
Adverse effects	Increased risk of adverse reactions with inappropriate use of CM products or when patients self-select CM products without professional advice. Increased risk if products used are not manufactured to pharmaceutical grade quality.
Drug interactions	Increased risk of drug interactions when patients: (a) self-select CM products without professional advice; (b) do not disclose use of CM products to their pharmacist or medical doctor; (c) do not disclose use of pharmaceutical drugs to their CM practitioner.
Financial cost	If an expensive medicine or therapy is not providing benefits and a patient continues to use it, this presents an unnecessary financial burden.
Lost opportunity to treat	Failure to undertake a different treatment with proven benefits, when the current treatment is ineffective but is being used to the exclusion of others.
False hope of a cure	When cure is unlikely, the use of any medicine or therapy that is associated with false hope may delay important considerations, such as attending to 'unfinished business'.

products, it is just as difficult to find reliable and understandable information about their safety and efficacy.

ADVERSE DRUG REACTIONS (ADRs)

The World Health Organization (WHO) defines an ADR as a 'response to a medicine which is noxious and unintended that occurs at doses normally used in humans'. When two medicines interact in a way that produces an unwanted effect, this is also referred to as an ADR. Adverse reactions have been classified into different types depending on severity and likelihood or onset of reaction, and do not always result in serious outcomes; however, an ADR is considered serious when it is suspected of causing death, danger to life, admission to hospital, prolongation of hospital stay, absence from productive activity, increased investigational or treatment costs, or birth defects.

Adverse reactions can arise from either an intrinsic or an extrinsic effect. An intrinsic effect refers to the active ingredient itself, such as the herbal medicine present within a product, whereas an extrinsic effect relates to product characteristics resulting from poor manufacturing processes or quality control, such as contamination and adulteration. Intrinsic adverse effects can be categorised in a similar way to pharmaceutical medicines and are mainly type A or type B reactions.

Type A reactions

Type A reactions are the most common form and are typically dose-related, predictable from the known pharmacology of the medicine, associated with high morbidity but low mortality, and potentially avoidable (Routledge et al 2004). People most at risk of a type A reaction are frail, older patients who are also likely to be receiving a combination of medicines and those with altered hepatic or renal function. There is now mounting evidence to indicate that some type A adverse reactions are due to genetic polymorphisms, which affect an individual's drug clearance rate and therefore toxicological response. This may explain why certain individuals taking medicines in the recommended doses experience adverse reactions, whereas the majority of the population do not. Examples related to pharmaceutical medicine are bleeding with anticoagulants and hypoglycaemia with the use of insulin. An example for

herbal medicine is licorice-associated hypertension, which is thought to be caused by increased renal sodium retention. The glycyrrhetinic acid in licorice inhibits renal 11-beta-hydroxysteroid dehydrogenase type 2 and, by that mechanism, increases the access of cortisol to the mineralocorticoid receptor that causes renal sodium retention and potassium loss. If continued for sufficient time, clinically significant changes in blood pressure and potassium status develop. This can be avoided by recommending that high-dose licorice herbal products not be used for longer than 2 weeks (Heilmann et al 1999). In recognition of this adverse effect, some manufacturers produce licorice products that do not contain glycyrrhetinic acid, so that they can be used more safely in the long term.

Table 7.2 gives some examples of known or suspected type A adverse reactions to herbs and natural supplements. For many herbal and natural medicines, there is insufficient reliable information about possible adverse reactions; where available, evidence from clinical trials, case reports and post-marketing surveillance

TABLE 7.2 EXAMPLES OF KNOWN OR SUSPECTED TYPE A ADVERSE REACTIONS TO HERBS AND NATURAL SUPPLEMENTS	
HERB OR NATURAL SUPPLEMENT	**ADVERSE EFFECT/S**
Andrographis paniculata	Vomiting, anorexia and gastrointestinal discomfort
Creatine	Nausea, vomiting, cramping, dehydration, fluid retention
Trigonella foenum (fenugreek)	Diarrhoea, flatulence
Fish oils	Gastrointestinal discomfort, diarrhoea
Allium sativum (garlic)	Breath and body odour, nausea, dyspepsia, flatulence, diarrhoea, increased bleeding
Zingiber officinale (ginger)	Gastric irritation, dyspepsia
Camellia sinensis (green or black tea)	CNS stimulation
Gymnema sylvestre	Hypoglycaemia
Paullinia cupana (guarana)	CNS stimulation
Selenium	Nausea, vomiting, irritability, fatigue, nail changes

systems are the main sources of information used in this book.

Type B reactions

Type B reactions are idiosyncratic and uncommon, difficult to predict and not dose related. They tend to have higher morbidity and mortality than type A reactions and are often immunologically mediated (Myers & Cheras 2004). Other factors contributing to type B reactions are receptor or drug metabolism abnormalities and the unmasking of a biological deficiency (e.g. glucose-6-phosphate dehydrogenase deficiency) (Bryant et al 2003). They do not appear to relate to genetic polymorphisms.

An example of a type B reaction to a pharmaceutical drug is interstitial nephritis with the use of NSAIDs. With regard to CMs, *Asteraceae* dermatitis provides a good example of a type B hypersensitivity reaction — specifically, an allergic contact dermatitis caused by exposure to allergens from the *Asteraceae* family or the daisy group of plants and plant extracts. Some examples of common plants that belong to this family are arnica (*Arnica montana*), chamomile (*Chamomilla recuita*), marigold (*Calendula officinalis*), echinacea (*Echinacea* spp), tansy (*Tanacetum vulgare*), feverfew (*Tanacetum parthenium*) and yarrow (*Achillea millefolium*). The most important allergens in the *Asteraceae* family are the sesquiterpene lactones, which are present in the oleoresin fraction of the leaves, stems, flowers and possibly pollen (Gordon 1999). The condition is most frequently seen in middle-aged and elderly people; it typically starts in summer and disappears in the autumn or winter. The dermatitis manifests as eczema and can develop from exposure to airborne particles, direct topical application (such as cosmetics, perfumes, essential oils) or oral ingestion of allergenic components. The diagnosis of allergy can be difficult to establish, because there are few completely reliable laboratory tests and sometimes symptoms can mimic infectious disease symptoms. Table 7.3 gives examples of known or suspected type B adverse reactions.

Extrinsic factors

Extrinsic factors are also a consideration and of particular relevance when medicinal products are not manufactured according to the standards of good manufacturing practice, such as

TABLE 7.3 EXAMPLES OF KNOWN OR SUSPECTED TYPE B ADVERSE REACTIONS TO HERBS AND NATURAL SUPPLEMENTS	
HERB OR NATURAL SUPPLEMENT	**ADVERSE EFFECT/S**
Andrographis paniculata	Urticaria
Aloe vera	Hypersensitivity and contact dermatitis
Chamomilla recutita	Asteraceae dermatitis
Echinacea spp	Asteraceae dermatitis and anaphylaxis
Tanacetum parthenium (feverfew)	Asteraceae dermatitis — lip swelling, mouth ulceration and soreness when the leaves are chewed
Zingiber officinale (ginger)	Contact dermatitis with topical use
Thymus vulgaris (thyme)	Contact dermatitis with topical use of the oil

some produced in the USA and various Asian countries. Problems can result from a lack of standardisation, contamination, substitution of raw materials, adulteration or incorrect extraction, preparation or dosage information.

REGULATION AND PRODUCT INFORMATION

Numerous regulations are in place in Australia and New Zealand to protect people from potentially unsafe and dubious therapeutic products. Both countries have an international best-practice, risk-based regulatory system that encompasses both complementary and pharmaceutical medicines. Currently the Therapeutic Goods Administration (TGA) regulates the system in Australia, and aims to ensure the safety and quality of products and the truthful labelling of therapeutic goods. All products are entered onto the Australian Register of Therapeutic Goods (ARTG) and allocated an AUST L number if considered low risk (most CM products) or AUST R number if considered high risk, or low risk with a high-level claim (prescription drugs and many OTC pharmaceutical medicines). Products with either an Aust L or an Aust R number have been evaluated for safety and quality, whereas those with an AUST R number have also been evaluated

THE 'BOTANICAL ADULTERANTS PROGRAM'

Three leading nonprofit organisations — the American Botanical Council (ABC), the American Herbal Pharmacopoeia (AHP), and the University of Mississippi's National Center for Natural Products Research (NCNPR) initiated a large-scale program to educate members of the herbal and dietary supplement industry about ingredient and product adulteration. This arose because of concerns within the herbal and dietary supplement community about the suspected and confirmed practice of adulteration of numerous ingredients. This raises questions about the identity and quality of some popular herbal ingredients sold in dietary supplements in the United States and in other botanical products (e.g. medicines, cosmetics, etc.) in global markets.

It is understood that adulteration of herbal ingredients can be accidental or deliberate. The ABC-AHP-NCNPR Botanical Adulterants Program will focus on both accidental adulteration that occurs as a result of poor quality-control procedures, as well as the intentional adulteration of plant-based products for financial gain. This industry-funded program aspires to serve as a self-regulatory mechanism for industry to address adulteration problems through education rather than federal regulation.

For more information go to: http://abc.herbalgram.org/site/PageNavigator/About_Adulterants_Program.html

It appears that many people are unclear about the TGA's role in this regard and think it has a greater capacity to monitor product quality than actually occurs. According to a survey of more than 3000 people living in South Australia, approximately half assumed that CMs were independently tested by a government agency (MacLennan et al 2006).

It is important to note that the regulation of therapeutic goods varies greatly between countries and is influenced by ethnological, medical and historical factors. For instance, CM products are treated as foods by the Food and Drug Administration in the USA and not required to be manufactured to the same quality-control standards as pharmaceutical medicines (Brownie 2005).

While the regulation of CM products in Australia can always be improved, the current system employed by the TGA is providing an important safeguard for the public. This was clearly demonstrated in a national survey of over 1100 pharmacy customers attending 60 community pharmacies across Australia (Braun et al 2010a). Of the entire sample, 72% had taken a complementary medicine in the previous 12 months. Of these 7% (n = 55) thought they had experienced a side effect to a CM product at some time. Most (71%) described their reaction as mild, 22% as moderate and four people as severe. That works out at less than 0.5% of CM product users suspecting they had a serious reaction. As further details were not provided about the suspected reaction, causality could not be determined and the figures serve as a guide only.

RELIABLE INFORMATION SOURCES

When it comes to sources of information about herbal and natural medicines, Australian consumer reports consistently put family and friends as people's main sources of information about CM. This was first seen back in a 1999 Australian consumer report which found that 51% of people surveyed ask their friends or relatives for advice, with their mothers ranked as number one for healthcare advice (and it is open to debate as to where the mothers get their information from). In 2001, an Australian rural survey produced similar results, finding that 64.5% of people first ask family and friends for advice (Wilkinson & Simpson 2001). Interestingly, 78% of nursing, pharmacy

for efficacy. Importantly, the TGA does not undertake the evaluation itself but relies on sponsors to provide the evidence.

The TGA also acts to ensure that all therapeutic products (complementary and pharmaceutical) are produced according to the code of Good Manufacturing Practice (GMP), and both licenses and audits manufacturers. Since the Pan Pharmaceuticals debacle in 2003, when more than 1000 CM products were recalled owing to quality control concerns, there have been calls for more frequent auditing of manufacturers in order to maintain closer control over product quality.

or biomedical science students had used CAM in the previous 12 months, and 56% had visited a CAM practitioner. They, too, cited friends and family as their main sources of information (Wilkinson & Simpson 2001). More recent studies keep confirming that people seek advice from their family and friends and medical doctors and pharmacists are never ranked higher.

In recent years information technology has revolutionised the availability of health information for both practitioners and their patients. Besides relying on traditional sources of health information, such as healthcare providers, family and friends, people now have easy access to a variety of sources, particularly since the advent of the internet, email and text messaging.

Advertising plays a role in informing consumers about therapeutic products and is regulated by the government. Advertisements must comply with the Therapeutic Products Advertising Code and Therapeutic Product Act(s) and Rules, which state that advertising must be truthful, balanced and not misleading, and promote responsible use, and that the claims must be substantiated. The regulations relate to advertisements disseminated in all forms of media, including emails, websites and SMS messages. However, some information routes are exempt: bona fide news, editorial, public interest or entertainment programs are not restricted by the code, allowing for freedom of speech, but also allowing for sensationalism and inaccuracies.

In 2000, a study published in the *New England Journal of Medicine* found that media coverage of new drugs often exaggerates their benefits and downplays the associated risks (Moynihan et al 2000). The study analysed a sample of 207 stories released by 40 media outlets (36 newspapers, 4 television networks), which appeared between 1994 and 1998. Of the stories reviewed, 40% did not report benefits quantitatively and, of those that did, 83% used statistics to exaggerate the beneficial effect of the drug. Potential harm associated with use of the drug was not mentioned in 53% of stories, and 70% failed to mention costs. Based on the results of this study, it was concluded that news media stories about medicines may be inadequate or incomplete regarding benefits, risks and costs, and may fail to disclose financial ties between researchers and pharmaceutical companies.

It is clear that a number of factors influence the way journalists report health issues in the news media. One important factor relates to the information provided (or not provided) to the journalist by a medical journal, researcher or company in a press release. The following case about the safety of echinacea provides a local example. In 2002, an article entitled 'Adverse reactions associated with echinacea — the Australian experience' was published in a scientific journal. It described in detail five allergic reactions to different echinacea preparations, further stating that 51 adverse reaction reports involving echinacea had been reported to the Adverse Drug Reactions Advisory Committee (ADRAC) (Mullins & Heddle 2002). This was then reported in the news media as alarming and drew much debate about the safety of herbal medicines in general. Inspection of the original article reveals that the reports were collected over a 21-year period, an important fact that failed to be included in the original press release (Flinders Medical Centre 2006).

A study published in the *Journal of the American Medical Association* suggests that incomplete or inaccurate press releases may be more common than once thought (Woloshin & Schwartz 2002). The study assessed the quality of press releases from seven high-profile journals, which were selected for their professional influence and because they are frequently cited by the news media. It was identified that for 544 articles published in the journals over the study period, 127 press releases were issued. Of these press releases, only 23% reported study limitations, 65% quantified study results and only 22% reported the source of funding.

Ideally, journalists, program researchers and writers involved in the media need to be able to assess the scientific information provided to them, and then present it accurately to consumers in a way that is easy to understand, unambiguous and not misleading, so that they can make better personal health decisions. Inaccurate, incomplete and inconsistent information not only confuses consumers, it also confuses healthcare providers and makes it difficult for them to determine which resource is useful and reliable.

A 2008 study by the National Prescribing Service in Australia found that both general practitioners (GPs) and pharmacists seek or need information regarding complementary medicines, and are particularly interested in information about drug interactions, adverse effects, contraindications and evidence of effectiveness. GPs tend to refer to trade journals, MIMS, the internet in general, and peer-reviewed medical journals for information about CMs. Pharmacists' most common sources were the internet, MIMS and the Australian Pharmaceutical Products (APP) guide, colleagues and complementary medicine textbooks (Brown et al 2008). Interestingly, when asked which information sources were considered moderately or highly useful, CM textbooks came out on top for both groups of healthcare professionals. This implies that practitioners who only used standard drug information sources were not accessing the most useful resources available. Another consequence is the assumption by these practitioners that either little evidence exists (because little is available in standard pharmaceutical or medical texts or journals), or that there are no good resources.

Similarly, a study funded by the Department of Health and Ageing and the Pharmacy Guild that investigated the quality use of medicines in relation to complementary medicines found that pharmacists have trouble locating information they consider credible, and are keen for standardised information to be endorsed by a reputable organisation and made widely available.

MEDICAL DATABASES AND TEXTS: INCONSISTENCY

Unfortunately, some medical databases and textbooks that are widely used in the hospital system and universities are not always up to date; authors don't critically examine the evidence from primary sources and sometimes overstate the safety issues without considering the wider perspective. This makes it extremely difficult for a busy clinician to find accurate information in a timely manner.

An example presented here is the purported interaction between *Ginkgo biloba* and warfarin. Ginkgolides found in ginkgo leaf inhibit platelet aggregation according to in vitro and ex vivo studies. As a result, it has been assumed that the effect is clinically relevant, and ginkgo has been implicated as the causative factor in case reports where haemorrhage has been described in association with ginkgo use (Koch

2005). It has also led many writers and clinicians to assume that a pharmacodynamic interaction exists between ginkgo and drugs affecting haemostasis at the platelet level (Bone 2008). Evidence from multiple controlled studies published over the last 5 years casts doubt on the clinical significance of this theoretical interaction, indicating it is unsubstantiated (see monograph on *Ginkgo biloba* for further details). Major databases and textbooks on complementary medicines provide quite different information to readers about this issue, adding to the confusion (Table 7.4).

ADR INCIDENCE

Alarmingly, the rates of ADR-related hospital admissions are rising and account for considerable morbidity, mortality and costs. One Australian study found that one in ten patients who visited a GP had experienced a significant ADR within the previous 6 months, and almost 50% of these were assessed as moderate to severe by the GP (Miller et al 2006). An ADR is more likely to be experienced with increasing age, peaking at 65 years and older, and by females rather than males. Children aged between 1 and 4 years are three times more likely to have an ADR than children in other age groups. At this rate, ADRs rank as one of the most important causes of morbidity. Anticoagulants, NSAIDs and cardiovascular medicines feature prominently as preventable, high-impact problems in Australia and other countries (Pirmohamed et al 2004, Runciman et al 2003).

Although ADRs also occur with CMs, relatively few reports have been collected through spontaneous post-marketing surveillance systems. The most extensive database of ADRs to herbal medicines is held by the Uppsala Monitoring Centre, the coordinating centre for the WHO Programme for International Drug Monitoring (see www.who-umc.org). It receives data from national centres in 72 countries and, over the past 20 years, 11,716 case reports of suspected herbal ADR have been collected. The most commonly reported non-critical effects were (from higher to lower incidence): pruritus, urticaria, rash, erythematous rash, nausea, vomiting, diarrhoea, fever, abdominal pain and dyspnoea. The most common critical effects were: facial oedema,

TABLE 7.4 EXAMPLES OF CURRENT DATABASES AND TEXTBOOKS REPORTING ON THE PURPORTED GINKGO–WARFARIN INTERACTION

RESOURCE	INTERACTION INFORMATION	COMMENTS
MIMS on CD	'Warfarin interacts with a wide range of complementary medicines, including vitamin and herbal preparations, e.g. Gingko biloba … have confirmed or potential interactions with warfarin.'	Accessed 10 July 2008 Ginkgo spelt incorrectly Insufficient information provided
eAMH (Australian Medicines Handbook)	No interaction information	Accessed 10 July 2008 Last updated Jan 2008
AltMedDex (Thomson Reuters 2008)	'Concomitant use of ginkgo and anticoagulants may increase the risk of bleeding complications. *Adverse effect:* increased risk of bleeding *Clinical management:* Avoid concomitant use of ginkgo and anticoagulants. *Severity:* major *Onset:* delayed *Documentation:* fair *Probable mechanism:* Ginkgolide B may inhibit platelet activating factor (PAF)-induced platelet aggregation'	Accessed 10 July 2008 Information does not reflect current evidence base.
The desktop guide to complementary and alternative medicine (Ernst et al 2006)	'Potentiation of anticoagulants is often mentioned, but a systematic review of the evidence refuted the notion.'	Published 2006 Succinct and evidence based
Herbs and natural supplements — an evidence based guide (Braun & Cohen 2007)	'Theoretically, ginkgo may increase bleeding risk when used together with warfarin; however, two randomised double-blind studies have found that *Ginkgo biloba* does not affect the pharmacokinetics or pharmacodynamics, INR or clinical effects of warfarin … and two clinical trials have not found evidence of significant effects on bleeding … Due to the potential seriousness of such an interaction, caution is still advised.'	Last updated 2006 Evidence based
The ABC clinical guide to herbs (Blumenthal 2003)	'Interaction with drugs inhibiting blood coagulation cannot be excluded.' Several case reports of bleeding reported, followed by RCTs showing no evidence of interaction with warfarin or aspirin.	Published 2003 Evidence based

hepatitis, angio-oedema, thrombocytopenia, hypertension, chest pain, convulsions, purpurea, dermatitis and death.

In Australia, the ADRAC database holds reports of suspected ADRs. From 1 November 1972 to 19 April 2005, it has only 1112 reports related solely to CMs. This is reassuring, when one considers that in 2004 approximately 52% of the population were identified as users of at least one non-medically prescribed CM product in the previous 12 months (MacLennan et al 2006). The relatively small number of case reports can be interpreted as indicative of the comparative safety of CMs and the effectiveness of pre-market checks; however, the impact of under-reporting should not be dismissed.

Research on under-reporting of serious ADRs in the USA and Canada suggests that formal reporting rates may be as low as 1.5% of total ADRs (Miller et al 2006). In the specific case of CMs, CAM practitioners and retail staff may not report such events because:
• they are unaware of ADR schemes
• they are not qualified or trained to consider the possibility of ADRs
• they are not motivated to report any ADR that comes to their notice.

In addition, herbal medicine consumers may not be motivated to report ADRs to their doctor, as one British study suggests (Barnes et al 1998), or they may not consider the possibility that their symptoms may be related to the CM products they use.

CASE REPORTS AND POST-MARKETING SURVEILLANCE SYSTEMS

Given that current knowledge about CMs is incomplete and that controlled studies are often lacking for CAM, well-documented case reports can serve as a critical early warning system until further research is undertaken, whereas poorly documented case reports can be misleading. Unfortunately, reports of ADRs with herbal medicines often cause some controversy and contain incomplete data; for example, one systematic review, which assessed information from four electronic databases, located 108 cases of suspected medicine–herb interactions. Of these, 68.5% were classified as 'unable to be evaluated' and only 13% were described as 'well-documented' (Fugh–Berman & Ernst 2001). Table 7.5 lists the elements that should be included in a report of an adverse reaction.

Besides improving the quality of reporting, the ideal would be to chemically analyse the product to authenticate the ingredients and make sure that quality control issues are not involved. This is particularly important when the implicated product has not been manufactured under a strict GMP code.

Much of the information obtained from the current spontaneous post-marketing surveillance systems about CM safety is of limited value, as it does not provide an estimate of the incidence of adverse reactions. Without understanding the level of incidence, case reports can easily be interpreted as cause for alarm or alternatively dismissed as irrelevant. Additionally, authorities discourage reporting of less severe ADRs, so many mild-to-moderate side effects remain undetected and are a hidden source of patient morbidity.

Post-marketing surveillance systems aim to detect trends in ADR and become useful when a large number of reports relating to a specific medicine are received. When evidence gathers to suggest a significant problem, the TGA may issue an alert on its website, impose new conditions on the product's listing or registration, suspend or cancel listing or registration, impose new manufacturing conditions and, if considered sufficiently serious, issue a mandatory product recall. Alerts in recent years have included warnings about drug interactions with St John's wort (*Hypericum perforatum*), suspected hepatotoxicity with products containing kava kava and renal toxicity with Chinese herbal medicines containing the herb *Aristolochia*. The Advisory Committee on Complementary Medicines (ACCM) advises the TGA on matters regarding CMs and is made up of people considered expert in this area.

The two cases involving black cohosh and kava kava provide examples of how post-marketing surveillance systems can alert government agencies of a potential safety issue and the ensuing steps taken and research conducted to identify what the issue is and its prevalence.

Black cohosh

Rare, spontaneous hepatotoxicity has been reported in at least 42 case reports world-wide with treatment by *Cimicifuga racemosa rhizoma* (Levitsky et al 2005, Lynch et al 2006, Nisbet & O'Connor 2007, Teschke & Schwarzenboeck 2009, Whiting et al 2002). As a result, several safety reviews have been conducted to evaluate the available data and determine what risk exists with the use of this herb.

A 2008 safety review of black cohosh products was conducted by the Dietary Supplement Information Expert Committee of the US Pharmacopeia's Council of Experts. All the reports of liver damage were assigned possible causality, and none were probable or certain causality. The clinical pharmacokinetic and animal toxicological information did not reveal

---

TABLE 7.5 IMPORTANT COMPONENTS OF AN ADVERSE REACTION REPORT

Patient demographics: male/female, age, social history if relevant

Suspected product details: formula as stated on label, batch number, expiry date and Aust L or Aust R number

Details of the person making the report

Manufacturer's details

Relevant medical history

Other medicines and treatments being used (including other complementary medicines)

Dose used, duration of use and administration form

Date and time of onset

Adverse effects: description of signs and symptoms

Outcome of event

Information regarding re-challenge, if applicable

Presence of confounding variables: e.g. additives

unfavourable information about black cohosh. The Expert Committee determined that in the United States black cohosh products should be labelled to include a cautionary statement, a change from their decision of 2002, which required no such statement (Mahady et al 2008).

Assessment of the 42 cases by European Medicines Agency (EMEA) has shown a possible or probable causality in only four out of 42 patients. A diagnostic algorithm has been applied in the four patients with suspected BC (Black cohosh) hepatotoxicity using several methods to allow objective assessment, scoring and scaling of the probability in each case. Due to incomplete data, the case of one patient was not assessable. For the remaining three patients, quantitative evaluation showed no causality for BC in any patient regarding the observed severe liver disease (Teschke & Schwarzenboeck 2009).

In Australia in February 2006, the TGA announced that based on the appraisal of case reports, a causal association between black cohosh and serious hepatitis exists; however, the incidence is very low considering its widespread use. As a result, products available in Australia containing black cohosh have to carry label warnings informing consumers of the risk. The conclusion made by the TGA is considered controversial by some experts because numerous confounding factors were present in many of the case reports, such as the use of multiple ingredient preparations, concurrent use of at least one pharmaceutical medicine and the presence of other medical conditions.

A 2008 study evaluated the effects of black cohosh extract on liver morphology and on levels of various hepatic function indices in an experimental model finding that at high doses, well above the recommended dosage, black cohosh appears quite safe (Mazzanti et al 2008).

More recently, Teschke (2010b) investigated data from 69 spontaneous or published case reports of suspected black cohosh-induced hepatotoxicity and found confounding variables such as uncertainty about the quality and authenticity of the black cohosh product, dose or insufficient adverse event description, missing or inadequate evaluation of a clear temporal association, the possible presence of other medications or comorbidities and lack of de-challenge or re-exposure. A clear causal relationship between black cohosh and hepatotoxicity was not found.

Even more recently, a 2011 meta-analysis investigated the potential hepatotoxicity of black cohosh (Remifemin) from published RCTs in perimenopausal and postmenopausal women. Liver function data (AST, ALT and γ-GT) from 1020 women was compared at baseline and after taking black cohosh (40–128 mg/day) for 3 to 6 months. No significant difference between the treatment and reference groups were found (Naser et al 2011).

Kava kava

Kava was well tolerated and considered as devoid of major side effects until 1998 when the first reports of kava hepatotoxicity appeared. Causality of hepatotoxicity for kava ± co-medicated drugs was evident after the use of predominantly ethanolic and acetonic kava extracts in Germany ($n = 7$), Switzerland ($n = 2$), United States ($n = 1$) and Australia ($n = 1$) as well as after aqueous extracts in New Caledonia ($n = 2$) (Teschke et al 2008a). Moreover, cases of tourists developing serious toxic liver disease after consumption of kava beverages in traditional Samoan kava ceremonies were reported (Christl et al 2009). For this reason, in 2002 the herb was withdrawn from various European countries (Sarris et al 2013), and the FDA issued a safety alert about kava and its liver problems (Teschke et al 2010a). In 2002 in Australia, the TGA posed a maximum limit of 125 mg kava lactones on kava tablets or capsules and a maximum of 3 g of dried rhizome per teabag with a maximum daily dose of 250 mg kava lactones allowed.

Various authors evaluated the reported cases. In an analysis of 36 cases of hepatotoxicity, the pattern of injury was both hepatocellular and cholestasis, the majority of patients were women, the culmative dose and latency were highly variable and liver transplant was necessary in eight of the cases (Stickel et al 2003). The WHO published a report in May 2007 entitled *Assessment of the risk of hepatotoxicity with kava products* (WHO 2007). It evaluated data from 93 case reports of which 8 were determined to have a close association between the use of kava kava and liver dysfunction; 53 cases were classified as having a possible relationship, but they could not be fully assessed due to insufficient data or other potential causes of liver damage; five cases had a positive rechallenge. Most of the other case reports could not be evaluated due to lack of information. It concluded that there is 'significant concern' for a cause and effect relationship between kava products and hepatotoxicity, especially for organic extracts. The report noted other risk factors such as heavy alcohol intake, preexisting liver disease, genetic polymorphisms of cytochrome P450 enzymes, excessive dosage and co-medication with other potentially hepatotoxic drugs and potentially interacting drugs.

Similarly, Teschke et al analysed 26 suspected cases of which causality was unassessable, unrelated or excluded for 16 cases owing to lack of temporal association and causes independent of kava or co-medicated drugs. Overall, the survey concluded that kava taken as recommended is associated with rare hepatotoxicity, whereas overdose, prolonged treatment and co-medication may carry an increased risk (Teschke et al 2008b, Teschke et al 2010a). However, several papers outlined pros and cons of the current methods of causality evaluation (Teschke et al 2011, Teschke & Wolff 2011).

The latest publications have accepted a causal relationship between the use of various kava extracts, including aqueous extracts, and liver injury, and have focused on an assessment of possible causes (Teschke et al 2009). Despite this, evidence is still lacking of in vivo hepatotoxicity in experimental animals under conditions similar to human kava use. Furthermore, in commercial Western kava extracts, pipermethystine was not detectable and flavokavain B was present as a natural compound in amounts much too low to cause experimental liver injury (Lechtenberg et al 2008).

More recent reports have postulated that mould hepatotoxins present in kava raw material may be the cause of hepatotoxicity (Teschke et al 2012, Teschke et al 2013). This could be the case given that aflatoxins have been detected in kava samples (Rowe & Ramzan 2012).

Strict guidelines for kava standardisation have now been suggested by several researchers. They include: (1) use of a noble kava cultivar such as Borogu, at least 5 years old at time of harvest, (2) use of peeled and dried rhizomes and roots, (3) aqueous extraction, (4) dosage recommendation of ≤ 250 mg kavalactones per day (for medicinal use), (5) systematic rigorous future research and (6) a Pan Pacific quality control system enforced by strict policing (Teschke et al 2011).

FACTORS THAT MAKE AN ADR MORE LIKELY

Although little investigation has been conducted into what factors influence the likelihood of ADRs with CMs, it can be assumed most factors that increase the risk of ADRs with pharmaceutical medicine will also apply to CMs. These factors can be grouped as patient-related or therapeutic.

Patient-related factors
- Older age. Declining liver and kidney function as a result of ageing can increase sensitivity to both therapeutic and adverse effects. During times of ill health, the elderly can experience a further loss of homeostatic reserve, once again increasing sensitivity to the effects of medicines and interactions (Atkinson et al 2001).
- Females appear to be more susceptible to ADRs.
- Concurrent disease, acute and/or severe.
- History of atopic disease.
- Confusion.
- Genetic factors: for example, variations in liver enzymes.
- Reduced renal or hepatic function. Altered metabolism or excretion of a medicine can increase the risk of toxicity.
- Self-medication. Prudent self-care can offer numerous benefits to the individual, society and the healthcare system if there is access to quality services, products and information. However, when people at higher risk of adverse effects self-medicate with OTC medicines, it can be potentially harmful. Additionally, interactions that do not produce a clinically obvious change, such as elevation in blood pressure, serum cholesterol or warfarin INR, can remain undetected and uncorrected unless professional advice is sought.
- Use of multiple healthcare practitioners. This is of concern when practitioners fail to communicate effectively with one another to ensure that interactions are avoided and identified.

Therapeutic factors

- Dose. Most ADRs are dose-related, with higher doses increasing risk.
- Route of administration (e.g. topical application) can cause delayed hypersensitivity.
- Prolonged and/or frequent therapy.
- Medicines not manufactured under a code of good manufacturing practice (GMP) have an increased risk of extrinsic effects.
- Use of concurrent high-risk medicines; for example, those with a narrow therapeutic index (NTI) such as warfarin, digoxin, lithium, cyclosporin, phenytoin, barbiturates, theophylline, many HIV medicines (e.g. saquinavir), antineoplastic agents (e.g. methotrexate) and anti-arrhythmic agents (e.g. quinidine). These medicines are particularly sensitive to pharmacokinetic alterations in which small changes to blood concentrations can cause a clinically significant change to drug activity. Depending on whether drug concentrations are reduced or increased, there is the potential to cause a loss of efficacy or induce toxic effects, respectively.
- Polypharmacy. This is of particular concern in the elderly, who may have chronic diseases and are known to use more medicines than any other age group, increasing the risk of interactions. Additionally, in many serious diseases such as cancer and HIV, multi-drug treatment is the standard of care.
- Use of medicines known to induce or inhibit cytochrome (CYP) enzymes, particularly CYP 3A4, which is responsible for the metabolism of many common pharmaceutical medicines.

STRATEGIES FOR PREVENTING AND LIMITING ADRs

Many countries are trying to cope with the growing problem of ADRs and their associated morbidity and mortality. Currently in Australia and New Zealand there are many structures and initiatives in place, such as regulatory agencies, the CMEC, 'quality use of medicines' organisations and information providers, safety and quality organisations and professional bodies; however, it is ultimately the practitioner and the patient who play the definitive roles.

Strategies for clinicians

- Encourage open and honest communication — between patient, carer and practitioner, and between fellow practitioners about treatments prescribed. One way of achieving this is for CM practitioners to label all dispensed herbal medicines with the botanical names of the herbs included in the product, together with suggested dosage, date of manufacture and practitioner's contact details.
- Take a careful medical and medicines history, including previous allergies and adverse effects.
- Consider non-medicinal treatments.
- Avoid polypharmacy and complicated treatment regimens.
- Become familiar with the potential safety issues associated with a medicine to avoid unnecessarily inducing an ADR or misdiagnosing one as a symptom of a new disease. An important adjunct to this is having access to reliable medical and CM information, and having a network of experts or informed colleagues to consult. Computer-generated prescriptions and decision-support systems are frequently advocated as possible solutions and can be useful if their information is accurate and updated frequently.
- Regularly review therapeutic goals and medicines being used. This provides an opportunity to promote patient compliance and ensure that the appropriate medicines are being taken safely.
- When problems do arise, practitioners need to be aware of their professional responsibility to report a suspected ADR to one of the following:
  - Adverse Drug Reactions Advisory Committee (Reporting is confidential, open to everyone and is now possible online at www.tga.gov.au.)
  - Relevant herbal and natural medicine associations such as the National Herbalists Association of Australia (www.nhaa.org.au)
  - Relevant manufacturer (Manufacturers keep their own records and are formally obliged to inform the TGA Prescriber, if applicable.)

Strategies for patients

Patients also play an important role in promoting a beneficial and harm-free outcome. They should ensure that they understand the benefits and potential risks associated with their treatment and be confident that they know how to take/use it appropriately. The Australian Commission on Safety and Quality in Health Care produced a patient information booklet entitled *10 tips for safer health care* (ACSQHC 2003) to encourage patients to become more active in their own healthcare while in hospital. Many of the steps outlined in the booklet are relevant to people taking CMs in the community or in hospital.

Below is a summary of recommendations for patients choosing to use or currently using CM, adapted from *10 tips for safer health care*.

- Choose a suitably experienced and qualified CM practitioner or ask for a referral from a trusted medical practitioner, pharmacist or other source.

- Become an active member of your own healthcare team. Help clinicians reach an accurate diagnosis, discuss appropriate management strategies, ensure treatment is administered and adhered to, identify side effects quickly and take appropriate action.

- Tell all healthcare practitioners about all the medicines being used (complementary and conventional). This includes telling doctors about complementary medicines and telling naturopaths and herbalists about pharmaceutical medicines.

- Make sure information given by the healthcare practitioner about the condition and the treatment options available is understood. In the case of lengthy explanations or recommendations, ask the practitioner to provide written information that can be taken home.

- Ask questions when you need more information because you are uncertain or the information provided is unclear.

- Be motivated to learn about the health condition being addressed, treatments being used and ways to improve wellbeing by referring to reliable information sources.

THE RATIONAL USE OF HERBAL AND NATURAL MEDICINES

Overall, when manufactured, prescribed and used appropriately, the safety of OTC CMs is high. Serious adverse effects and dangerous interactions are rare, particularly in comparison with the thousands of reports attributed to pharmaceutical medicines. Even so, the assessment of likely adverse reactions or interactions should remain integral to patient management.

Currently, there are few large-scale clinical studies confirming and clarifying the clinical significance of most suspected adverse reactions and interactions associated with CMs, and much remains unknown. It is important to recognise that the information presented in this book requires individual interpretation, because the clinical effects of any medicine or any potential interaction, no matter how well documented, will not occur consistently in each patient, each time or to the same degree of intensity.

Ultimately, the ideal in clinical practice is to combine knowledge about the medicine and the disease, experience of both, and information about the patient and the individual's circumstance in order to make wise treatment choices (Table 7.6). This requires the

TABLE 7.6 FACTORS TO CONSIDER IN THE RATIONAL USE OF COMPLEMENTARY MEDICINES	
FACTORS TO CONSIDER	**RATIONALE**
Products that are not produced under a code of GMP **should not be used.**	The quality of the product cannot be guaranteed.
Know the benefits, risks, potential adverse reactions and interactions and seek out reliable information. Additional training and/or access to accurate and updated information is important.	More than half the population use CMs and there is no sign of their popularity abating. Some CMs have proven benefits and offer cost-effective treatment options; however, safety issues also exist. Marketing/sales and company information is not sufficient, and education in the area of CM efficacy and safety may be limited.

(Continued)

TABLE 7.6 FACTORS TO CONSIDER IN THE RATIONAL USE OF COMPLEMENTARY MEDICINES *(continued)*	
FACTORS TO CONSIDER	**RATIONALE**
Do not rely on label claims alone.	Although manufacturers must hold the evidence to support the claims made on a product label, often the label claims do not provide enough information to make an informed judgement.
Do not rely on label dose recommendations alone.	Some manufacturers state the lowest effective dose on the label to ensure that a patient's general requirements will be met; however, in practice, practitioners should prescribe a dose to meet the individual's needs, which may be higher than label doses, yet still be within safe limits.
Take care when high-risk medicines are involved.	In combination with drugs that have a narrow therapeutic index and many anticancer and HIV medicines, screen for interactions. In the case of herbal medicines, any product containing St John's wort (*Hypericum perforatum*) should be considered higher risk. Screen for interactions.
Take care with people considered to be at higher risk of adverse reactions or in 'at risk' circumstances.	Older age; reduced renal or liver function; acute or severe disease; polypharmacy; history of atopy and/or confusion; when drugs with a narrow therapeutic index are involved; during pregnancy or lactation; in children; before major surgery
Ensure that all health professionals involved in a patient's care are aware of CM use.	Effective communication will foster appropriate and safe use.
Do not assume all healthcare professionals have the knowledge to monitor safe use.	Few medical practitioners have had formal training in the safety issues of CM, and not all health practitioners have ready access to evidence-based safety data.
Know the manufacturer and supplier details.	If in doubt about a product, call the manufacturer or supplier for more information.
Know the prescriber's details (if relevant).	The original prescriber may have valuable information about the patient and the medicine, which may assist informed decision making.
Medicines should be stored appropriately.	Appropriate storage will depend on the patient's circumstance (e.g. at home, in hospital or in a hospice), level of vigilance and the type of medicine used.

application of current knowledge, as well as good observational skills, open communication and clinical experience to reduce the risk of adverse reactions and maximise successful outcomes.

REFERENCES

ACSQHC (Australian Commission on Safety and Quality in Health Care). 10 tips for safer health care. Commonwealth of Australia. 2003.

Aronson JK et al. Adverse drug reactions: keeping up to date. Fundam Clin Pharmacol 16 (2002): 49–56.

Atkinson AJ et al. Principles of clinical pharmacology. London: Academic Press, 2001.

Barnes J et al. Different standards for reporting ADRs to herbal remedies and conventional OTC medicines: face-to-face interviews with 515 users of herbal remedies. Br J Clin Pharmacol 45 (1998): 496–500.

Blumenthal M. ABC clinical guide to herbs. Austin: American Botanical Council, 2003.

Bone KM. Potential interaction of Ginkgo biloba leaf with antiplatelet or anticoagulant drugs: What is the evidence? Mol Nutr Food Res 52.7 (2008): 764–771.

Braun L. The integration of complementary medicine in Victorian hospitals — a focus on surgery and safety. Melbourne: RMIT, 2007.

Braun L, Cohen MM. Herbs and natural supplements: An evidence based guide, 2nd edn. Sydney: Elsevier, 2007.

Braun LA et al. Adverse reactions to complementary medicines: the Australian pharmacy experience. Int J Pharm Pract, 18.4 (2010a): 242–244.

Braun LA et al. Perceptions, use and attitudes of pharmacy customers on complementary medicines and pharmacy practice. BMC Complement Altern Med 10 (2010b): 38.

Broom AF et al. Use of complementary and alternative medicine by mid-age women with back pain: a national cross-sectional survey. BMC Complement Altern Med 12 (2012): 98.

Brown J et al. General practitioners and pharmacists. Complementary medicines information use and needs of health professionals. Sydney: National Prescribing Service, 2008.

Brownie S. The development of the US and Australian dietary supplement regulations: What are the implications for product quality? Complement Ther Med 13 (2005): 191–198.

Bryant B et al. Pharmacology for health professionals. Sydney: Elsevier, 2003.

Burgess CL et al. Adverse drug reactions in older Australians, 1981–2002. Med J Aust 182 (2005): 267–270.

Christl SU et al. Toxic hepatitis after consumption of traditional kava preparation. J Travel Med. Jan–Feb 16.1 (2009): 55–56.

Davis SR et al. Use of complementary and alternative therapy by women in the first 2 years after diagnosis and treatment of invasive breast cancer. Menopause 17.5 (2010): 1004–1009.

Ernst E et al. The desktop guide to complementary and alternative medicine, 2nd edn. London: Mosby, Elsevier, 2006.

Flinders Medical Centre, Government of South Australia. Media release 2006.

Fugh-Berman A, Ernst E. Herb–drug interactions: review and assessment of report reliability. Br J Clin Pharmacol 52 (2001): 587–595.

Gordon LA. Compositae dermatitis. Aust J Dermatol 40 (1999): 123–128.

Grant SJ et al. The use of complementary and alternative medicine by people with cardiovascular disease: a systematic review. BMC Public Health 12 (2012): 299.

Heilmann P et al. Administration of glycyrrhetinic acid: significant correlation between serum levels and the cortisol/cortisone-ratio in serum and urine. Exp Clin Endocrinol Diabetes 107 (1999): 370–378.

Ilan R, Fowler R. Brief history of patient safety culture and science. J Crit Care 20 (2005): 2–5.

Jamison JR. Herbal and nutrient supplementation practices of chiropractic patients: an Australian case study. J Manipulative Physiol Ther 26 (2003): 242.

Koch E. Inhibition of platelet activating factor (PAF)-induced aggregation of human thrombocytes by ginkgolides: considerations on possible bleeding complications after oral intake of Ginkgo biloba extracts. Phytomedicine 12.1–2 (2005): 10–16.

Langman LJ, Kapur BM. Toxicology: then and now. Clin Biochem 39.5 (2006): 498–510.

Lechtenberg M, et al. Is the alkaloid pipermethystine connected with the claimed liver toxicity of Kava products? Pharmazie. 63.1 (2008): 71–74.

Levitsky J et al. Fulminant liver failure associated with the use of black cohosh. Dig Dis Sci 50.3 (2005): 538–539.

Lynch CR et al. Fulminant hepatic failure associated with the use of black cohosh: a case report. Liver Transpl 12.6 (2006): 989–992.

MacLennan A et al. The escalating cost and prevalence of alternative medicine. Prev Med 35 (2002): 166–173.

MacLennan AH et al. The continuing use of complementary and alternative medicine in South Australia: costs and beliefs in 2004. Med J Aust 184 (2006): 27–31.

Mahady GB et al. United States Pharmacopeia review of the black cohosh case reports of hepatotoxicity. Menopause 15.4 Pt 1 (2008): 628–638.

Manya, K et al. The use of complementary and alternative medicine among people living with diabetes in Sydney. BMC Complement Altern Med 12 (2012): 2.

Mazzanti G et al. Effects of Cimicifuga racemosa extract on liver morphology and hepatic function indices. Phytomedicine 15.11 (2008): 1021–1024.

Miller GC et al. Adverse drug events in general practice patients in Australia. Med J Aust 184 (2006): 321–324.

Moynihan R et al. Coverage by the news media of the benefits and risks of medications. N Engl J Med 342 (2000): 1645–1650.

Mullins RJ, Heddle R. Adverse reactions associated with echinacea: the Australian experience. Ann Allergy Asthma Immunol 88 (2002): 42–51.

Myers SP, Cheras PA. The other side of the coin: Safety of complementary and alternative medicine. Med J Aust 181 (2004): 222–225.

Naser B et al. Suspected black cohosh hepatotoxicity: no evidence by meta-analysis of randomized controlled clinical trials for isopropanolic black cohosh extract. Menopause 18.4 (2011): 366–375.

Nisbet BC, O'Connor RE. Black cohosh-induced hepatitis. Del Med J 79.11 (2007): 441–444.

Pirmohamed M et al. Adverse drug reactions as cause of admission to hospital: prospective analysis of 18,820 patients. BMJ 329 (2004): 15–19.

Routledge PA et al. Adverse drug reactions in elderly patients. Br J Clin Pharmacol 57 (2004): 121–126.

Rowe A, Ramzan I. Are mould hepatotoxins responsible for kava hepatotoxicity? Phytother Res. 26.11 (2012):1768–1770.

Runciman WB et al. Adverse drug events and medication errors in Australia. Int J Qual Health Care 15 (Suppl 1) (2003): i49–i59.

Sarris J et al. Kava in the treatment of generalized anxiety disorder: a double-blind, randomized, placebo-controlled study. J Clin. Psychopharmacol. 33 (2013): 643–648.

Stickel F et al. Hepatitis induced by Kava (Piper methysticum rhizoma). J Hepatol. 39.1 (2003): 62–67.

Teschke R et al. Kava hepatotoxicity — a clinical review. Ann Hepatol. 9.3 (2010a): 251–265.

Teschke R. Black cohosh and suspected hepatotoxicity: inconsistencies, confounding variables, and prospective use of a diagnostic causality algorithm. A critical review. Menopause 17.2 (2010b): 426–440.

Teschke R, Schwarzenboeck A. Suspected hepatotoxicity by Cimicifugae racemosae rhizoma (black cohosh, root): critical analysis and structured causality assessment. Phytomedicine 16.1 (2009): 72–84.

Teschke R et al. Kava hepatotoxicity: regulatory data selection and causality assessment. Dig Liver Dis. 41.12 (2011): 891–901.

Teschke R et al. Contaminant hepatotoxins as culprits for kava hepatotoxicity — fact or fiction? Phytother Res. 27.3 (2013): 472–474.

Teschke R et al. Kava hepatotoxicity in traditional and modern use: the presumed Pacific kava paradox hypothesis revisited, Br J Clin Pharmacol. 73.2 (2012): 170–174.

Teschke R et al. Herbal hepatotoxicity by kava: update on pipermethystine, flavokavain B, and mould hepatotoxins as primarily assumed culprits. Dig Liver Dis. 43.9 (2011): 676–681.

Teschke R et al. Kava hepatotoxicity: comparison of aqueous, ethanolic, acetonic kava extracts and kava-herbs mixtures. J Ethnopharmacol. 123.3 (2009): 378–384.

Teschke R et al. Kava hepatotoxicity: a European view. NZ Med J 3.121 (2008a): 90–98.

Teschke R et al. Kava hepatotoxicity: a clinical survey and critical analysis of 26 suspected cases. Eur J Gastroenterol Hepatol 20.12 (2008b): 1182–1193.

Teschke R. Kava hepatotoxicity: pathogenetic aspects and prospective considerations. Liver Int. 30.9 (2010b):1270–1279.

Thomson Reuters publishers. Micromedex Health Care Series, AltMedDex 2008.

Watson KD. Toxicology, history of. In: Philip W (ed). Encyclopedia of toxicology. New York: Elsevier, 2005, pp 364–370.

Whiting PW et al. Black cohosh and other herbal remedies associated with acute hepatitis. Med J Aust 177 (2002): 440–443.

WHO. Assessment of the risk of hepatotoxicity with kava products. World Health Organization, May 2007.

Wilkinson JM, Simpson MD. Complementary therapy use by nursing, pharmacy and biomedical science students. Nurs Health Sci 3 (2001): 19–27.

Woloshin S, Schwartz LM. Press releases: translating research into news. JAMA 287 (2002): 2856–2858.

CHAPTER 8

INTERACTIONS WITH HERBAL AND NATURAL MEDICINES

A pharmacological interaction is said to occur when the response to one medicine varies from what is usually predicted because another substance has altered the response. Usually the term 'interaction' has a negative connotation when referring to medicines, because it can lead to drug toxicity or a loss of drug effect, and it may be difficult to predict. However, interactions can also benefit the patient by improving outcomes, reducing side effects or reducing costs. In order for healthcare professionals to interpret interaction data and avoid or beneficially manipulate an interaction, or deal with an adverse effect due to an interaction, it is essential to have an understanding of the mechanisms involved.

Although thousands of drug interactions are studied each year, there has been far less scientific investigation into interactions with herbal and natural medicines. Research conducted with pharmaceutical medicines can provide some theoretical insights into the mechanisms of drug–herb interactions, but predicting clinical significance is difficult. Unlike conventional medicines, herbs and food-based supplements contain a complex mixture of bioactive chemicals, some of which may contribute to the overall therapeutic effect of the substances. The chemical composition is also variable and depends on factors such as the plant part used, seasonality, growing and harvesting conditions and extraction and manufacturing processes. Furthermore, some plant constituents have poor oral bioavailability, so in vitro screening for interactions will produce misleading results.

Evidence from controlled human studies has been steadily increasing in recent years; however, most information is still derived from in vitro and animal experiments. This approach is not without its limitations, as using evidence to predict what will happen in humans from studies not conducted in humans is bound to contain inaccuracies and therefore must be interpreted cautiously.

It must be mentioned that even when evidence from a controlled human study is available, predicting the likelihood and severity of a real-life interaction in a specific patient is still difficult and prone to error. Ultimately, the clinical importance of a herb–drug interaction depends on factors that relate to the medicines involved and the patients themselves. The chief medicinal factors will be dose, duration and frequency of use and administration route. Individual patient factors include age, gender, food intake, gastric and urinary pH, current state of health, preexisting disease and genetic polymorphism.

INTERACTION MECHANISMS

When one considers the great variation in physical properties and pharmacological effects of the numerous substances used as medicines, together with the variable nature of herbal medicines, it is apparent that a virtually endless number of interactions are possible. It is generally accepted, however, that there are two major interaction mechanisms, namely pharmacokinetic and pharmacodynamic interactions.

A third minor category of physicochemical or pharmaceutical interactions also exists. Regardless of the mechanism involved, there can be three possible outcomes from an interaction:
1. increased therapeutic or adverse effects (additive or synergistic)
2. decreased therapeutic or adverse effects (additive or synergistic)
3. a unique response that does not occur when either agent is used alone.

PHARMACOKINETIC INTERACTIONS

Pharmacokinetics refers to the quantitative analysis of the absorption, distribution, metabolism and excretion of a medicine. Pharmacokinetic interactions occur when there is an alteration to any of these four processes, causing a change in the amount and persistence of available drug at receptor sites or target tissues. As a result, a change in the magnitude of effect or the duration of effect can occur without a change in the type of effect. Interactions of this type may have multiple mechanisms, making clinical predictions difficult. Additionally, there are many patient factors that influence the pharmacokinetics of a drug, such as age, liver and renal function, degree of physiological stress and the presence of other diseases such as hyperthyroidism.

Factors affecting absorption

Drug absorption is determined by the physicochemical properties of a drug, as well as by its formulation and route of administration. Because most herbal and nutritional medicines are administered orally, as tablets, capsules, teas and tinctures, this discussion will focus on interactions associated with these dose forms.

Most absorption of orally administered medicines occurs in the small intestine, which has a larger surface area than the stomach and greater membrane permeability. If a slow-release dosage form is taken and it continues to release the drug for more than 6 hours, then absorption will also occur in the large intestine. The absorption of oral dose forms is influenced by differences in pH along the gastrointestinal tract, surface area per luminal volume, blood perfusion, the presence of bile and mucus and the nature of epithelial membranes. Changes to gastrointestinal flora, transport systems, chelation and ion exchange also influence absorption.

Interactions at this level can alter the rate of absorption and/or extent of absorption of a medicine.

Changes in relative rate of absorption

Although a medicine may eventually be fully absorbed, a significantly slowed absorption rate may mean that it never reaches effective serum levels, or that an unwanted 'sustained release' effect causes prolonged activity or a delay in prompt relief. In some clinical situations, decreased rates of absorption are of no concern; however, in others it may be important. Generally, a decreased rate of absorption is less important for medicines that are given in multiple-dose regimens to achieve a steady state serum level than for those that are given as single doses or are required to produce a rapid effect (e.g. analgesics).

Changes in extent of absorption

Altering the extent of absorption may also have significant consequences. Increasing the amount of medicine absorbed may produce higher plasma levels and a higher risk of adverse reactions or toxicity. Alternatively, reducing the amount of medicine absorbed may result in reduced efficacy or therapeutic failure. This is of particular concern for medicines with a narrow therapeutic index, such as warfarin and digoxin.

Mucilaginous herbs

Although little research has been conducted to determine the effects of herbal medicines on the absorption of other medicines, one double-blind study found that guar gum slowed the absorption rate of digoxin, but did not alter the extent of absorption, whereas penicillin absorption was both slowed and reduced (Huupponen et al 1984). This brings into question the effects of other gums and highly mucilaginous herbal medicines, such as *Ulmus fulvus* (slippery elm), *Althea officinalis* (marshmallow) and *Plantago ovata* (psyllium). Poorly lipid soluble, the mucilaginous content forms an additional physical barrier to absorption, but whether this will have a clinically significant effect on rate and/or extent of absorption of other medicines is uncertain and remains to be tested.

Nutrients

More research has been conducted into the way nutrients interact and alter the absorption of pharmaceutical medicines than with herbal medicines. The interactions between iron and many minerals provide a useful example. Aluminium, calcium bicarbonate or magnesium trisilicate taken in antacid preparations are known to reduce the extent of iron absorption owing to an alteration in gastric pH. This type of interaction is easily avoided by separating the intake of iron by at least 2 hours from the last dose of antacid.

Intrinsic drug transporters

Until recently, when an orally administered medicine exhibited poor absorption, it was generally assumed that this was because of either physicochemical problems or significant first-pass hepatic metabolism. Recently, it has been recognised that for many medicines poor oral bioavailability could be related to the influence of transporter proteins (Benet & Cummins 2001). Transporter proteins are associated with the transfer of some medicines from the intestinal lumen, through the biological barrier of the intestinal mucosa, into the systemic circulation and back again. Transporters fall into two main categories: carriers and pumps. Carriers are involved in three types of transport processes: facilitated diffusion, co-transport and counter-transport. Pumps are distinguished from carriers by the linkage of transport to an external source of energy. Examples of transporters in the intestine are P-glycoprotein (P-gp), members of the multi-drug-resistance-associated protein family (breast-cancer resistance protein, organic cation and anion transporters) and members of the organic anion polypeptide family (Wagner et al 2001). Of these, P-gp is the most studied (see *Clinical note*).

Herbal and natural medicines affecting P-gp

The influence of herbal and natural medicines on P-gp expression has only recently been considered, so much is still unknown and speculative. To date, most research has centred on St John's wort, although clinical testing with other herbs has now gained momentum: every few months more studies investigating the likelihood and clinical significance of proposed interactions are published.

In 1999, clinical testing found that St John's wort significantly reduces serum levels of digoxin after 10 days' co-administration (Johne et al 1999). The suspected mechanism of interaction was chiefly liver enzyme induction; however, the magnitude of effect seen in this study, and in others, suggested that P-gp induction was involved (Hennessy et al 2002). More recently, several clinical tests have confirmed that St John's wort has significant P-gp induction effects. One study found up to a 4.2-fold increase in P-gp expression compared with a placebo after 16 days' administration.

CLINICAL NOTE — P-GLYCOPROTEIN: AN IMPORTANT DRUG TRANSPORTER

P-glycoprotein was first studied in the context of cancer research, where its over-expression in tumour cells is associated with multi-drug resistance (Jodoin et al 2002). In cancer cells, P-gp is one of the transporters responsible for actively expelling chemotherapeutic drugs from cells, thereby decreasing intracellular concentrations and thus drug efficacy. As a result, identification of those substances that reduce P-gp expression and can be administered safely with chemotherapeutic agents is being investigated.

P-gp is found on the surface of hepatocytes, and epithelial cells of the renal tubules, the intestine, placenta and capillaries in the brain (Lin 2003). It plays an important role in the processes of absorption, distribution, metabolism and excretion of medicines. P-gp has a counter-transport activity, meaning it can transport medicines from the blood back into the gastrointestinal tract, thereby reducing bioavailability.

In humans, P-gp demonstrates genetic polymorphism, which may partly account for the inter-individual variability seen in drug absorption. One study conducted in 25 volunteers supports this idea and found that a greater than eight-fold difference in expression of intestinal P-gp is possible (Lown et al 1997).

The expression of P-gp can be altered by a number of factors, such as everyday foods, herbs and pharmaceutical medicines. In the case of P-gp inhibition, there will be an increase in absorption, systemic exposure and tissue distribution of medicines that are P-gp substrates, whereas P-gp induction produces the opposite effect.

(Continued)

Interactions with substances that inhibit P-gp are of great interest, as they can potentially enhance the absorption of important medicines that are generally poorly absorbed, such as chemotherapeutic medicines. Alternatively, P-gp inhibition may theoretically increase the incidence of side effects or the toxicity of some medicines, producing unwanted effects.

Some important P-gp substrates are:

Berberine	Methotrexate
Colchicine	Morphine
Cortisol	Nifedipine
Cyclosporin	Progesterone
Digoxin	Protease inhibitors
Erythromycin	Taxol
Indinavir	Tamoxifen
Loperamide	*Vinca* alkaloids

Similar results were seen in another study in which 14 days' administration of St John's wort resulted in a 1.4-fold increased expression of duodenal P-gp (Durr et al 2000). Induction of P-gp is attributed to pregnane X receptor activation by the hyperforin constituent (Lin 2003). Low hyperforin products are therefore less likely to induce P-gp.

St John's wort is not the only natural substance found to influence P-gp. Other studies suggest that rosemary extract may have the opposite effect, inhibiting P-gp. Treating multi-drug-resistant mammary tumour cells with rosemary extract produced an increase in intracellular concentrations of doxorubicin and vinblastine (both P-gp substrates) (Plouzek et al 1999). The same effects were not seen in cells that lack P-gp expression, suggesting that rosemary extract inhibits P-gp activity. The isoflavone genistein has also been investigated, with some results suggesting inhibition of P-gp-mediated drug transport (Castro & Altenberg 1997). Other studies have found that different polyphenols, such as green tea polyphenols, resveratrol (a polyphenol from red wine), curcumin, caffeine, theanine and methoxyflavones from orange, may inhibit drug transport via P-gp (Jodoin et al 2002).

Grapefruit juice is well known to interact with a number of medicines, so it is not surprising that it has also been investigated for effects on P-gp. Currently, evidence is conflicting, as several studies have found that components in grapefruit juice inhibit P-gp (Eagling et al 1999, Ohnishi et al 2000, Soldner et al 1999, Spahn-Langguth & Langguth 2001), whereas a randomised, crossover clinical study found no significant effects (Becquemont et al 2001). A more recent in vitro study produced similar results with 5% normal concentration of grapefruit, orange and apple juices; however, inhibition of other transporter proteins was observed (Dresser et al 2002).

Research suggests that quercetin inhibits P-gp expression (Choi & Li 2005, Chung et al 2005, Kitagawa et al 2005, Wang et al 2004). Studies with experimental models have demonstrated that pretreatment with quercetin increases the bioavailability of the calcium-channel blocker, diltiazem (Choi & Li 2005), and of digoxin (Wang et al 2004). Intriguingly, one in vivo study found quercetin significantly decreased the oral bioavailability of cyclosporin, which is the opposite of what would be expected, suggesting that other mechanisms may also be involved (Hsiu et al 2002).

Although in vitro studies have also identified an inhibitory effect on P-gp for silymarin, the active constituent group in St Mary's thistle (Chung et al 2005, Zhang & Morris 2003), recent clinical testing found no significant effect in vivo (Gurley et al 2006). Additionally, the herb schisandra inhibits P-gp (Jin et al 2010). Table 8.1 lists herbal and natural medicines that have suspected or known effects on P-gp, together with the research that gives evidence for these effects.

Factors affecting metabolism

Metabolism can occur before and during absorption, thereby limiting the amount of drug reaching the systemic circulation. In the intestinal lumen, digestive enzymes and bowel flora are capable of causing a wide range of metabolic reactions. The intestinal mucosa is also capable of metabolising drugs, with new research suggesting it is a major metabolic organ for some medicines (Doherty & Charman 2002).

For many medicines, metabolism chiefly occurs in the liver in two apparent phases, known as phase I or functionalisation reactions and phase II or conjugation reactions. Phase I reactions include oxidation, hydroxylation, dealkylation and reduction. Examples of Phase I reactions include conversion of an active drug to an inactive, less active, more active

TABLE 8.1 HERBAL AND NATURAL MEDICINES WITH SUSPECTED OR KNOWN EFFECTS ON P-GLYCOPROTEIN		
HERBAL/NATURAL MEDICINE	**EFFECT**	**EVIDENCE**
St John's wort	Induction	Clinical studies (Hennessy et al 2002, Johne et al 1999) In vivo and clinical study (Durr et al 2000) In vitro (Perloff et al 2001), also positive for hypericin Case report (Barone et al 2000)
Grapefruit juice	Inhibition	Clinical studies (Di Marco et al 2002, Edwards et al 1999) In vivo (Spahn-Langguth & Langguth 2001, Tian et al 2002) In vitro (Eagling et al 1999, Ohnishi et al 2000, Soldner et al 1999, Takanaga et al 1998)
Grapefruit juice	No effect	Clinical study (Becquemont et al 2001)
Orange and apple juice	Inhibition	Clinical study: Seville orange (Di Marco et al 2002) In vivo: orange (Tian et al 2002) In vitro (Ikegawa et al 2000, Takanaga et al 2000)
Rosemary extract	Inhibition	In vitro (Plouzek et al 1999)
Genistein and daidzein	Inhibition	In vitro (Evans 2000, Castro & Altenberg 1997)
Genistein and daidzein	Possible induction	In vitro (den Boer et al 1998)
Resveratrol	Inhibition	In vitro (Jodoin et al 2002)
Curcumin	Inhibition	In vitro (Anuchapreeda et al 2002, Romiti et al 1998)
Quercetin	Inhibition	In vitro and in vivo (Choi & Li 2005, Chung et al 2005, Kitagawa et al 2005, Scambia et al 1994, Wang et al 2004)
Green tea polyphenols, especially epigallocatechin gallate	Inhibition	In vitro (Jodoin et al 2002, Sadzuka et al 2000)
Piperine (a major component of black pepper)	Inhibition	In vivo (Bhardwaj et al 2002)
St Mary's thistle	Inhibition	In vitro tests (Chung et al 2005, Zhang & Morris 2003)
St Mary's thistle	No effect	Human study (Gurley et al 2006)

or toxic metabolite, and conversion of an inactive prodrug to an active metabolite. Phase II reactions include glucuronidation, sulfation, acetylation and methylation glutathionation, glycination and other amino acid conjugations (taurine, glutamine, carnitine, arginine), and usually result in the formation of inactive compounds that are water-soluble and easily excreted (Blower et al 2005).

Although there are many enzymes responsible for phase I reactions, the most important enzyme group is the cytochrome P450 system (CYP), which comprises more than 50 enzymes and is responsible for the metabolism of many drugs, nutrients, endogenous substances and environmental toxins.

Cytochromes

Cytochrome P450 is a generic term for a super-family of enzymes (haem containing mono-oxygenases) that have existed throughout nature since the beginning of life more than 3.5 billion years ago (Pirmohamed & Park 2003). The P450s are found chiefly in the liver, but also to a lesser extent in the intestines, kidneys, skin and lungs. These enzymes are responsible for foreign compound metabolism, which evolved about 400–500 million years ago to enable animals to detoxify chemicals in plants. The cytochrome P450 (CYP) enzymes are the most powerful in vivo oxidising agents and are able to catalyse the oxidative biotransformation of a wide range of chemically and biologically unrelated exogenous and endogenous substrates. They are named by a root symbol CYP, followed by a number for family, a letter for subfamily, and another number for the specific gene. For example, CYP3A4 would refer to a specific enzyme from the cytochrome P450 system, family 3, subfamily

A and gene 4. Three main CYP families (CYP1, 2, 3) are responsible for metabolism of therapeutic drugs. The different P450 isoforms vary in their abundance within the liver. Of these, the cytochromes CYP2C9, CYP2D6 and CYP3A4 are the most abundant in the human body (Pirmohamed & Park 2003).

The CYP2C sub-family accounts for 15–20% of the total P450 content of the liver, and metabolises approximately 20% of all drugs (Pirmohamed & Park 2003). The main member of this sub-family is CYP2C9, which is responsible for the metabolism of a number of compounds, including warfarin, phenytoin and various NSAIDs. Cytochrome 2D6 is responsible for the metabolism of approximately 25% of therapeutically used drugs, although it accounts for only <5% of the total P450 content. The CYP3A sub-family accounts for 30% of the total P450 content and is responsible for metabolism of about 50% of therapeutic drugs. Table 8.2 provides examples of common drugs and the cytochromes chiefly responsible for their metabolism. For a more complete list that is frequently updated, see Flockhart 2007.

The expression and activity of many CYP isoenzymes vary enormously between individuals. Part of the inter-individual variability is environmentally determined by the concomitant intake of drugs and foodstuffs that cause induction and inhibition of the different P450 isoforms. P450 gene polymorphism may also influence expression and activity of CYP enzymes, as this can lead to:
- abolished activity of a CYP enzyme (e.g. CYP2C9, CYP2C19 and CYP2D6 can be genetically absent in some livers [USFDA 2014])

- reduced activity
- altered activity
- increased activity where there is gene duplication.

For example, one study identified that 30% of Ethiopians had multiple copies of the 2D6 gene (up to 13), resulting in ultra-rapid metabolism of CYP2D6 substrates (Aklillu et al 1996). As a result, standard doses of CYP2D6 substrates (e.g. beta-blockers, some opioids and tricyclic antidepressants) will not produce anticipated or adequate responses, and higher drug doses are necessary to produce therapeutic effects. It has also been estimated that 7% of Caucasians lack CYP2D6. These individuals will not experience the anticipated therapeutic effects of prodrugs that are CYP2D6 substrates, such as codeine, and will appear more sensitive to the side effects of CYP2D6 substrates (e.g. beta-blockers, some opioids and tricyclic antidepressants) (USFDA 2014).

Another example is the polymorphic distribution of CYP2C9, which is absent in 1% of Caucasians. More than 100 drugs in current use are known substrates of CYP2C9, corresponding to approximately 10–20% of commonly prescribed drugs. Of note, CYP2C9 is chiefly responsible for the metabolism of NSAIDs and COX-2-specific inhibitors (e.g. celecoxib).

Many other factors affect CYP activity, such as the ingestion of foreign compounds (e.g. environmental contaminants) or the ingestion of certain constituents found in food, beverages and medicines.

Because of overlapping substrates, many drug interactions involve both P-gp and CYP3A4.

TABLE 8.2 SELECTED DRUGS THAT ACT AS SUBSTRATES FOR CYP ENZYMES	
CYP ENZYME	**DRUGS**
CYP1A2	amitriptyline, caffeine, melatonin, naproxen, paracetamol, tacrine, theophylline, verapamil, R-warfarin
CYP2B6	amitriptyline, diazepam, methadone, midazolam, tamoxifen, temazepam, testosterone
CYP2C9	amitriptyline, celecoxib, diclofenac, fluoxetine, ibuprofen, tamoxifen, S-warfarin
CYP2C19	amitriptyline, imipramine, indomethacin, omeprazole, progesterone, propranolol, R-warfarin
CYP2D6	amitriptyline, beta blockers, codeine, fluoxetine, flecainide, haloperidol, nicotine, ondansetron, paroxetine, sertraline, tamoxifen, tramadol
CYP3A4	alprazolam, caffeine, codeine, cyclosporin, erythromycin, HIV antivirals (e.g. indinavir), lovastatin, midazolam, oestradiol, ondansetron, progesterone, simvastatin, tamoxifen, taxol, testosterone

Enzyme inhibition

Competitive CYP inhibition is dose-dependent and occurs when inhibitors compete with other substances for a particular enzyme. Non-competitive inhibition is also possible and occurs when a substance either destroys or binds irreversibly to a CYP enzyme. In both instances, serum levels of those drugs chiefly metabolised by the affected enzyme will become elevated and the inhibition process is rapid. This is of particular concern with medicines that have a narrow therapeutic index, as very small changes in dose or blood levels can produce significant changes in activity. In the case of enzyme inhibition, raised blood levels can lead to increased side effects and toxicity.

Although inhibition of a CYP enzyme is generally regarded as raising the serum levels of an active drug, this is not always the case. If the drug involved is a prodrug, then it is inactive in its administered form and must be converted to its active form, usually via metabolic processes. If metabolism is slowed, then the production of active metabolites will also be slowed. An example is codeine, which is primarily metabolised by CYP2D6 into its active analgesic metabolite morphine; therefore, CYP2D6 inhibition has the potential to slow or reduce its analgesic activity.

Inhibitors do not all have the same strength and can be classified as strong, moderate or weak, depending on their effect on drug clearance compared to normal values. For example, Flockhart describes a strong inhibitor as one that causes more than 80% decrease in clearance, a moderate inhibitor as one that causes a 50–80% decrease in drug clearance and a weak inhibitor as one that causes a 20–50% decrease in drug clearance (Flockhart 2007).

Enzyme inhibition is not always harmful and has been manipulated to raise serum drug levels without the need to increase the dose administered. The result has obvious cost advantages when extremely expensive drugs are involved and has been used in some hospitals for medicines such as cyclosporin.

To date, the most studied natural substance capable of significantly inhibiting CYP enzymes is grapefruit. The finding that grapefruit juice markedly increases the bioavailability of some orally administered medicines was based on an unexpected observation from an interaction study between the calcium-channel antagonist felodipine and ethanol. In the study, grapefruit juice was used to mask the taste of ethanol, but actually affected the results by reducing CYP3A4 by 62% and significantly raising felodipine levels (Bailey et al 1998). Since then, the constituents of grapefruit juice have been extensively studied and found to affect the transport and metabolism of many other medicines (Eagling et al 1999, Kane & Lipsky 2000).

Increasingly, research is being conducted to determine whether other commonly used herbal medicines have an affect on CYP activity in vivo. For example, one research group in the United States screened *Citrus aurantium*, *Echinacea purpurea*, milk thistle (*Silybum marianum*) and saw palmetto (*Serenoa repens*) extracts for effects on CYP1A2, CYP2D6, CYP2E1 and CYP3A4 activity in healthy subjects (Gurley et al 2004). Of the four herbs, only *E. purpurea* was found to have any effect on the CYP enzymes tested, with a minor influence on CYP1A2 and CYP3A4. Using the same method, extracts of the herbs goldenseal (*Hydrastis canadensis*), black cohosh (*Cimicifuga racemosa*), kava kava (*Piper methysticum*) and valerian (*Valeriana officinalis*) were tested for effects on CYP1A2, CYP2D6, CYP2E1 or CYP3A4/5 activity (Gurley et al 2005). Goldenseal strongly inhibited CYP2D6 and CYP3A4/5 activity in vivo, whereas kava kava inhibited CYP2E1, black cohosh weakly inhibited CYP2D6 and no effect was observed for valerian. In a separate study, testing *Panax ginseng* and *Ginkgo biloba*, no effect was observed on CYP activity; however, garlic oil inhibited CYP2E1 activity by 39% (Gurley et al 2002). More recently, a 2012 review considering which herbs are likely to induce clinically relevant drug interactions concluded that the herb schisandra is likely to inhibit CYP3A4 in humans, as is golden seal (Gurley et al 2012).

There are many other examples to be found in the individual monographs of this book.

Enzyme induction

Alternatively, many different medicines and everyday substances have been found to induce the CYP enzymes (e.g. broccoli, Brussels sprouts, char-grilled meat, high-protein diets, tobacco and alcohol). Research is now identifying a number of herbal medicines that cause CYP induction to various degrees; however, the most studied to date is St John's wort.

Clinical tests have confirmed that long-term administration of St John's wort has significant CYP inducer activity, particularly CYP3A4 (Durr et al 2000, Roby et al 2000, Ruschitzka et al 2000, Wang et al 2001). It appears that the hyperforin component is a potent ligand for the pregnane X receptor, which regulates expression of CYP3A4 mono-oxygenase. In this way, hyperforin increases the availability of CYP3A4, resulting in enzyme induction (Moore et al 2000).

Lack of in vitro–in vivo correlation

It is interesting to observe an apparent lack of in vitro–in vivo correlation with some studies of CYP. For example, in vitro investigations implicate milk thistle extract and/or silibinin as inhibitors of human CYP3A4, CYP2C9, CYP2D6 and CYP2E1; however, in vivo evidence for CYP-mediated interactions by milk thistle is less compelling (Gurley et al 2004). This may be owing to poor bioavailability of key constituents, large inter-individual differences in absorption of constituents, inter-product variability in the ratios of constituent, poor dissolution of dosage forms or other mechanisms.

Factors affecting excretion

The kidneys are the major organs of excretion, but it also occurs to a lesser extent via other routes such as saliva, sweat, faeces, breast milk and the lungs. If a medicine is chiefly eliminated by one pathway, then alterations to that particular pathway can theoretically have a significant influence on its excretion.

With regard to urinary excretion, factors that alter renal function can interfere with the excretion of medicines and their metabolites. There are three main ways that renal function can be modified (Blower et al 2005):
- altered renal tubular reabsorption by substances that affect urinary pH
- changes in renal tubular secretion by agents that either compete for active secretion or that alter the activity of membrane transporter proteins
- changes in glomerular filtration induced by agents that alter cardiac output.

Alterations to urinary pH are easily achieved with regard to herbal and natural substances; for example, the half-life of an acidic medicine,

---

CLINICAL NOTE — PHARMACOGENETICS

Pharmacogenetics largely deals with genes encoding drug transporters, drug-metabolising enzymes and drug targets (Ingelman-Sundberg 2004). It is now well established that the polymorphism of metabolising enzymes, and in particular that of P450 cytochromes, has the greatest effect on inter-individual variability of drug response, as evidenced by many studies. These polymorphisms affect the response of individuals to drugs used in the treatment of depression, psychosis, cancer, cardiovascular disorders, ulcer and gastrointestinal disorders, pain and epilepsy, among others. The costs of genotyping are reducing and our knowledge about the benefits of predictive genotyping for more effective and safe drug therapy is increasing. This means that in future predictive genotyping for CYP enzymes will become routine, allowing individualised prescribing to produce better clinical outcomes with less risk of side effects.

---

such as a salicylate, can be increased with acidification of urine — for example, with high doses of ascorbic acid, because less is eliminated. Alternatively, the half-life of a weakly basic drug, such as amphetamine, may be decreased when urine is acidified. Alkalisation of urine produces the opposite effects and can occur with low-protein diets or the ingestion of substances such as potassium citrate.

PHARMACODYNAMIC INTERACTIONS

Pharmacodynamic interactions result when one substance alters the sensitivity or responsiveness of tissues to another. This type of interaction results in additive, synergistic or antagonistic drug effects and is of particular concern when medicines used simultaneously have overlapping toxicities.

In practice, clinicians frequently use additive or synergistic pharmacodynamic interactions to improve clinical outcomes. For example, medical doctors may prescribe a combination of antibiotics against difficult-to-eradicate microorganisms, or several antihypertensive drugs to one patient. Herbalists widely prescribe combinations of herbs with similar actions to strengthen clinical effects, and naturopaths may combine nutritional and herbal supplements in a similar way.

Pharmacodynamic interactions do not always produce wanted results, such as when several medicines with overlapping adverse effects or toxicities are used together, leading to more serious adverse effects. An example is the combined use of an opioid analgesic, which can induce drowsiness, and an antiemetic drug such as metoclopramide, which can also induce drowsiness. Other unwanted effects include potentiating drug activity to a clinically uncomfortable or dangerous level, or reducing activity and therefore the effectiveness of treatment.

Although pharmacodynamic interactions involving herbal and natural medicines and pharmaceutical medicines have not been thoroughly investigated, theoretical predictions are easy to produce. For example, case reports suggest that kava kava may have dopamine receptor antagonist activity and therefore theoretically can interact with dopamine agonists (e.g. L-dopa), opposing their effect (Meseguer et al 2002, Spillane et al 1997). Predicting real-life responses is difficult, because the evidence does not come from a controlled clinical study and individual factors such as dose, administration route and patient health further influence outcomes.

PHYSICOCHEMICAL INTERACTIONS

Physicochemical interactions occur when two substances come into contact and are either physically or chemically incompatible. This type of interaction can take place during the manufacture or administration of medicines and can affect both the rate and the extent of absorption of one or both medicines. Physicochemical interactions are a well-known concern among medical herbalists and naturopaths who prescribe and dispense their own herbal combinations.

Reduced absorption

Tannins

Herbs with significant tannin content have the potential to be involved in physicochemical interactions with other medicines, both outside and within the body, because they form precipitates with proteins, nitrogenous bases, polysaccharides and some alkaloids and glycosides (Mills 1991). Additionally, tannins will form complexes with metal ions such as iron, inhibiting their absorption (Glahn et al 2002). To avoid this interaction, herbal extracts containing tannins are traditionally not mixed with extracts containing alkaloids (Bone & Mills 2000).

In practice, herbal medicines containing tannins are used both internally and externally. When used internally, it is recommended that they be taken between meals or on an empty stomach to minimise precipitation of dietary proteins and digestive enzymes in the gut (Baxter et al 1997). Additionally, tannins can reduce the absorption of some minerals, so should not be taken at the same time. For example, the absorption of iron is significantly reduced in the presence of tannins, with one study finding amounts as small as 5 mg of tannic acid are able to inhibit iron absorption by 20% and higher levels of 100 mg by 88% (Brune et al 1989). Tannins are widely found in the plant kingdom, as shown in Table 8.3.

Chelation

Physicochemical interactions can also occur via a process of chelation, which is the chemical interaction of a metal ion and other substance that results in the formation of a molecular complex in which the metal is firmly bound and isolated. In other words, the metal ion irreversibly binds to a second molecule, leading to reduced activity or inactivation of that metal. A common example is the interaction between iron and various drugs, including tetracycline antibiotics.

TABLE 8.3 COMMON HERBS WITH SIGNIFICANT TANNIN CONTENT	
COMMON NAME	**BOTANICAL NAME**
Agrimony	*Agrimony eupatorium*
Bearberry	*Arctostaphylus uva-ursi*
Bistort	*Polygonum bistorta*
Meadowsweet	*Filipendula ulmaria*
Raspberry	*Rubus idaeus*
Rhubarb	*Rheum* spp. root
Spinach	*Chenopodium* spp.
Tea	*Camellia sinensis*
Tormentil	*Potentilla tormentilla*

A number of compounds found naturally in food have the potential to interact with medicines in this way. For example, oxalic acid found in spinach and rhubarb or phytic acid found in bran can form insoluble complexes with calcium, thereby reducing its absorption.

Increased absorption

Not all physicochemical interactions result in reduced absorption. It is widely accepted that interactions between plant components can enhance clinical effects by increasing the bioavailability of key pharmacologically active constituents.

The results of continuing investigation into the chemistry of St John's wort provide a good example. In vivo studies using hypericin and pseudohypericin found that the solubility of these two active constituents increases by approximately 60% in the presence of natural procyanidins (Butterweck et al 1998). Further research has isolated naturally occurring hyperoside, rutin and quercetin as some of the key components responsible for this interaction.

Although still largely speculative, the interaction between naturally occurring surfactant constituents, such as saponins, and poorly lipid soluble active constituents could feasibly result in increased absorption through a micellisation process. Besides improving oral bioavailability, the interaction could also improve dermal penetration.

Different forms of saponins are widely found in the plant kingdom and are used either internally or externally, depending on the particular herb (Table 8.4).

SYNERGY HERBAL RESEARCH

In practice, herbalists use inter-herbal interactions to produce better outcomes. This practice is much the same as that of medical practitioners employing multi-target drug therapy in the treatment of cancer, hypertension and antibiotic resistance. Owing to the chemical complexity of herbal medicines, intra-herbal interactions are also being identified that largely explain the therapeutic superiority of many herbal drug extracts over single constituents isolated from the same herbal extracts. Synergistic effects can be produced if the constituents of an extract affect different targets or interact with one another in order to improve the solubility and thereby enhance the bioavailability

TABLE 8.4 COMMON HERBS CONTAINING SAPONINS	
COMMON NAME	**BOTANICAL NAME**
Astragalus	*Astragalus membranaceus*
Bupleurum	*Bupleurum falcatum*
Horsechestnut	*Aesculus hippocastanum*
Japanese ginseng	*Panax japonicus*
Licorice	*Glycyrrhiza glabra*
Poke root	*Phytolacca decandra*
Soybean	*Glycine max*
Withania	*Withania somnifera*

of one or several substances of an extract. Synergy research in phytomedicine has established itself as a new activity in recent years and focuses on studying intra-herbal and inter-herbal interactions to better understand how therapeutic benefits can be harnessed.

INTERACTION SCREENING TOOLS

Information about interactions is derived from in vitro tests, studies with experimental animal models and, increasingly, clinical studies. Most studies of interactions conducted to date have focused on herbal constituents and their effects on cytochrome (CYP) enzymes and, increasingly, P-glycoprotein (P-gp), with few studies investigating effects on drug transport or phase II metabolism.

In vitro tests

Most studies conducted to investigate herb–drug interactions have used in vitro testing of herbal constituents in microsomal systems, supersomes, cytosols, expressed enzymes or cell-culture systems such as transfected cell lines, primary cultures of human hepatocytes and tumour-derived cells. While in vitro models provide a quick screening method for potential herb–drug interactions they do not always correlate with in vivo findings. One problem frequently encountered in the existing in vitro literature is the use of inappropriately high concentrations of single, isolated constituents obtained from commercial sources, and utilisation of these in experiments when only a small fraction of the compound may actually be bioavailable. Many natural products are generally subject to first-pass metabolism and to a much larger extent than conventional pharmaceutical agents, which are in most cases specifically developed to be substantially bio-available or otherwise formulated as prodrugs. In addition, many are less bioavailable because of their hydrophilic nature or large molecular size (Markowitz et al 2008).

Animal studies

These studies may give important information on herb interactions. Probe substrates/inhibitors can be used to explore the effects of herbs on the activity of specific CYP enzyme in vivo, e.g. caffeine for CYP1A2, tolbutamide for CYP2C9, mephenytoin for CYP2C19, dextromethorphan or debrisoquine for CYP2D6, chlorzoxazone for CYP2E1 and midazolam or erythromycin for CYP3A4. In addition, a cocktail of probe drugs have been used to explore the activities of multiple CYPs in the same experiment. Ultimately, in vivo clinical studies are more reliable than in vitro tests as a means of determining the clinical importance of herb–drug interactions, although these studies can quickly be confounded by the documented variability found in specific constituents between individual botanical products as well as by the choice of probe substrates administered (Markowitz et al 2008).

Relying solely on in vitro or animal model experiments to predict clinically relevant herb–drug interactions is problematic and can provide inaccurate information. The herbs *Ginkgo biloba* and saw palmetto will be used here as examples to illustrate this point.

In vitro and/or tests with animal models have shown both cytochrome induction and inhibition for *Ginkgo biloba* (Chatterjee et al 2005, Chang et al 2006a, 2006b, Gaudineau et al 2004, He & Edeki 2004, Kubota et al 2004, Kuo et al 2004, Mohutsky et al 2006, Ohnishi et al 2003, Ryu & Chung 2003, Shinozuka et al 2002, Sugiyama et al 2004a, 2004b, von Moltke et al 2004, Zhao et al 2006). In contrast, four clinical studies have failed to identify a clinically significant effect on a variety of cytochromes. In one clinical study, Gurley et al (2002) demonstrated that *Ginkgo biloba* had no significant effect on CYP1A2, CYP2D6 or CYP3A4 activity. Markowitz et al (2003b) also conducted a human study and found no significant effects on CYP2D6 or CYP3A4 activity. Two further clinical studies found no significant effect for

Ginkgo biloba on CYP2C9 activity (Greenblatt et al 2006, Mohutsky et al 2006). Overall, there have been at least 29 human studies investigating whether *Ginkgo biloba* alters the pharmacokinetics of multiple drugs (e.g. warfarin and digoxin) and affects various cytochromes. Of these, 23 studies found no observable effect, three a modest effect and three provided some evidence of CYP induction. However, when compared to FDA guidelines, these three studies do not suggest a clinically significant or important drug interaction potential (Gurley et al 2012).

Saw palmetto showed potent inhibition of CYP3A4, CYP2D6 and CYP2C9 in vitro (Yale & Glurich 2005); however, no significant effect was observed on CYP2D6 or CYP3A4 activity according to a clinical study by Markowitz et al (2003a). Gurley et al (2004) also found no significant effect for saw palmetto on CYP1A2, CYP2D6, CYP2E1 or CYP3A4 activity in healthy subjects.

To add to the complexity of the problem, in some instances researchers have conducted testing with individual herbal components or different forms of a herb and found different effects on CYPs. For example, using animal models Fukao et al (2004) demonstrated that diallyl sulphide (100 micromol/kg) increased cytochrome CYP2E1 activity slightly but significantly (1.6-fold versus control), whereas diallyl disulfide and diallyl trisulfide did not affect CYP2E1 activity or the hepatic total CYP level or CYP1A1/2 activity. The significance of these results in clinical practice is difficult to determine, as the overall effect on CYP activity will depend on the concentrations of these various constituents present in a garlic product. The example also highlights the general difficulty in extrapolating results for one herbal extract to another, as there may be a significant chemical variation between batches of the same herbal product and between different products of the same herb grown and produced by various manufacturers.

Clinical studies

These studies provide the most relevant information; however, they are costly to produce and are mostly conducted with young, healthy males, which may or may not accurately reflect the responses of other populations (e.g. women, the elderly).

TABLE 8.5 ADVANTAGES AND LIMITATIONS OF HERB–DRUG INTERACTION STUDIES		
STUDY TYPE	ADVANTAGES	LIMITATIONS
In vitro	Provides information about specific mechanisms under controlled conditions. Relatively simple to conduct compared with clinical studies. Inexpensive tests to conduct compared with clinical studies. Relatively quick to conduct.	Does not account for poor bioavailability of the test compound. May use one isolated constituent, whereas herbal extracts contain multiple constituents. Does not account for human genetic polymorphism. May use clinically irrelevant concentration. Metabolites of botanical extracts are poorly characterised for most extracts and may contribute to the net inhibitory or inductive effects observed, which will not be detected with in vitro testing.
In vivo using animal models	Can address some of the issues relating to bioavailability. Can produce quicker results than clinical studies. Can provide information when clinical studies are not able to be conducted.	Species variations make results difficult to interpret. Selection of appropriate dosage can be difficult and very large doses are often used. Does not account for human genetic polymorphism.
Clinical studies	Provide the most relevant information and are the most definitive.	Most studies conducted in healthy male subjects; however, most relevant results are obtained when conducted with the population that will be using the product. Inter-product variability in constituent ratios means tested product may not accurately represent effects of other products. Cannot differentiate between gut and liver effects (e.g. cytochromes). Does not provide information about mechanisms. Are costly and time consuming. May never be done for ethical reasons (e.g. safety studies in pregnancy).

Table 8.5 presents a summary of the strengths and limitations relevant to different types of research into interactions.

PUTTING THEORY INTO PRACTICE

It is clear that many patients will be taking herbal and natural medicines and pharmaceutical medicines at some stage of their lives. In some instances, use will overlap, so a patient will be taking several medicines at the same time. In order to promote the safe use of all medicines, the following section provides ideas for consideration and discussion, practical tools to aid in reducing the risk of interactions and in detection of adverse reactions and general recommendations.

INTERACTION MECHANISMS

Predicting the clinical importance of a herb–drug interaction is difficult and largely depends on factors that relate to the medicines administered and the individual patient. Having an understanding of the interaction mechanisms involved is also essential.

Medicine factors

Consider the types of medicines involved, administration route, dosage and duration of use. Drugs with a narrow therapeutic index are of most concern, as minor changes to serum levels can have clinically significant outcomes. Drugs that are administered intravenously will not always be subject to the same concerns as orally ingested drugs. In the case of herbal medicines, some preparations contain multiple CYP or transporter-modulating constituents, with some constituents causing induction and others inhibition. This means the overall outcome will depend on the amount of inducer/inhibitor constituents present, the CYPs or transporters affected and the relative strengths of inducers/inhibitors. Since herbal medicines naturally vary in constituent ratios owing to environmental and process factors, their effects on CYPs and transporters are more difficult to predict than for single-entity drugs.

Individual patient factors

The severity of the interaction is also influenced by factors such as age, gender, preexisting medical conditions and comorbidities, environmental influences and diet. Genetic polymorphism is increasingly becoming recognised as another significant factor that can alter a patient's risk of experiencing adverse drug reactions. The importance an interaction is given is also related to some extent to the setting in which it occurs. Risk can be minimised or managed when patients openly discuss their use of herbal and pharmaceutical medicines with all their healthcare providers and they are carefully supervised.

Problems and pitfalls interpreting the evidence

Firstly, understanding the basic mechanisms involved is essential, as is keeping in mind the type of evidence that might suggest the possibility of an interaction. It is important to note the general lack of correlation between in vitro and in vivo tests, and the inaccuracies of extrapolating data from animal models to predict clinical significance in humans. In many cases, interaction studies are absent, so clinicians must use their professional judgement to evaluate what is known about the medicines and the patient, and then the likelihood of a clinically relevant interaction.

A PREDICTIVE ALGORITHM

The METOPIA algorithm provides a framework for healthcare professionals when making rational decisions about the introduction of a second, potentially interacting medicine. In this chapter, it is assumed that a herbal medicine is involved. METOPIA stands for:

Medication and mechanisms

- What types of medicines are involved? High-risk medicines such as those with a narrow therapeutic index require closer monitoring.
- Is an interaction theoretically possible? This needs to be based on a fundamental understanding of the pharmacokinetic parameters and pharmacodynamic effects of the medicines involved.

Evidence available?

- Is there supportive evidence for an anticipated interaction?

- If so, what is the weight of that evidence (theoretical, in vitro, in vivo, case reports or clinical trials)?

If the information gathered so far suggests an interaction is possible, continue with the following steps.

Timing and dose — introducing which, when and for how long?

- When are the medicines being taken — at the same time or are doses separated by several hours? It is particularly important to determine the timing if a physicochemical interaction is anticipated.
- What is the duration of use? Interaction mechanisms may develop only over several days or weeks (such as CYP induction), or may occur more rapidly.

Outcomes possible

- What is the potential clinical outcome of an interaction — major, minor or neutral? In regard to herbal medicine, this is often speculative.

Practitioner considerations

- Is the practitioner in a position to monitor and manage an interaction should it become significant? In a hospital setting, an interaction is generally considered important if something must be done to relieve patient symptoms or if it will have a significant impact on critical therapy. Practitioners and nursing staff are in an ideal position to monitor for interactions and respond quickly should this be necessary. In a community setting, general practitioners, pharmacists, naturopaths and herbalists are better placed, and adequate patient self-monitoring becomes more important.

Individual considerations

- What are the patient's individual preferences and ability to self-monitor a potential interaction should it arise?

Action required

- Having established the criteria so far, five actions are possible:
  - *Avoid* — consider an alternative treatment that is unlikely to produce undesirable interaction effects.

– *Avoid unless adequate medical monitoring is possible* — changing the dose and regimen may be required for safe combined use.

– *Caution* — tell patients to be aware that a particular event is possible and to seek advice if they are concerned.

– *Observe* — the practitioner is alert to the possibility of an interaction, even though it is unlikely to have clinical consequences and is likely to be a neutral interaction.

– *Prescribe* — the outcome of the interaction is beneficial and can be used to improve clinical outcomes.

ASSESSING THE LIKELIHOOD OF AN ADVERSE DRUG–HERB INTERACTION

The likelihood that an adverse reaction is responsible for a patient's presenting signs and symptoms should always be considered. If suspicious, then it is essential to take appropriate steps to clarify the likelihood of an adverse reaction.

Patient evaluation

Factors to consider are:
• detailed description of the event — severity of symptoms, signs, onset, duration, frequency
• differential diagnoses (e.g. non-medicinal causes, such as exacerbation of condition, laboratory error or an interaction).

Causality and probability

Determining a cause-and-effect relationship between a medicine and an adverse reaction can be difficult. The degree of certainty that links a medicine to a specific reaction can be classified as definite, probable, possible, conditional or doubtful, and must be assessed in each individual case. Several algorithms exist to help clinicians determine the likelihood of an adverse reaction. Table 8.6 shows the Naranjo algorithm adapted for use as an interaction detection tool (Naranjo et al 1981). The adverse drug reaction possibility classification is based on the total score:

>8	highly probable
4–7	probable
1–3	possible
0	doubtful

NEXT STEPS IF INTERACTION IS LIKELY
Analysis of the medicine

If an interaction involving a herbal or natural medicine is highly likely, then it must be authenticated, botanically verified and analysed for the presence of contaminants. These essential steps will establish whether the interaction is due to an intrinsic property of the medicine itself, and therefore reproducible, or to extrinsic factors such as poor manufacturing processes.

Case reporting

All suspected adverse reactions should be reported to several authorities:
• The local government agency responsible for post-marketing surveillance and collecting adverse drug reaction case reports. In Australia this is the Adverse Drug Reactions Advisory Committee (ADRAC). (Reporting is confidential, open to everyone and is now possible online at www.tga.gov.au.)
• Relevant local herbal and natural medicine associations such as the National Herbalists Association of Australia (www.nhaa.org.au).
• Relevant product manufacturer. (Manufacturers keep their own records and are obligated to inform the TGA.)
• Prescriber, if applicable.

Chapter 7 provides further practical information about the safe use of CAM and risk factors for adverse events and interactions.

TWO MEDICINES REQUIRING SPECIAL ATTENTION
DIGOXIN

Digoxin is a drug indicated for the treatment of numerous cardiac ailments, such as atrial fibrillation and severe heart failure. It has a positive inotropic effect on both normal and failing hearts, although its primary benefit is mediated by neurohormonal modulation. It has a narrow therapeutic index and therefore minor changes in dose or serum levels can have clinically significant consequences. Digoxin is subject to pharmacokinetic and pharmacodynamic interactions with pharmaceutical, herbal and natural medicines, resulting in possible therapeutic failure or toxicity (Table 8.7).

TABLE 8.6 ASSESSING THE LIKELIHOOD THAT AN ADVERSE REACTION IS CAUSED BY AN INTERACTION				
QUESTION	YES	NO	DON'T KNOW	SCORE
Do previous conclusive reports of this interaction exist?* It is suggested that several resources are examined to determine whether the report is a possible, probable or confirmed interaction.	+1	0	0	
Did the adverse event appear after the suspected medicine/herb/nutrient was co-administered?	+2	−1	0	
Did the adverse reaction improve after the suspected medicine/herb/nutrient was discontinued?	+1	0	0	
Did the adverse reaction reappear when the medicine/herb/nutrient was readministered?	+2	−1	0	
Are there alternative causes (other than the suspected medicine/s) that could produce this reaction?	−1	+2	0	
Was the medicine detected in the blood (or other fluids) at levels known to be toxic or subtherapeutic, when previous levels were within the normal range?	+1	0	0	
Was the reaction more severe when the dose of medicine/herb/nutrient was increased, or less severe when decreased?	+1	0	0	
Has the patient had a similar reaction to the same or similar medicine in any previous exposure, when concomitant complementary medicines were not used?	−2	+1	0	
Was the event confirmed by objective evidence?	+1	0	0	
TOTAL score				

*Although a rechallenge provides important evidence, this is not always appropriate.

TABLE 8.7 SUSPECTED OR KNOWN INTERACTIONS BETWEEN DIGOXIN AND HERBAL MEDICINES	
INCREASED DIGOXIN EFFECTS POSSIBLE	DECREASED DIGOXIN EFFECTS POSSIBLE
Herbs that induce potassium loss with long-term use: • *Glycyrrhiza glabra* (licorice) • *Paullinia cupana* (guarana) • Anthraquinone-containing herbal laxatives (senna, cascara, aloes and buckthorn) Some herbal diuretics may also induce some degree of potassium loss; however, clinical significance is unknown.	Herbs currently known to induce P-gp and/or CYPs in a clinically significant manner: • *Hypericum perforatum* (St John's wort)
Herbs containing cardiac glycosides: • *Nerium oleander* (oleander) • *Adonis autumnalis* (false hellebore) • *Convallaria majalis* (lily of the valley)	Herbs containing > 50,000 ppm potassium: • *Avena sativa* (oats) • *Taraxacum officinale* (dandelion) • *Apium graveolens* (celery)
Pharmacodynamic interaction theoretically possible, although not seen in one clinical study: • *Crataegus oxyacantha* (hawthorn)	Foods containing >50,000 ppm potassium: • asparagus • beetroot • bok choy • cucumber • lettuce • rhubarb • spinach
Herbs and natural constituents known or suspected to inhibit P-gp or CYPs: • apple juice • curcumin • daidzein • genistein • grapefruit • green tea polyphenols • orange juice (seville oranges) • piperine • quercetin • resveratrol • rosemary extract	

Potassium changes

Potassium states are of special concern with digoxin because hypokalaemia lowers the threshold for drug toxicity. It is well known that pharmaceutical medicines such as thiazide diuretics and corticosteroids have the potential to induce a state of hypokalaemia. There are several herbal medicines that require attention such as *Glycyrrhiza glabra* (licorice), *Paullinia cupana* (guarana) and anthraquinone laxatives (e.g. aloes, buckthorn, cascara and senna). As with potassium-depleting drugs, adequate potassium intake should be recommended and potassium levels monitored together with clinical signs and symptoms.

Alternatively, there are a number of herbal medicines and foods that contain significant amounts of potassium that could increase the threshold for drug efficacy. Some of the common herbs and foods containing greater than 50,000 ppm of potassium include asparagus, beetroot, bok choy, cucumber, lettuce, rhubarb, *Avena sativa* (oats), *Taraxacum officinale* (dandelion) and *Apium graveolens* (celery).

P-gp and changes to metabolism

Digoxin is a substrate for P-gp, therefore serum digoxin levels are altered when P-gp induction or inhibition occurs. It is known that drugs such as verapamil and quinidine, which affect P-gp, can significantly interact with digoxin and in recent years several herbal and natural medicines have also been identified with the potential to alter P-gp activity. Of these, the herb St John's wort has been investigated under controlled clinical conditions and found to decrease the digoxin area-under-the-curve by 25% after 10 days' treatment (Johne et al 1999). Monitoring of plasma digoxin concentration and clinical effects is required when patients commence or cease St John's wort while taking digoxin. As discussed earlier, several other herbs affect P-gp expression and concurrent use should be supervised.

Pharmacodynamic interactions

Pharmacodynamic interactions are theoretically possible when herbs containing naturally occurring cardiac glycoside constituents, such as oleander (*Nerium oleander*), false hellebore (*Adonis autumnalis*) and lily of the valley (*Convallaria majalis*), are ingested at the same time. Although not commonly prescribed for internal use,

theoretically these plants may reinforce drug activity and induce symptoms of toxicity. Signs and symptoms of digoxin toxicity include anorexia, nausea, vomiting, diarrhoea, weakness, visual disturbances and ventricular tachycardia.

It has been speculated that the herb hawthorn (*Crataegus oxyacantha*) could potentiate the effects of cardiac glycosides, as both in vitro and in vivo studies indicate it has positive inotropic activity. Furthermore, the flavonoid components of hawthorn also affect P-gp function and cause interactions with drugs that are P-gp substrates, such as digoxin. In practice, however, results from a randomised crossover trial that evaluated co-administration of digoxin 0.25 mg with *Crataegus* special extract WS 1442 (hawthorn leaves with flowers) 450 mg twice daily for 21 days found no significant difference to any measured pharmacokinetic parameters (Tankanow et al 2003). Although this is reassuring, combined use should be supervised by a healthcare professional and drug requirements monitored.

In practice, the likelihood and significance of these interactions varies considerably, and the response required to ensure safe use of medicines can be multifaceted. For example, if Mr A has been taking St John's wort for several months and then digoxin is introduced, routine monitoring of digoxin levels enables appropriate doses to be determined and ensures the safe use of both medicines. However, it is essential to advise Mr A to inform his healthcare professional when use of St John's wort is going to be ceased or the dosage changed, as digoxin levels will require closer monitoring during the change. On the other hand, if Mrs B has been taking digoxin for some time and then St John's wort is to be introduced, additional monitoring is required for at least 3 weeks to determine whether a new effective digoxin dose is required. Once again, if there is to be an alteration to St John's wort use, Mrs B should be advised to see a healthcare professional for monitoring during the transition.

Interference with therapeutic drug monitoring for digoxin

In 1996, a case was reported of a possible interaction between Siberian ginseng and digoxin (McRae 1996). More specifically, it involved an elderly man whose serum digoxin levels rose (but did not produce toxic symptoms) when he concurrently took a Siberian ginseng product, fell when the product was stopped and then rose again when use was resumed. Unfortunately, the report was inaccurate, as the product was later analysed and found to contain digitalis. Additionally, no case reports suggesting drug toxicity were published over the following years. Research published in 2010 suggests that eleutherosides found in the herb are chemically related to cardiac glycosides and may interfere with digoxin assays. Furthermore, several other herbal medicines have been identified with the ability to interfere with drug monitoring for digoxin, such as Dan Shen, Chan Su, *Uzara* root and Asian ginseng (Dasgupta 2003). According to Dasgupta, monitoring free digoxin eliminates the interference from Dan Shen and Chan Su, but is not useful in overcoming interference by Siberian or Asian ginseng. For these herbs, using the EMIT urine test or the Bayer, Randox, Roche or Beckman assays is appropriate.

WARFARIN

Warfarin is an important anticoagulant drug with a narrow therapeutic index. If blood levels become elevated, potentially serious consequences can arise if bleeding complications develop, whereas reduced blood levels can result in failure to protect the patient from thromboembolic events. Pharmacologically, the anticoagulant effect is dependent on its ability to interfere with hepatic synthesis of vitamin K-dependent clotting factors. As such, any significant changes to vitamin K ingestion can alter the drug's activity. Common foods with high vitamin K levels (>100 micrograms/100 g) are: beef (liver), broccoli, cabbage, cauliflower, egg yolk, kale, lettuce, spinach, canola oil (rapeseed) and soybean oil.

Pharmacodynamic interactions

Pharmacodynamic interactions can theoretically occur when other medicines with coagulant or anticoagulant activity are used concurrently. Medicines with antiplatelet activity, such as ginger and garlic, can theoretically increase the risk of bruising or bleeding when taken concurrently with warfarin. Other herbal medicines suspected to potentiate the pharmacological effects of warfarin include guarana and bilberry in very high doses. Alternatively, herbs containing naturally occurring coumarins exhibit weak anticoagulant activity, if any at all (unless converted to dicoumarol as a result of improper storage), so do not necessarily pose an additional bleeding risk (see also Chapter 9).

The case of *Ginkgo biloba* is a curious one, as there is evidence that one of its components, ginkgolide B, is a potent platelet-activating factor antagonist (Smith et al 1996). However, multiple placebo-controlled studies have failed to detect a significant effect on platelet function or coagulation (see monograph for more details). One was an escalating dose study, which found that 120 mg, 240 mg or 480 mg given daily for 14 days did not alter platelet function or coagulation (Bal Dit et al 2003). Interaction studies have further found that the INR does not increase when patients are concurrently taking *Ginkgo biloba* with warfarin (Engelsen et al 2002, Jiang et al 2005). Owing to the serious nature of such potential interactions, a cautious approach is advised.

Pharmacokinetic interactions

Warfarin consists of a pair of enantiomers and is extensively metabolised by CYP1A2, 3A4 and 2C9. Metabolism of the more biologically active isomer, the S form, occurs chiefly by CYP2C9, whereas a minor metabolic pathway is CYP3A4. The less potent R isomer is chiefly metabolised by CYP1A2. Therefore, any alteration to the expression or activity of these specific enzymes can affect the drug's pharmacokinetics.

As is the case with nearly all herbal medicines, predicting the clinical significance of these theoretical interactions is difficult because most evidence currently comes from in vitro and in vivo tests and case reports.

THE RATIONAL USE OF HERBAL AND NATURAL MEDICINES

Since the first few human studies were conducted back in the late 1990s suggesting serious herb-drug interactions could occur, hundreds of further studies have been performed to test whether commonly used herbal medicines have the potential to interact with pharmaceutical drugs. At the time, the media touted the first studies as being the 'tip of the iceberg' and headlines of 'dangerous drug-herb cocktails' were commonplace.

TABLE 8.8 RATIONAL USE OF HERBAL AND NATURAL MEDICINES

- Be informed and seek out unbiased information — do not rely on label claims alone.
- Know the benefits, risks, potential adverse reactions and interactions — additional training and/or access to accurate and updated information is important.
- Do not assume all healthcare professionals have the knowledge to monitor safe use.
- Be aware that medical practitioners' and pharmacists' knowledge of herbal and natural medicines may be limited.
- Ensure that all healthcare professionals involved in a patient's care stay informed of herbal and natural medicine use.
- Take care with children, the elderly and pregnant or lactating women.
- Take care when high-risk medicines are being taken.
- Take care with HIV, cancer or other serious illnesses.
- Know the manufacturer or supplier details.
- Store medicines appropriately.

Over the last 15 years, it has become apparent that the metaphorical iceberg has not emerged and there are, in fact, only a handful of commonly used herbal medicines with the potential to cause serious drug interactions. Medicines with a narrow therapeutic window are of greatest concern (such as warfarin), as are medications used in serious diseases and life-threatening situations such as anti-rejection, anticancer and anti-HIV medication.

As with all drug interactions, safety is greatly improved when patients openly discuss all the medications they are taking, clinicians are informed about the potential for interactions and appropriate steps are taken to avoid or minimise the interaction via separating doses, altering dosage regimens, ceasing some treatments or altering drug dosages. Often careful supervision is all that is required by an informed clinician and diligent patient.

The two algorithms presented in this chapter provide a general guide to help in clinical practice and make sure the key factors are considered. As always, it is important to recognise that using this information in practice requires individual interpretation, because the clinical effects of any interaction, no matter how well documented, will not occur consistently in each patient, each time or to the same degree of intensity. Ultimately, it is the application of current knowledge, together with good observational skills, open communication and clini-

cal experience that will reduce the risk of unwanted interactions and maximise successful outcomes. Table 8.8 lists key steps towards the rational use of herbal and natural medicines.

REFERENCES

Aklillu E et al. Frequent distribution of ultrarapid metabolizers of debrisoquine in an Ethiopian population carrying duplicated and multiduplicated functional CYP2D6 alleles. J Pharmacol Exp Ther 278.1 (1996): 441–446.

Anuchapreeda S et al. Modulation of P-glycoprotein expression and function by curcumin in multidrug-resistant human KB cells. Biochem Pharmacol 64.4 (2002): 573–582.

Bailey DG et al. Grapefruit juice–drug interactions. Br J Clin Pharmacol 46.2 (1998): 101–110.

Bal Dit SC et al. No alteration in platelet function or coagulation induced by EGb761 in a controlled study. Clin Lab Haematol 25.4 (2003): 251–253.

Barone GW et al. Drug interaction between St. John's wort and cyclosporine. Ann Pharmacother 34.9 (2000): 1013–1016.

Baxter NJ et al. Multiple interactions between polyphenols and a salivary proline-rich protein repeat result in complexation and precipitation. Biochemistry 36.18 (1997): 5566–5577.

Becquemont L et al. Effect of grapefruit juice on digoxin pharmacokinetics in humans. Clin Pharmacol Ther 70.4 (2001): 311–316.

Benet LZ, Cummins CL. The drug efflux–metabolism alliance: biochemical aspects. Adv Drug Deliv Rev 50 Suppl 1 (2001): S3–11.

Bhardwaj RK et al. Piperine, a major constituent of black pepper, inhibits human P-glycoprotein and CYP3A4. J Pharmacol Exp Ther 302.2 (2002): 645–650.

Blower P et al. Drug–drug interactions in oncology: why are they important and can they be minimized? Crit Rev Oncol Hematol 55.2 (2005): 117–142.

Bone K, Mills S. Principles and practice of phytotherapy. London: Elsevier, 2000.

Brune M et al. Iron absorption and phenolic compounds: importance of different phenolic structures. Eur J Clin Nutr 43.8 (1989): 547–557.

Butterweck V et al. Solubilized hypericin and pseudohypericin from Hypericum perforatum exert antidepressant activity in the forced swimming test. Planta Med 64.4 (1998): 291–294.

Castro AF, Altenberg GA. Inhibition of drug transport by genistein in multidrug-resistant cells expressing P-glycoprotein. Biochem Pharmacol 53.1 (1997): 89–93.

Chang TK et al. Distinct role of bilobalide and ginkgolide A in the modulation of rat CYP2B1 and CYP3A23 gene expression by Ginkgo biloba extract in cultured hepatocytes. Drug Metab Dispos 34.2 (2006a): 234–42.

Chang TK et al. Effect of Ginkgo biloba extract on procarcinogen-bioactivating human CYP1 enzymes: identification of isorhamnetin, kaempferol, and quercetin as potent inhibitors of CYP1B1. Toxicol Appl Pharmacol 213.1 (2006b): 18–26.

Chatterjee SS et al. Influence of the Ginkgo extract EGb 761 on rat liver cytochrome P450 and steroid metabolism and excretion in rats and man. J Pharm Pharmacol 57.5 (2005): 641–650.

Choi JS, Li X. Enhanced diltiazem bioavailability after oral administration of diltiazem with quercetin to rabbits. Int J Pharm 297.1–2 (2005): 1–8.

Chung SY et al. Inhibition of P-glycoprotein by natural products in human breast cancer cells. Arch Pharm Res 28.7 (2005): 823–828.

Dasgupta A. Review of abnormal laboratory test results and toxic effects due to use of herbal medicines. Am J Clin Pathol 120.1 (2003): 127–137.

Den Boer ML et al. The modulating effect of PSC 833, cyclosporin A, verapamil and genistein on in vitro cytotoxicity and intracellular content of daunorubicin in childhood acute lymphoblastic leukemia. Leukemia 12.6 (1998): 912–920.

Di Marco MP et al. The effect of grapefruit juice and Seville orange juice on the pharmacokinetics of dextromethorphan: the role of gut CYP3A and P-glycoprotein. Life Sci 71.10 (2002): 1149–1160.

Doherty MM, Charman WN. The mucosa of the small intestine: how clinically relevant as an organ of drug metabolism? Clin Pharmacokinet 41.4 (2002): 235–253.

Dresser GK et al. Fruit juices inhibit organic anion transporting polypeptide-mediated drug uptake to decrease the oral availability of fexofenadine. Clin Pharmacol Ther 71.1 (2002): 11–20.

Durr D et al. St John's Wort induces intestinal P-glycoprotein/MDR1 and intestinal and hepatic CYP3A4. Clin Pharmacol Ther 68.6 (2000): 598–604.

Eagling VA et al. Inhibition of the CYP3A4-mediated metabolism and P-glycoprotein-mediated transport of the HIV-1 protease inhibitor saquinavir by grapefruit juice components. Br J Clin Pharmacol 48.4 (1999): 543–552.

Edwards DJ et al. 6′,7′-Dihydroxybergamottin in grapefruit juice and Seville orange juice: effects on cyclosporine disposition, enterocyte CYP3A4, and P-glycoprotein. Clin Pharmacol Ther 65.3 (1999): 237–244.

Engelsen J et al. Effect of coenzyme Q10 and Ginkgo biloba on warfarin dosage in stable, long-term warfarin treated outpatients: A randomised, double blind, placebo-crossover trial. Thromb Haemost 87.6 (2002): 1075–1076.

Evans AM. Influence of dietary components on the gastrointestinal metabolism and transport of drugs. Ther Drug Monit 22.1 (2000): 131–136.

Flockhart DA. Drug interactions: cytochrome P450 drug interaction table. Indiana University School of Medicine (2007). Available: http://medicine.iupui.edu/flockhart/table.htm 23/7/2014.

Fukao T et al. The effects of allyl sulfides on the induction of phase II detoxification enzymes and liver injury by carbon tetrachloride. Food Chem Toxicol 42.5 (2004): 743–749.

Gaudineau C et al. Inhibition of human P450 enzymes by multiple constituents of the Ginkgo biloba extract. Biochem Biophys Res Commun 318.4 (2004): 1072–1078.

Glahn RP et al. Inhibition of iron uptake by phytic acid, tannic acid, and ZnCl2: studies using an in vitro digestion/Caco-2 cell model. J Agric Food Chem 50.2 (2002): 390–395.

Greenblatt DJ et al. Ginkgo biloba does not alter clearance of flurbiprofen, a cytochrome P450-2C9 substrate. J Clin Pharmacol 46.2 (2006): 214–221.

Gurley BJ et al. Cytochrome P450 phenotypic ratios for predicting herb–drug interactions in humans. Clin Pharmacol Ther 72.3 (2002): 276–287.

Gurley BJ et al. Effect of milk thistle (Silybum marianum) and black cohosh (Cimicifuga racemosa) supplementation on digoxin pharmacokinetics in humans. Drug Metab Dispos 34.1 (2006): 69–74.

Gurley BJ et al. In vivo assessment of botanical supplementation on human cytochrome P450 phenotypes: Citrus aurantium, Echinacea purpurea, milk thistle, and saw palmetto. Clin Pharmacol Ther 76.5 (2004): 428–440.

Gurley BJ et al. In vivo effects of goldenseal, kava kava, black cohosh, and valerian on human cytochrome P450 1A2, 2D6, 2E1, and 3A4/5 phenotypes. Clin Pharmacol Ther 77.5 (2005): 415–426.

Gurley BJ et al. Pharmacokinetic herb-drug interactions (part 2): drug interactions involving popular botanical dietary supplements and their clinical relevance. Planta Med, 78.13 (2012): 1490–1514.

He N, Edeki T. The inhibitory effects of herbal components on CYP2C9 and CYP3A4 catalytic activities in human liver microsomes. Am J Ther 11.3 (2004): 206–212.

Hennessy M et al. St John's wort increases expression of P-glycoprotein: implications for drug interactions. Br J Clin Pharmacol 53.1 (2002): 75–82.

Hsiu SL et al. Quercetin significantly decreased cyclosporin oral bioavailability in pigs and rats. Life Sci 72.3 (2002): 227–235.

Huupponen R et al. Effect of guar gum, a fibre preparation, on digoxin and penicillin absorption in man. Eur J Clin Pharmacol 26.2 (1984): 279–281.

Ikegawa T et al. Inhibition of P-glycoprotein by orange juice components, polymethoxyflavones in adriamycin-resistant human myelogenous leukemia (K562/ADM) cells. Cancer Lett 160.1 (2000): 21–28.

Ingelman-Sundberg M. Pharmacogenetics of cytochrome P450 and its applications in drug therapy: the past, present and future. Trends Pharmacol Sci 25.4 (2004): 193–200.

Jiang X et al. Effect of ginkgo and ginger on the pharmacokinetics and pharmacodynamics of warfarin in healthy subjects. Br J Clin Pharmacol 59.4 (2005): 425–432.

Jin et al. Enhancement of oral bioavailability of paclitaxel after oral administration of Schisandrol B in rats. Biopharmaceutics & Drug Disposition 31.4 (2010): 264–268.

Jodoin J et al. Inhibition of the multidrug resistance P-glycoprotein activity by green tea polyphenols. Biochim Biophys Acta 1542.1–3 (2002): 149–159.

Johne A et al. Pharmacokinetic interaction of digoxin with an herbal extract from St John's wort (Hypericum perforatum). Clin Pharmacol Ther 66.4 (1999): 338–345.

Kane GC, Lipsky JJ. Drug–grapefruit juice interactions. Mayo Clin Proc 75.9 (2000): 933–942.

Kitagawa S et al. Structure–activity relationships of the inhibitory effects of flavonoids on P-glycoprotein-mediated transport in KB-C2 cells. Biol Pharm Bull 28.12 (2005): 2274–2278.

Kubota Y et al. Pretreatment with Ginkgo biloba extract weakens the hypnosis action of phenobarbital and its plasma concentration in rats. J Pharm Pharmacol 56.3 (2004): 401–405.

Kuo I et al. Effect of Ginkgo biloba extract on rat hepatic microsomal CYP1A activity: role of ginkgolides, bilobalide, and flavonols. Can J Physiol Pharmacol 82.1 (2004): 57–64.

Lin JH. Drug–drug interaction mediated by inhibition and induction of P-glycoprotein. Adv Drug Deliv Rev 55.1 (2003): 53–81.

Lown KS et al. Role of intestinal P-glycoprotein (mdr1) in interpatient variation in the oral bioavailability of cyclosporine. Clin Pharmacol Ther 62.3 (1997): 248–260.

Markowitz JS et al. Multiple doses of saw palmetto (Serenoa repens) did not alter cytochrome P450 2D6 and 3A4 activity in normal volunteers. Clin Pharmacol Ther 74.6 (2003a): 536–542.

Markowitz JS et al. Multiple-dose administration of Ginkgo biloba did not affect cytochrome P-450 2D6 or 3A4 activity in normal volunteers. J Clin Psychopharmacol 23.6 (2003b): 576–581.

Markowitz JS et al. Predicting interactions between conventional medications and botanical products on the basis of in vitro investigations. Mol Nutr Food Res 52.7 (2008): 747–754.

McRae S. Elevated serum digoxin levels in a patient taking digoxin and Siberian ginseng. Can Med Assoc J 155.3 (1996): 293–295.

Meseguer E et al. Life-threatening parkinsonism induced by kava-kava. Mov Disord 17.1 (2002): 195–196.

Mills S. The essential book of herbal medicine. Arkana: Penguin Books, 1991.

Mohutsky MA et al. Ginkgo biloba: evaluation of CYP2C9 drug interactions in vitro and in vivo. Am J Ther 13.1 (2006a): 24–31.

Mohutsky MA et al. Ginkgo biloba: evaluation of CYP2C9 drug interactions in vitro and in vivo. Am J Ther 13.1 (2006b): 24–31.

Moore LB et al. St. John's wort induces hepatic drug metabolism through activation of the pregnane X receptor. Proc Natl Acad Sci USA 97.13 (2000): 7500–7502.

Naranjo CA et al. A method for estimating the probability of adverse drug reactions. Clin Pharmacol Ther 30.2 (1981): 239–245.

Ohnishi A et al. Effect of furanocoumarin derivatives in grapefruit juice on the uptake of vinblastine by Caco-2 cells and on the activity of cytochrome P450 3A4. Br J Pharmacol 130.6 (2000): 1369–1377.

Ohnishi N et al. Studies on interactions between functional foods or dietary supplements and medicines. I. Effects of Ginkgo biloba leaf extract on the pharmacokinetics of diltiazem in rats. Biol Pharm Bull 26.9 (2003): 1315–1320.

Perloff MD et al. Saint John's wort: an in vitro analysis of P-glycoprotein induction due to extended exposure. Br J Pharmacol 134.8 (2001): 1601–1608.

Pirmohamed M, Park BK. Cytochrome P450 enzyme polymorphisms and adverse drug reactions. Toxicology 192.1 (2003): 23–32.

Plouzek CA et al. Inhibition of P-glycoprotein activity and reversal of multidrug resistance in vitro by rosemary extract. Eur J Cancer 35.10 (1999): 1541–1545.

Roby CA et al. St John's Wort: effect on CYP3A4 activity. Clin Pharmacol Ther 67.5 (2000): 451–457.

Romiti N et al. Effects of curcumin on P-glycoprotein in primary cultures of rat hepatocytes. Life Sci 62.25 (1998): 2349–2358.

Ruschitzka F et al. Acute heart transplant rejection due to Saint John's wort. Lancet 355.9203 (2000): 548–549.

Ryu SD, Chung WG. Induction of the procarcinogen-activating CYP1A2 by a herbal dietary supplement in rats and humans. Food Chem Toxicol 41.6 (2003): 861–866.

Sadzuka Y et al. Efficacies of tea components on doxorubicin induced antitumor activity and reversal of multidrug resistance. Toxicol Lett 114.1–3 (2000): 155–162.

Scambia G et al. Quercetin potentiates the effect of adriamycin in a multidrug-resistant MCF-7 human breast-cancer cell line: P-glycoprotein as a possible target. Cancer Chemother Pharmacol 34.6 (1994): 459–464.

Shinozuka K et al. Feeding of Ginkgo biloba extract (GBE) enhances gene expression of hepatic cytochrome P-450 and attenuates the hypotensive effect of nicardipine in rats. Life Sci 70.23 (2002): 2783–2792.

Smith PF et al. The neuroprotective properties of the Ginkgo biloba leaf: a review of the possible relationship to platelet-activating factor (PAF). J Ethnopharmacol 50.3 (1996): 131–139.

Soldner A et al. Grapefruit juice activates P-glycoprotein-mediated drug transport. Pharm Res 16.4 (1999): 478–485.

Spahn–Langguth H, Langguth P. Grapefruit juice enhances intestinal absorption of the P-glycoprotein substrate talinolol. Eur J Pharm Sci 12.4 (2001): 361–367.

Spillane PK et al. Neurological manifestations of kava intoxication. Med J Aust 167.3 (1997): 172–173.

Sugiyama T et al. Ginkgo biloba extract modifies hypoglycemic action of tolbutamide via hepatic cytochrome P450 mediated mechanism in aged rats. Life Sci 75.9 (2004a): 1113–1122.

Sugiyama T et al. Induction and recovery of hepatic drug metabolizing enzymes in rats treated with Ginkgo biloba extract. Food Chem Toxicol 42.6 (2004b): 953–957.

Takanaga H et al. Inhibition of vinblastine efflux mediated by P-glycoprotein by grapefruit juice components in Caco-2 cells. Biol Pharm Bull 21.10 (1998): 1062–1066.

Takanaga H et al. Polymethoxylated flavones in orange juice are inhibitors of P-glycoprotein but not cytochrome P450 3A4. J Pharmacol Exp Ther 293.1 (2000): 230–236.

Tankanow R et al. Interaction study between digoxin and a preparation of hawthorn (Crataegus oxyacantha). J Clin Pharmacol 43.6 (2003): 637–642.

Tian R et al. Effects of grapefruit juice and orange juice on the intestinal efflux of P-glycoprotein substrates. Pharm Res 19.6 (2002): 802–809.

USFDA (United States Food and Drug Administration). [Cytochrome enzymes]. Available online: www.fda.gov/ 23/7/2014.

Von Moltke LL et al. Inhibition of human cytochromes P450 by components of Ginkgo biloba. J Pharm Pharmacol 56.8 (2004): 1039–1044

Wagner D et al. Intestinal drug efflux: formulation and food effects. Adv Drug Deliv Rev 50 (Suppl 1) (2001): S13–S31.

Wang YH et al. Lethal quercetin-digoxin interaction in pigs. Life Sci 74.10 (2004): 1191–1197.

Wang Z et al. The effects of St John's wort (Hypericum perforatum) on human cytochrome P450 activity. Clin Pharmacol Ther 70.4 (2001): 317–326.

Yale SH, Glurich I. Analysis of the inhibitory potential of Ginkgo biloba, Echinacea purpurea, and Serenoa repens on the metabolic activity of cytochrome P450 3A4, 2D6, and 2C9. J Altern Complement Med 11.3 (2005): 433–439.

Zhang S, Morris ME. Effect of the flavonoids biochanin A and silymarin on the P-glycoprotein-mediated transport of digoxin and vinblastine in human intestinal Caco-2 cells. Pharm Res 20.8 (2003): 1184–1191.

Zhao LZ et al. Induction of propranolol metabolism by Ginkgo biloba extract EGb 761 in rats. Curr Drug Metab 7.6 (2006): 577–587.

CHAPTER 9

PREOPERATIVE CARE: CONSIDERATIONS

Reducing the risk of surgery and maximising successful outcomes is the common effort of surgeons, anaesthetists, doctors, nurses and other healthcare professionals. However, few consider the influence of herbal and natural medicines and whether this has the potential to alter outcomes. Even fewer consider the effects of these medicines after surgery. This chapter explores the potential of herbal and natural medicines to hinder surgical outcomes and also introduces the concept of using these medicines beneficially.

EXTENT OF CM USE

According to a number of hospital surveys conducted in the United States and in Australia, use of complementary medicines (CMs) is well established among surgical patients (Braun & Cohen 2011, Braun et al 2006a, Grauer 2004, Kaye et al 2000, Leung et al 2001, Norred 2002, Norred et al 2000, Silverstein & Spiegel 2001, Tsen et al 2000).

One survey of 3106 patients attending pre-operative clinics in the USA found that 51% were using CMs, and that women were more likely users than men (Tsen et al 2000). Age was also a factor, with patients aged between 40 and 60 years greater consumers of CMs. Overall, only 21% of patients sought advice from a healthcare provider about supplement use, whereas the majority cited friends and family or their own decision as reasons for taking these medicines.

Another survey of 1017 patients presenting for pre-anaesthetic evaluation found that approximately one in three were taking one or more herb-related compounds (Kaye et al 2000). Disturbingly, nearly 70% of these patients did not report use when they were asked during routine anaesthetic assessment. Lack of communication was also detected in a review of 2560 patients, which identified that 39% were taking natural supplements, with herbal medicines being the most popular (Leung et al 2001). Of these, 44% did not consult with their primary-care doctor and 56% did not inform their anaesthetist before surgery.

Similar trends have also been identified among Australian surgical patients (Braun et al 2006a, Grauer 2004). A survey of 508 presurgical inpatients at two tertiary hospitals found that in the 2 weeks before admission, 46% had used CMs, of which 38% were self-prescribed (Braun et al 2006a). Just over half these patients planned to continue using them while in hospital. During the 2 weeks before admission, 64% had not discussed use with any community-based or hospital-based healthcare professional. Similar to findings of other studies, patients using CMs were most likely to be female, and to have pursued higher education and earn above-average incomes. Interestingly, this study found that age was not predictive of use, and that older patients were just as likely as young patients to be using CM. Importantly, 58% of surgical patients did not discuss their use with a hospital doctor, nurse or pharmacist. When patients were asked why they did not tell hospital staff, it was not because they feared being judged negatively, but overwhelmingly because they were not asked. This was also the first Australian study to ask patients about their interest in hospital-based CM therapies; 85% expressed an interest.

A recent study of cardiothoracic surgical patients at a private hospital in Melbourne also revealed that CM use is widespread by this population before surgery. Nearly half (51%) took CMs in the two weeks before admission and, interestingly, medical doctors were the main prescribers. The most popular supplements were fish oils and multivitamins, and use was not significantly associated with gender, education or income. Many patients did not tell hospital staff about use, not because of fear of being judged negatively, but, similarly, mainly because they were not asked (Braun & Cohen 2011).

Poor communication was identified again at two other hospitals whereby 20% of surgical patients had used vitamin supplements and 14% herbal medicines in the previous 6 weeks, but only 28% had informed hospital staff (Grauer 2004). Once again, the majority of patients had self-selected their treatment.

These findings pose several important questions, such as whether surgeons, anaesthetists, doctors or pharmacists are aware of the potential safety issues associated with CMs, routinely ask patients about herbal and natural medicines in a way that encourages open dialogue and have the knowledge and resources to interpret the answers. Survey results published in 2001 found that, although doctors did ask about herbal and natural medicine use, most did not check with reference texts for more information (Silverstein & Spiegel 2001). Disturbingly, the survey also detected an obvious lack of knowledge about common herbal medicines among doctors. A more extensive study was conducted with hospital doctors and pharmacists at an Australian tertiary hospital (Braun et al 2006b). The study of 127 surgeons, anaesthetists, doctors and pharmacists found that 68% thought CMs could be dangerous and that patients' use needed to be monitored; however, only 28% routinely asked patients about CM use. All groups lacked knowledge and confidence in dealing with

CM, and 81% felt they had insufficient knowledge to be able to identify whether a CM product could adversely affect patient care. Despite this, few checked for side effects or interactions when patients using CMs were identified.

When patients do report using herbal and natural medicines, hospital doctors and pharmacists do not routinely document this information in patients' charts, making effective communication even more difficult (Braun et al 2006b, Cohen et al 2002). Cohen et al (2002) found the prevalence of supplement use was 64% in a group of 212 patients, but only 35% of all supplements were recorded on patients' charts.

ASSESSING POTENTIAL FOR ADVERSE EFFECTS

The use of CM by surgical patients should not pose any serious concern, unless they have the potential to cause adverse events that would negatively affect the outcome of surgery and impede recovery. Potential unwanted effects, such as increased bleeding risk, sympathomimetic effects or detrimental interactions with medicines commonly used in the perioperative period, are some examples.

Developing a list of herbal and natural supplements with a realistic potential to cause adverse effects in surgery is difficult at the current time, as the pharmacology of many of these medicines, including pharmacodynamic and pharmacokinetic properties, has yet to be fully elucidated. Until evidence from controlled clinical studies is available, other evidence will be used but should be interpreted cautiously.

SAFETY, SIDE EFFECTS AND INTERACTIONS WITH OTHER MEDICINES

The risk of harm associated with the use of CMs is largely unknown; however, it is likely to be greatest in high-risk surgery; that is, when the surgical procedure to be undertaken and the patient's health status put the patient at real risk of serious complications. Factors such as preexisting fluid and electrolyte status, cardiorespiratory performance, comorbidities and medical pretreatments need to be considered when assessing safety in patients (Girbes 2000). Additionally, the type of surgical procedure should be considered; in particular, those procedures in which increased bleeding would be a serious complication (e.g. orthopaedics or neurosurgery) or those that put significant physical strain on the patient (e.g. coronary bypass) would be considered high risk.

BLEEDING RISK

Surgery is often associated with some degree of blood loss, but this is usually limited by the body's haemostatic mechanisms, which finely regulate interactions between components on the blood vessel walls, circulating platelets and plasma proteins. A retrospective survey of adverse surgical outcomes in several US hospitals found that postoperative bleeding accounted for 10.8% of all surgical adverse events, making it the third most frequent adverse surgical event (Gawande et al 1999). In practice, whether bleeding risk is a serious concern is usually dictated by the type of surgery to be undertaken. For example, minor dental procedures would not be as seriously affected by increased bleeding as neurosurgery.

A number of explanations may account for increased bleeding, such as undiagnosed clotting disorders, liver disease or the preoperative use of certain medicines such as antiplatelet agents. Over time, it has become recognised that some CMs also have the potential to influence the body's haemostatic response. Initially evidence was derived from case reports suggesting CM use was associated with bleeding or from in vitro tests indicating antiplatelet activity; however, an increasing number of clinical studies are now being published to more rigorously determine which CM products cause clinically significant bleeding.

Herbal medicines and food supplements

Whether preoperative use of herbal medicine alters bleeding risk is difficult to determine because few controlled trials are available for this specific population. Evidence is usually extrapolated from other sources to identify those medicines with suspected antiplatelet or anticoagulant activity and, while still largely speculative, this will continue to provide a guide until more robust evidence is available. However, care should be taken not to assume that when a CM-drug interaction exists with an anticoagulant drug (e.g. warfarin) it is always due to a pharmacodynamic interaction and therefore the CM alone has significant bleeding activity. Glucosamine provides a good example of this conundrum.

Glucosamine

Glucosamine products are extremely popular and mainly used for the symptomatic relief of osteoarthritis in the shorter term and for chondroprotection when used long-term. In 2007, Knudsen and Sokol searched the US Food and Drug Administration (FDA) MedWatch database and identified 20 case reports suggesting that D-glucosamine or glucosamine-chondroitin sulfate use with warfarin was associated with altered coagulation (manifested by increased INR, or increased bleeding or bruising) (Knudsen & Sokol 2008). This is a relatively small number of cases given the great popularity of glucosamine supplementation, particularly in older adults and the number of prescriptions written for warfarin.

Of the 20 case reports, four included use of warfarin and glucosamine alone and in 15 cases, use was also combined with chondroitin sulphate. In three cases, consumers were also using agents known to affect INR, thereby discounting their value in determining causality. Serious outcomes such as hospitalisation were reported in five of 20 cases and six others reported excessive bruising or bleeding. Most of the reports were from consumers and lacked important details, such as use of other medications, time frames for use and also follow up observations when glucosamine was stopped.

In addition, the WHO-adverse drug reaction database contains 21 more detailed reports of possible warfarin–glucosamine interactions. The reports tend to come from industry or healthcare professionals and are more comprehensive than the consumer reports in the United States (Knudsen & Sokol 2008). These reports more strongly suggest that glucosamine potentiates the anticoagulant effects of warfarin. Of the 21 cases, 11 described people on long-term warfarin therapy with a stable INR before taking glucosamine. Eight patients experienced a change to INR within 3 weeks and for 5 patients, this happened within 1–3 months. Importantly, the change in INR resolved in 81% of the 21 individuals when glucosamine was stopped.

Regarding safety in surgery, the question remains, does glucosamine used on its own increase the risk of serious bleeding? Until further research can be conducted to determine whether the interaction is pharmacodynamic or pharmacokinetic, it is recommended that patients cease use at least 1 week prior to major surgery and then recommence glucosamine treatment when it is safe to do so. Considering this is a long-term therapy, suspending use for several weeks should not pose any major issue for patients.

Besides the problems arising from extrapolating information from drug–CM interaction reports, difficulties also arise when evidence is contradictory, making clinical recommendations even more difficult. The herb *Tanacetum parthenium*, also known as feverfew, provides a good example. Several test-tube studies and animal models have observed inhibition of platelet aggregation (Heptinstall et al 1988, Jain & Kulkarni 1999, Makheja & Bailey 1982); however, no significant effects were seen in a small study of 10 patients receiving feverfew (Biggs et al 1982).

The problem of inconsistent information can add to practitioners' confusion, as some databases are infrequently updated or give undue weight to case reports and seemingly less consideration of safety information derived from clinical studies. The case of ginkgo biloba illustrates this point.

Ginkgo biloba

Ginkgo biloba is a popular herbal medicine used mainly for cognitive decline and peripheral vascular diseases. Concern over whether G. *biloba* significantly increases bleeding first arose in response to several case reports describing haemorrhage during or after surgery (Hauser et al 2002, Schneider et al 2002), and evidence that one of its components, ginkgolide B, is a platelet-activating factor antagonist (Smith et al 1996). In the following years, at least 10 clinical studies were conducted that found no evidence of significant bleeding or platelet effects due to G. *biloba* ingestion (Aruna & Naidu 2007, Bal Dit et al 2003, Beckert et al 2007, Carlson et al 2007, Engelsen et al 2003, Gardner et al 2007, Kohler et al 2004, Jiang et al 2005, Lovera et al 2007, Wolf 2006). Studies have included young healthy volunteers, older adults, people with multiple sclerosis and people using warfarin or aspirin at the same time as G. *biloba*. An escalating-dose study found that 120 mg, 240 mg or 480 mg given daily for 14 days did not alter platelet function or coagulation (Bal Dit et al 2003). Only one clinical study demonstrated that EGb761 (80 mg/day) produced a significant reduction in blood viscosity after 30 days' treatment (Galduroz et al 2007). In 2011, a meta-analysis of 18 RCTs was conducted and concluded that standardised G. *biloba* therapy was not associated with a higher bleeding risk, thereby providing level 1 evidence that *ginkgo biloba* is safe.

Food supplements contain concentrated forms of dietary foods, such as fish oils or fibre. Herbal and food supplements overlap in many cases because various herbs are also eaten as foods (e.g. ginger). Keeping this in mind, it is not unusual to find evidence that suggests normal dietary intake of a food does not appreciably alter bleeding risk, whereas ingesting concentrated products will. For example, 4 g ginger daily does not alter platelet aggregation or fibrinogen levels according to one clinical study, whereas a dose of 10 g/day significantly reduces platelet aggregation according to another (Bordia et al 1997).

Commonly used herbal medicines and food supplements available over the counter (OTC) that have been found to inhibit platelet aggregation under clinical test conditions include garlic, ginger root, onion, policosanol and pine bark extract (Araghi-Niknam et al 2000, Arruzazabala et al 2002, Bordia et al 1975, 1997, Harris et al 1990, Jung et al 1991). Often, very high doses above normal dietary intakes are required to produce these results.

Fish oils

Fish oil supplements are extremely popular and considered by some healthcare professionals to increase the risk of bleeding in surgery. A search through the Medline database reveals several case reports where bleeding episodes are attributed to fish oil ingestion (Buckley et al 2004, Jalili & Dehpour 2007, McClaskey & Michalets 2007). In each of these cases, the person affected was elderly and also taking warfarin.

In contrast to this, numerous clinical intervention studies indicate no increased risk of bleeding. In 2008, Harris examined 19 clinical studies that used doses of fish oil varying from 1 g/day to 21 g/day in patients undergoing major vascular surgery (coronary artery bypass grafting, endarterectomy) or femoral artery puncture for either diagnostic cardiac catheterisation or percutaneous transluminal coronary angioplasty. Of note, in 16 studies patients were taking aspirin and in three studies patients were taking heparin. The review concluded that the risk of bleeding was virtually non-existent. Frequent comments accompanying the studies were 'no difference in clinically significant bleeding noted' or 'no patient suffered from bleeding complications'. The same conclusion was reached in a 2008 review that stated no published studies had reported clinically significant bleeding episodes among patients treated with antiplatelet drugs and fish oils (3–7 g/day) (Harris et al 2008).

Similarly, in 2013, a clinical audit of over 900 elective cardiothoracic surgical patients at the Alfred Hospital (Australia) found the use of 3000 mg of omega-3 EFAs before surgery did not significantly increase the incidence of re-admission to theatre due to bleeding or alter blood transfusion requirements (Braun et al 2014).

In light of this body of evidence, it is apparent that fish oil supplementation does not significantly increase serious bleeding risk.

Salicylate-containing herbs

Many salicylate-containing herbs, such as willowbark and meadowsweet, are suspected of having blood-thinning activity based on their chemical relationship to aspirin. When these herbs are ingested, salicylic acid is formed, which accounts for some of their anti-inflammatory and antipyretic activity. The synthesis of aspirin involves adding an acetyl group to salicylic acid, which not only reduces the irritant effect of the salicylic acid but also confers an antiplatelet effect. The conversion of salicylic acid to acetylsalicylic acid does not occur in the body, so it is unlikely that these herbs will have an appreciable effect on bleeding (Forrelli 2003). This has been borne out in a clinical study that found a therapeutic dose of *Salicis cortex* extract (willowbark containing 240 mg salicin per daily dose) produced a total serum salicylate concentration bioequivalent to 50 mg acetylsalicylate, which

had a minimal effect on platelet aggregation (Krivoy et al 2001).

Coumarin-containing herbs

A similar confusion has arisen surrounding the presence of naturally occurring coumarin compounds in herbs. Coumarin compounds are benzo-alpha-pyrones and are found in popular herbal medicines such as dong quai, alfalfa, celery, fenugreek and red clover. Nearly all natural coumarin compounds contain a hydroxyl or methoxy group in position 7, whereas dicoumarol and related anticoagulants are hydroxlated in the 4 position (Bone & Mills 2000). This difference in chemical structure is important because it influences the entity's potential to induce significant anticoagulant activity. It has been estimated that natural coumarins, which naturally are not substituted at the 4 position, have one-thousandth the anticoagulant activity of dicoumarol, so are unlikely to cause significant bleeding episodes (Bone & Mills 2000). As an example, a placebo-controlled study failed to identify significant changes to platelet aggregation, fibrinolytic activity or fibrinogen for the herbal medicine fenugreek, even though it contains naturally occurring coumarins (Bordia et al 1997).

Nutritional supplements

The safety of using preoperative nutritional supplements is also largely based on suspected antiplatelet or anticoagulant activity and is poorly researched. As such, identifying key supplements that increase bleeding risk is not straightforward and contradictory evidence also exists. Vitamin E provides a good example.

Although widely cited as affecting bleeding times, clinical studies with vitamin E supplements have produced conflicting results in recent years. According to one clinical study, a daily dose of 1200 IU of vitamin E (800 mg of D-alpha-tocopherol) taken for 28 days had no effect on platelet aggregation or coagulation compared with controls (Morinobu et al 2002). A dose of 600 mg (900 IU) of RRR-alpha-tocopherol taken for 12 weeks did not alter coagulation activity compared with placebo in another clinical study (Kitagawa & Mino 1989). However, doses of 75 IU and 450 IU have been shown to decrease platelet aggregation in human subjects in other studies (Calzada et al 1997, Mabile et al 1999).

ELECTROLYTE STATUS AND BLOOD-PRESSURE EFFECTS

Whether preoperative use of CM products significantly alters electrolyte status or blood pressure and thus increases the surgical risk is unknown and still largely speculative. Controlled trials are unavailable, so evidence is extrapolated from other sources to identify those medicines with suspected activity.

Glycyrrhiza glabra

There are a small number of OTC herbal medicines with the potential to induce hypokalaemia, sodium retention or significant cardiovascular effects. The best documented of these is probably *Glycyrrhiza glabra* (licorice), which has significant pharmacological activity and the potential to cause adverse effects when used long-term in high doses. Determining a dose that is safe for all is difficult, as there is a great deal of individual variation in susceptibility to the herb's effects. One dose-response study that tested licorice in a variety of individuals has identified that doses as low as 50 g (75 mg glycyrrhetinic acid) taken daily for 2 weeks are capable of raising blood pressure in sensitive individuals (Sigurjonsdottir et al 2001). A return to baseline levels may take several weeks according to Commission E (Blumenthal et al 2000) and is also likely to vary between individuals.

G. glabra raises blood pressure and produces oedema by significantly decreasing serum concentrations of cortisol, ACTH and aldosterone, and increasing renin and sodium levels in a dose-dependent manner (Al Qarawi et al 2002). Glycyrrhetinic acid is the main constituent responsible, causing an 11-beta-hydroxylase deficiency secondary to an inability to convert 11-deoxycortisol or deoxycorticosterone into active glucocorticoids, cortisol and corticosterone (Heilmann et al 1999).

Paullinia cupana

Based on the herb's caffeine content and diuretic activity, *Paullinia cupana* (guarana) may potentially induce hypokalaemia and unwanted cardiovascular effects when used in excessive doses. Although these effects have not been tested in controlled clinical settings, results obtained for caffeine and the following case report provide some evidence of cardiovascular activity. A 25-year-old woman with preexisting mitral valve prolapse was reported as developing intractable ventricular fibrillation after consuming a 'natural energy' guarana health drink containing a high concentration of caffeine (Cannon et al 2001).

Panax ginseng

Despite *Panax ginseng*'s reputation for altering blood pressure, current evidence is contradictory and difficult to assess. Both hypotensive and hypertensive effects have been observed in animal studies with this herb, also known as Korean ginseng. However, interpreting the significance of these results is difficult, because injectable forms are sometimes used. Clinical observations are also contradictory, with both elevations and reductions in blood pressure reported (Valli et al 2002).

TISSUE PERFUSION AND REPERFUSION INJURY

Unfortunately, many critically ill surgical patients survive surgery only to die of infection or organ dysfunction over the ensuing days or weeks (Nathens et al 2002). The precise mechanism by which organ dysfunction occurs is unclear; however, there is increasing evidence that tissue injury is mediated at least in part by reactive oxygen species derived from inflammatory cells and the vascular damage caused by ischaemia–reperfusion injury. Based on this theory, research has begun to investigate the effects of pre- and postsurgical treatment with several medicines, such as antioxidant supplements. Probably the most research conducted to date has involved coenzyme Q10.

Coenzyme Q10 pretreatment

Clinical studies investigating the effects of oral coenzyme Q10 (CoQ10) supplementation before cardiac surgery suggest it may improve postoperative cardiac function, efficiency of mitochondrial energy production, reduce intraoperative myocardial structural damage and significantly reduce hospital stays (Chello et al 1996, Chen et al 1994, Judy et al 1993, Rosenfeldt et al 2002, Taggart et al 1996, Tanaka et al 1982, Zhou et al 1999).

One placebo-controlled study involving 100 patients investigated the effects of oral CoQ10 (30–60 mg) taken 6 days before surgery and found that treatment significantly lowered the incidence of low cardiac output during recovery (Tanaka et al 1982). These results suggested that presurgical treatment with CoQ10 increased myocardial tolerance to ischaemia during surgery. A smaller, randomised double-blind study also found reduced incidence of low cardiac output during recovery with CoQ10 pretreatment and a lowered incidence of elevated left atrial pressure (Chen et al 1994). Additionally, ventricular myocardial structure was better preserved in patients receiving CoQ10 before surgery, as measured by electron microscopy.

Besides having beneficial effects on cardiac output, pretreatment with CoQ10 has a number of other effects. A randomised, placebo-controlled study of 40 patients undergoing elective coronary artery bypass found that CoQ10 (150 mg/day) taken for 7 days before surgery produced a significantly lower incidence of ventricular arrhythmias during the recovery period compared with placebo (Chello et al 1994). Additionally, mean dopamine dosage required to maintain stable haemodynamics was significantly lower with CoQ10 pretreatment. One placebo-controlled study involving high-risk surgical patients used 100 mg/day CoQ10 for 14 days before surgery and for 30 days afterwards (Judy et al 1993). This treatment regimen dramatically hastened the recovery to 3–5 days, compared with 15–30 with a placebo, and significantly reduced the incidence of complications.

Another double-blind RCT investigated the effects of preoperative high-dose CoQ10 therapy (300 mg/day) in patients undergoing elective cardiac surgery (mainly coronary artery bypass graft surgery or valve replacement) (Rosenfeldt et al 2005). The study of 121 patients found that approximately 2 weeks of active treatment resulted in significantly increased CoQ10 levels in the serum, atrial myocardium and mitochondria compared to a placebo; however, no effects on duration of hospital stay were seen. Active treatment improved subjective assessment of physical QOL (+13%) in the CoQ10 group compared with the placebo; however, the authors point out that physical quality of life does not necessarily indicate improved cardiac pump function and further studies are required with larger sample sizes to clarify the role of CoQ10 in cardiac surgery.

CLINICAL NOTE — ALFRED HOSPITAL'S INTEGRATIVE CARDIAC WELLNESS PROGRAM

The increasing incidence of high-risk and elderly patients presenting for major surgery has presented a challenge for surgeons, due to the associated increased mortality and complication rate and costs. Over the last few years at the Alfred Hospital Melbourne, Australia, researchers in the Cardiothoracic Surgical Research Unit, led by Professor Frank Rosenfeldt, have developed regimens of metabolic therapy with the pyrimidine precursor orotic acid, and the antioxidant and mitochondrial respiratory chain component CoQ10. These regimens improve the response of the ageing and failing heart to hypoxia, ischaemia/reperfusion injury and aerobic stress such as occur during cardiac surgery. Omega-3 fatty acids and the antioxidant alpha-lipoic acid have been added to the metabolic cocktail, in light of emerging research showing benefits for this population. The metabolic regimen is now being combined with holistic therapy comprising inpatient and outpatient wellness education to create a novel integrative program of 'perioperative rehabilitation'. This approach is known as the Integrative Cardiac Wellness Program and officially commenced at the Alfred Hospital in 2008, and has been led by Professor Frank Rosenfeldt and Dr Lesley Braun..

For more information, see www.thealfred.org .au/icwg/.

Most recently, a 3-year prospective randomised clinical trial was completed at the Alfred Hospital in Melbourne. This involved 117 patients of mean age 65 years who were undergoing elective coronary artery bypass graft and/or valve surgery with or without coronary bypass (Leong et al 2007). Coenzyme Q10 (300 mg/day) was administered together with other natural metabolic agents (magnesium orotate 1200 mg/day, alpha lipoic acid 100 mg/day, omega-3 fatty acids 3000 mg/day and selenium 200 mcg/day) or identical placebos for a minimum of 2 weeks before and 1 month after surgery. Active treatment produced a highly significant reduction in the release of plasma troponin I at 24 hours ($P = 0.003$) postoperatively, indicating reduced cardiac muscle damage. Additionally, patients undergoing coronary artery bypass surgery experienced a significant 50% reduction in postoperative atrial fibrillation. It was also found that patients in the placebo group stayed 17% (6%–30%) longer in hospital than those in the metabolic group ($P = 0.002$). This result equates to an extra 1.3 days. These findings have major implications for patients' long-term mortality, quality of life and hospital costs.

The encouraging results obtained from CoQ10 in cardiac surgery may have special significance for the elderly, because recovery of cardiac function in this group is inferior to younger patients. It has been suggested that the aged myocardium is more sensitive to stress, and may therefore not be as well equipped to deal with the physical stress sustained during surgery. Rosenfeldt et al (1999) confirmed this theory, demonstrating an age-related deficit in myocardial performance after aerobic and ischaemic stress and the capacity of CoQ10 treatment to correct age-specific diminished recovery of function.

Although most clinical research has been conducted in patients undergoing cardiac surgery, one study suggested that pretreatment may have benefits in other situations. The effects of randomly assigned supplemental oral CoQ10 (150 mg/day) in 30 patients undergoing elective vascular surgery for abdominal aortic aneurysm or obstructive aorto-iliac disease abdominal clamping also produced positive results (Chello et al 1996). Pretreatment for 7 days before surgery reduced the degree of peroxidative damage during abdominal aortic cross-clamping compared with that seen in the placebo group.

Although CoQ10 is the most studied nutritional supplement for cardiac surgery support, investigation into others has also begun.

INTERACTIONS WITH MEDICINES COMMONLY USED DURING SURGERY

An interaction is said to have occurred if there is an alteration to the predicted effect of one substance when it has been given together with another. Owing to this lack of predictability, the term 'interaction' often has a negative connotation, but interactions can also be manipulated to advantage and offer potential benefits to patients.

As discussed in Chapter 8, herb–drug interactions have not been as extensively researched in clinical studies as pharmaceutical drug interactions. As such, recommendations are based on the best available evidence at the time of writing, chiefly sourced from primary biomedical literature. Furthermore, clinicians using this information in practice are advised that it requires individual interpretation, as the clinical effects of any interaction, no matter how well documented, will not occur consistently in each patient, each time or to the same degree of intensity.

Although there are a myriad of different surgical procedures currently being performed in hospitals and day-surgery centres, the same general drug classes tend to be used. These are analgesics and anaesthetics. In both cases, concurrent use of herbal and natural medicines theoretically has the potential to produce unwanted interactions or, alternatively, beneficial interactions.

ANALGESICS AND ANTI-INFLAMMATORIES

Pain is a complex phenomenon involving both an alteration to normal neuronal activity and an individual's perception of that alteration. As such, the sensation of pain is largely subjective and greatly influenced by psychological factors. A number of different medicines are used to relieve pain in the hospital setting.

Opioid analgesics, such as pethidine and morphine, are effective for most kinds of pain, inducing a sense of calm. Unfortunately, their use is associated with a number of unwanted effects such as nausea and vomiting, reduced gastrointestinal motility, constipation, drowsiness and the development of physical and psychological dependence.

Currently, controlled clinical trials to identify significant interactions are lacking; however, it is possible to make some theoretical predictions. From a pharmacodynamic perspective, concurrent use of another medicine that can further induce constipation, nausea or sedation has the potential to make these symptoms more troublesome (e.g. supplements containing calcium, iron, phytostanols or sterols). Medicines that have mild laxative effects, such as dandelion root and herb, psyllium husks, probiotics and yellow dock root, may be beneficial. Besides using CM products to reduce adverse effects, techniques that can reduce the perception of pain have the potential to augment analgesic effectiveness (e.g. acupuncture, massage, biofeedback, meditation and possibly aromatherapy).

In regards to potential pharmacokinetic interactions, the medicines tramadol and oxycodone are metabolised by CYP 2D6. The herb goldenseal (*Hydrastis canadensis*) contains isoquinoline alkaloids which significantly inhibit CYP 2D6 activity with the potential to raise serum drug levels if used at the same time (Gurley et al 2012). It will also reduce the conversion of codeine to morphine which is mediated by CYP 2D6. This botanical medicine is taken to treat and prevent common respiratory tract infections and often included together with *Echinacea* species in combination products that rank among the top-selling products in the United States.

Naproxen is chiefly metabolised by CYPs 2C9 and 1A2, paracetamol by CYPs 2E1 and 1A2. A variety of common substances can induce CYP 1A2 such as tobacco smoking, Brussels sprouts and char-grilled meats and therefore reduce serum levels, whereas grapefruit juice can inhibit CYP 1A2. Clinical studies in both young and elderly adults show that garlic oil products taken at a dose of 500 mg three times daily will inhibit CYP 2E1 (Gurley et al 2012). The anxiolytic herb kava kava also exhibits inhibition of CYP 2E1 clinically (Gurley et al 2005b), which mean serum levels of paracetamol can theoretically be increased with this combination.

ANAESTHETICS

Local anaesthesia is often used to eliminate pain during minor surgery. Local anaesthetics tend to have an intense and short-lived effect, although this depends largely on the technique of administration and whether a vasoconstrictor agent has been co-administered. General anaesthesia can involve the use of several medicines in addition to the anaesthetic agent, in order to dry secretions (e.g. antimuscarinic agents), reduce anxiety (e.g. benzodiazepines), produce amnesia and provide postoperative pain relief.

Whether CM products significantly interact with anaesthetics is largely unknown and still speculative because controlled clinical studies are lacking. Evidence extrapolated from other sources can identify those medicines with pharmacological actions that suggest an interaction is theoretically possible, but clinical significance remains uncertain. For instance, medicines with sedative activity can theoretically prolong or potentiate the sedation induced by the anaesthetic drug combination.

Valeriana officinalis

Both in vivo and numerous clinical studies confirm sedative or hypnotic activity for the herb valerian (see Valerian monograph). Furthermore, valerian has been compared with benzodiazepine drugs in at least three human trials and has been found to be an effective treatment for insomnia (Dorn 2000, Gerhard et al 1996). One double-blind randomised trial involving 202 patients found that valerian extract 600 mg/day (Sedonium) was as effective as 10 mg oxazepam in improving sleep quality over 6 weeks (Ziegler et al 2002). Two clinical studies found that valerian use is not associated with next morning somnolence, suggesting that the herb is short-acting (Gerhard et al 1996, Kuhlmann et al 1999). While a pharmacodynamic interaction is possible, leading to increased sedation, its short duration of action makes a clinically significant interaction between valerian and general anaesthetics unlikely.

Kava kava

Kava kava produces a significant reduction in anxiety compared with a placebo according to a 2003 Cochrane review, which analysed results from 12 clinical studies involving 700 subjects (Pittler & Ernst 2003). Preliminary evidence suggests it may be equivalent to benzodiazepines in non-psychotic anxiety. It is also used in insomnia, with some clinical evidence supporting its use. With regard to surgery, kava kava may produce beneficial effects for the anxious patient; however, it could theoretically increase CNS sedation when used with benzodiazepines. Additionally, clinical testing found that kava kava significantly inhibits ($\approx$ 40%) CYP2E1, which may have implications when used together with CYP2E1 substrates such as halothane, isoflurane and methoxyflurane, causing a rise in drug serum levels (Gurley et al 2005b). Kava kava should be used under professional supervision to avoid adverse outcomes.

St John's wort

Based on theoretical considerations, response to agents such as midazolam, diazepam and fentanyl may be reduced with *Hypericum perforatum* (St John's wort) because of pharmacokinetic interactions, whereas a pharmacodynamic interaction may occur with tramadol (Alfaro & Piscitelli 2001). These interactions are based on evidence that St John's wort (products containing the hyperforin constituent) induces cytochrome 3A4 and P-glycoprotein, as well as upregulating both 5-HT_{1A} and 5-HT_{2A} receptors and exerting a SSRI-like effect (see St John's wort monograph for more detail).

RECOMMENDATIONS BEFORE HIGH-RISK SURGERY

Appendix 3 (Vol 2, p. 1306) provides clinicians with guidance when advising patients due for surgery about the safe use of CMs. It is limited to the 132 CMs reviewed in this book and focuses on those that are known or suspected to increase bleeding or interact with drugs commonly used in the perioperative period. The recommendations are conservative and not likely to be relevant to many low-risk patients or those undergoing minor surgical procedures; however, it is imperative that each patient is individually assessed before surgery.

CMs are listed alphabetically by common name. The comments section includes a brief description of the type of evidence available to support the recommendation; more detailed information is given in individual monographs. Several different recommendations are possible. Sometimes there is a recommendation to suspend use 1–2 weeks before surgery, which should provide ample time for bleeding rates to return to normal or potential interactions to be avoided. This is most likely an overestimation of the actual time required. Please note that coumarin-containing and salicylate-containing herbs have not been included in Appendix 3 unless they have demonstrated antiplatelet or anticoagulant effects in animal or human studies. In some cases, the recommendations are dose-dependent; in others, CM use appears safe but there is a theoretical concern.

It is acknowledged that, in practice, not all surgical patients will be able to follow these recommendations. In situations where bleeding would be a serious complication and a 1-week minimum deferment is not possible, tests of haemostasis before surgery should be considered.

It must be reiterated that the clinical relevance of some interactions and adverse effects is unknown and controlled studies in surgical patients are not available. However, it would seem prudent for healthcare providers to become familiar with these medicines, in order to advise patients appropriately and anticipate, manage or avoid adverse events during the perioperative period.

PATIENT-CENTRED ASSESSMENT AND MANAGEMENT DURING PERIOPERATIVE CARE

The term 'evidence-based patient choice' (EBPC) is the merging together of two important modern movements in Western healthcare, namely evidence-based medicine and patient-centred care. Evidence-based medicine requires the use of the best available evidence to make decisions about medical management. However, the individual qualities, needs and preferences of patients have sometimes been neglected as relevant factors in the decision-making process. Models of EBPC advocate shared decision making, in which patients have received the appropriate evidence for their situation and are able to communicate their personal preferences (Ford et al 2003).

QUALITY USE OF MEDICINES

Inspired by the WHO, countries around the world are developing and instigating policies to ensure medicines are of acceptable safety, quality and efficacy and are accessible. At the end of 1999, Australia launched its National Medicines Policy. In order to achieve one of the key goals of this policy, the National Strategy for the Quality Use of Medicines was developed (see www.health.gov.au).

The goal of the Quality Use of Medicines (QUM) strategy is to optimise the use of medicines to improve health outcomes. It attempts to adopt EBPC into its framework, recognising that QUM requires the collaborative effort of a 'medication team' made up of doctors, pharmacists, nurses and patients. It advises also that CM products be included in assessing a patient's medication situation. In practice, this step appears to be problematic and handled very differently by hospitals.

AUSTRALIAN HOSPITALS: POLICIES AND PROBLEMS

Although the task of getting the right medicine to the right patient should be straightforward, it is rarely the case, according to an editorial in the *Journal of Pharmacy Practice and Research* (Ryan 2003). It has been suggested that many participants are involved in the process. Some of these are obvious, such as surgeons, doctors and pharmacists, while some less obvious, such as the manufacturer, pharmacy wholesaler, hospital nurse and medical educators. In the case of CMs, it is very complicated. Although hospitals should ideally respect the autonomy of patients who make informed decisions about the interventions they feel are in their best interests, they also have a duty of care. They are generally reluctant to administer herbal medicines or other substances that are not part of the standard hospital formulary, are of unknown quality and may have potential adverse effects with variable evidence of efficacy or require specific knowledge in their preparation or administration.

As a result, a number of hospitals have developed local policies that range from disallowing use of CMs (which includes herbal and natural medicines by definition) to treating these medicines as the 'patient's own'. Both approaches are problematic. Advising patients to discontinue taking all herbal and natural medicines before surgery may not free patients from risk relating to their use because withdrawal may be detrimental, in much the same way that withdrawal of some pharmaceutical medicines is associated with increased morbidity after surgery. Treating these medicines as 'the patient's own' may also provide false security, because their use may not be adequately monitored or considered in treatment and discharge plans.

The development of hospital policy and guidelines that take into account the principles of EBPC and QUM in regard to the use of CMs is no doubt challenging, and finding consensus among all members of the 'medication team', administration bodies and patients is a difficult task.

RECOMMENDATIONS

At various stages of the preoperative course, different healthcare professionals can intervene to ensure the patient is optimally prepared for surgery.

If anaesthesia is to be performed, a preoperative consultation is conducted by the attending anaesthetist. According to the Australian and New Zealand College of Anaesthetists (ANZCA), the consultation consists of a concise medical history, physical examination, a review of results of relevant investigations and current medications (see http://www.anzca.edu.au). Although not officially stated, this includes CMs. Currently in the United States, the American Society of Anesthesiologists recommends the discontinuation of all herbal medicines 2 weeks before elective surgery. In Australia and New Zealand, the situation is different because the ANZCA does not make the same general recommendation, instead relying on each anaesthetist to make an individual assessment.

Increasingly, hospital pharmacists are taking on the role of conducting presurgical medication reviews to improve patient safety. Although the focus is on the use of pharmaceutical medicines, the use of CMs is increasingly recognised and included in the medication discussion. Eight practice tips to promote patient safety and welfare are provided as a guide for all healthcare providers managing patients taking herbs and natural supplements during the preoperative period.

UNMANAGED INTEGRATED HEALTHCARE

Currently it appears that a number of patients are already receiving what could be described as unmanaged integrated healthcare, because they are taking herbal and natural medicines and sometimes consulting with a non-medical practitioner while being prescribed pharmaceutical medicines and consulting medical practitioners.

The ultimate aim of surgery is to improve a patient's quality of life by increasing their perception of health and their happiness in life, and reducing limitations so that they will ideally be able to participate in life in a more spirited way (Yun et al 1999). Surveys have identified that up to 50% of surgical patients are using CMs, no doubt as a means of

EIGHT PRACTICE TIPS TO PROMOTE PATIENTS' WELFARE AND SAFETY

1. **Ask all patients about the use of CMs.**

   According to the literature, many patients fail to disclose use of CMs to hospital staff; however, disclosure is more likely to occur if they are asked directly. Some patients may not understand what is meant by the term 'complementary medicine', so consider using phrases such as 'vitamins, minerals or herbal medicines' or 'natural medicines'. It will also be useful to determine whether the product was professionally prescribed or self-selected.

2. **Suspend use of CMs known or suspected to pose a safety risk 5–7 days before surgery, where appropriate.**

   According to the literature, a washout period of 5–7 days should be sufficient to ensure most CMs no longer present a safety concern (Ang-Lee et al 2001). If this is not possible or advisable, be aware of the potential problems and manage accordingly.

3. **If in doubt, refer to drug information centres, peer-reviewed literature or reputable resources for further information.**

   Evidence is accumulating about CM at a rapid rate, and it would be unreasonable to expect all healthcare professionals to keep up to date with these changes. However, referring to reputable information sources when unsure about patient safety is essential for best practice. This may involve referring to CM practitioners with the appropriate training and expertise.

4. **Document information and recommendations in the patient's chart.**

   A patient's CM use should be documented in the medication history and/or discharge summary as appropriate. The name, strength, brand and dose should be recorded.

5. **To continue use of CMs or not?**

   If a patient is experiencing benefits from the use of a CM, and the available evidence indicates safety, use should be continued, but monitored. If a patient is using a CM with known or suspected potential to cause adverse outcomes, an honest discussion about what is known and not known about the risks should ensue. If the patient still wishes to continue using the CM against professional advice, they should be asked to sign an acknowledgment form that informs them of the potential adverse effects and that their attending doctor or pharmacist has recommended against continued use. This should also be documented in the patient's medication history and/or discharge summary.

6. **Consider if and when a patient can resume taking the CM.**

   If use of an effective CM has been withdrawn, recommencement will be required to restore the patient's response. This should be discussed when taking the medication history.

7. **Recommend CMs with known safety and benefit.**

   If research indicates a CM has significant benefits during the perioperative period, then evidence-based practice dictates it should be considered in the patient's management.

8. **If an adverse event does occur, report this through the relevant channels.**

   Little research is available to determine the clinical significance of CMs in the perioperative period. As such, case reports provide useful clues that can guide future research to better determine factors affecting patients' safety.

achieving the same outcomes. While judicious self-care can offer numerous benefits to the individual, society and the healthcare system, there is clearly the potential for serious adverse outcomes, such as bleeding or drug interactions. The withholding of CMs because of lack of knowledge, fear or misinformation can also be problematic and result in patients being deprived of a therapeutic benefit or in the induction of withdrawal effects. It is not unreasonable to expect that, at some time in the future, unnecessarily withdrawing CMs or failing to properly advise patients against the use of a potentially harmful product will give rise to serious adverse events resulting in litigation.

Until further clinical testing has been conducted to determine whether the herbal and natural medicines discussed here will adversely affect or beneficially influence the outcome of surgery, a collaborative yet cautious approach is recommended.

REFERENCES

Alfaro C, Piscitelli S. Drug interactions. In: Atkinson A et al (eds). Principles of clinical pharmacology. San Diego: Academic Press, 2001: 167–80.

Al Qarawi AA et al. Liquorice (Glycyrrhiza glabra) and the adrenal–kidney–pituitary axis in rats. Food Chem Toxicol 40.10 (2002): 1525–1527.

Ang-Lee MK, Moss J, Yuan CS. Herbal medicines and perioperative care. JAMA 286 (2001): 208–216.

Araghi-Niknam M et al. Pine bark extract reduces platelet aggregation. Integ Med 2.2 (2000): 73–77.

Arruzazabala ML et al. Antiplatelet effects of policosanol (20 and 40 mg/day) in healthy volunteers and dyslipidaemic patients. Clin Exp Pharmacol Physiol 29.10 (2002): 891–897.

Aruna D, Naidu MU. Pharmacodynamic interaction studies of Ginkgo biloba with cilostazol and clopidogrel in healthy human subjects. Br J Clin Pharmacol 63.3 (2007): 333–338.

Bal Dit C et al. No alteration in platelet function or coagulation induced by EGb761 in a controlled study. Clin Lab Haematol 25.4 (2003): 251–253.

Beckert BW et al. The effect of herbal medicines on platelet function: An in vivo experiment and review of the literature. Plast Reconstr Surg 120.7 (2007): 2044–2050.

Biggs MJ et al. Platelet aggregation in patients using feverfew for migraine. Lancet 2.8301 (1982): 776.

Blumenthal M et al (eds). Herbal Medicine: Expanded Commission E Monographs. Austin, TX: Integrative Medicine Communications, 2000.

Bone K, Mills S. Principles and Practice of Phytotherapy. London: Elsevier. 2000.

Bordia A et al. Effect of the essential oils of garlic and onion on alimentary hyperlipemia. Atherosclerosis 21.1 (1975): 15–19.

Bordia A et al. Effect of ginger (Zingiber officinale Rosc.) and fenugreek (Trigonella foenumgraecum L.) on blood lipids, blood sugar and platelet aggregation in patients with coronary artery disease. Prostaglandins Leukot Essent Fatty Acids 56.5 (1997): 379–384.

Braun LA, Cohen M. Use of complementary medicines by cardiac surgery patients; undisclosed and undetected. Heart Lung Circ 20.5 (2011): 305–311.

Braun L et al. Wellness Program for Cardiac Surgery Improves Clinical Outcomes. Adv Integrat Med 1.1 (2014): 32–37.

Braun L et al. Use of complementary medicines by surgical patients: undetected and unsupervised. In: Proceedings of the 4th Australasian Conference on Safety and Quality in Health Care, Melbourne. Canberra: National Medicines Symposium, National Prescribing Service, 2006a.

Braun L et al. Perceptions and knowledge of complementary medicines within hospitals: is patient safety compromised? In: Proceedings of 4th Australasian Conference on Safety and Quality in Health Care, Melbourne. Canberra: National Medicines Symposium, National Prescribing Service, 2006b.

Buckley MS et al. Fish oil interaction with warfarin. Ann Pharmacother 38.1 (2004): 50–52.

Calzada C et al. The influence of antioxidant nutrients on platelet function in healthy volunteers. Atherosclerosis 128.1 (1997): 97–105.

Cannon ME et al. Caffeine-induced cardiac arrhythmia: an unrecognised danger of healthfood products. Med J Aust 174.10 (2001): 520–521.

Carlson JJ et al. Safety and efficacy of a ginkgo biloba-containing dietary supplement on cognitive function, quality of life, and platelet function in healthy, cognitively intact older adults. J Am Diet Assoc 107.3 (2007): 422–432.

Chello M et al. Protection by coenzyme Q10 from myocardial reperfusion injury during coronary artery bypass grafting. Ann Thorac Surg 58.5 (1994): 1427–1432.

Chello M et al. Protection by coenzyme Q10 of tissue reperfusion injury during abdominal aortic cross-clamping. J Cardiovasc Surg (Torino) 37.3 (1996): 229–35.

Chen YF et al. Effectiveness of coenzyme Q10 on myocardial preservation during hypothermic cardioplegic arrest. J Thorac Cardiovasc Surg 107.1 (1994): 242–247.

Cohen RJ et al. Complementary and alternative medicine (CAM) use by older adults: a comparison of self-report and physician chart documentation. J Gerontol A Biol Sci Med Sci 57.4 (2002): M223–M227.

Dorn M. Efficacy and tolerability of Baldrian versus oxazepam in non-organic and non-psychiatric insomniacs: a randomised, double-blind, clinical, comparative study. Forsch Komplementarmed Klass Naturheilkd 7.2 (2000): 79–84.

Engelsen J et al. [Effect of Coenzyme Q10 and Ginkgo biloba on warfarin dosage in patients on long-term warfarin treatment. A randomized, double-blind, placebo-controlled cross-over trial]. Ugeskr Laeger 165.18 (2003): 1868–1871.

Ford S et al. What are the ingredients for a successful evidence-based patient choice consultation? A qualitative study. Soc Sci Med 56.3 (2003): 589–602.

Forrelli T. Understanding herb–drug interactions. Tech Orthopaed 18.1 (2003): 37–45.

Galduroz JC et al. Gender- and age-related variations in blood viscosity in normal volunteers: a study of the effects of extract of Allium sativum and Ginkgo biloba. Phytomedicine 14.7–8 (2007): 447–451.

Gardner CD et al. Effect of Ginkgo biloba (EGb 761) and aspirin on platelet aggregation and platelet function analysis among older adults at risk of cardiovascular disease: a randomized clinical trial. Blood Coagul Fibrinolysis 18.8 (2007): 787–793.

Gawande AA et al. The incidence and nature of surgical adverse events in Colorado and Utah in 1992. Surgery 126.1 (1999): 66–75.

Gerhard U et al. Vigilance-decreasing effects of 2 plant-derived sedatives. Schweiz Rundsch Med Prax 85.15 (1996): 473–481.

Girbes AR. The high-risk surgical patient and the role of preoperative management. Neth J Med 57.3 (2000): 98–105.

Grauer RP. Preoperative use of herbal medicines and vitamin supplements. Anaesth Intensive Care 32.2 (2004): 173–177.

Gurley BJ et al. In vivo effects of goldenseal, kava kava, black cohosh, and valerian on human cytochrome P450 1A2, 2D6, 2E1, and 3A4/5 phenotypes. Clin Pharmacol Ther 77.5 (2005b): 415–426.

Gurley BJ et al. Pharmacokinetic herb-drug interactions (part 2): drug interactions involving popular botanical dietary supplements and their clinical relevance. Planta Med 78.13 (2012): 1490–1514.

Harris WS et al. Fish oils in hypertriglyceridemia: a dose-response study. Am J Clin Nutr 51.3 (1990): 399–406.

Harris WS et al. Omega-3 fatty acids and coronary heart disease risk: clinical and mechanistic perspectives. Atherosclerosis 197.1 (2008): 12–24.

Hauser D et al. Bleeding complications precipitated by unrecognized Ginkgo biloba use after liver transplantation. Transpl Int 15.7 (2002): 377–379.

Heilmann P et al. Administration of glycyrrhetinic acid: significant correlation between serum levels and the cortisol/cortisone-ratio in serum and urine. Exp Clin Endocrinol Diabetes 107.6 (1999): 370–378.

Heptinstall S et al. Inhibition of platelet behaviour by feverfew: a mechanism of action involving sulphydryl groups. Folia Haematol Int Mag Klin Morphol Blutforsch 115.4 (1988): 447–449.

Jain NK, Kulkarni SK. Antinociceptive and anti-inflammatory effects of Tanacetum parthenium L. extract in mice and rats. J Ethnopharmacol 68.1–3 (1999): 251–259.

Jalili M, Dehpour AR. Extremely prolonged INR associated with warfarin in combination with both trazodone and omega-3 fatty acids. Arch Med Res 38.8 (2007): 901–904.

Jiang X et al. Effect of ginkgo and ginger on the pharmacokinetics and pharmacodynamics of warfarin in healthy subjects. Br J Clin Pharmacol 59.4 (2005): 425–432.

Judy WV et al. Myocardial preservation by therapy with coenzyme Q10 during heart surgery. Clin Invest 71.8 (Suppl) (1993): S155–S161.

Jung EM et al. Influence of garlic powder on cutaneous microcirculation: A randomized placebo-controlled double-blind cross-over study in apparently healthy subjects. Arzneimittelforschung 41.6 (1991): 626–630.

Kaye AD et al. Herbal medicines: current trends in anesthesiology practice: a hospital survey. J Clin Anesth 12.6 (2000): 468–471.

Kitagawa M, Mino M. Effects of elevated d-alpha(RRR)-tocopherol dosage in man. J Nutr Sci Vitaminol (Tokyo), 35.2 (1989): 133–42.

Knudsen JF, Sokol GH. Potential glucosamine-warfarin interaction resulting in increased international normalized ratio: case report and review of the literature and MedWatch database. Pharmacother 28.4 (2008): 540–548.

Kohler S et al. Influence of a 7-day treatment with Ginkgo biloba special extract EGb 761 on bleeding time and coagulation: A randomized, placebo-controlled, double-blind study in healthy volunteers. Blood Coagul Fibrinolysis 15.4 (2004): 303–309.

Krivoy N et al. Effect of salicis cortex extract on human platelet aggregation. Planta Med 67.3 (2001): 209–212.

Kuhlmann J et al. The influence of valerian treatment on 'reaction time, alertness and concentration' in volunteers. Pharmacopsychiatry 32.6 (1999): 235–241.

Leong JY et al. Preoperative metabolic therapy improves outcomes from cardiac surgery: a prospective randomised clinical trial. [Conference Abstract] Heart Lung Circ 16 (Suppl 2) (2007): S178.

Leung JM et al. The prevalence and predictors of the use of alternative medicine in presurgical patients in five California hospitals. Anesth Analg 93.4 (2001): 1062–1068.

Lovera J et al. Ginkgo biloba for the improvement of cognitive performance in multiple sclerosis: a randomized, placebo-controlled trial. Mult Scler 13.3 (2007): 376–385.

Mabile L et al. Moderate supplementation with natural alpha-tocopherol decreases platelet aggregation and low-density lipoprotein oxidation. Atherosclerosis 147.1 (1999): 177–185.

Makheja AN, Bailey JM. A platelet phospholipase inhibitor from the medicinal herb feverfew (Tanacetum parthenium). Prostaglandins Leukot Med 8.6 (1982): 653–660.

McClaskey EM, Michalets EL. Subdural hematoma after a fall in an elderly patient taking high-dose omega-3 fatty acids with warfarin and aspirin: case report and review of the literature. Pharmacotherapy 27.1 (2007): 152–160.

Morinobu T et al. The safety of high-dose vitamin E supplementation in healthy Japanese male adults. J Nutr Sci Vitaminol (Tokyo), 48.1 (2002): 6–9.

Nathens AB et al. Randomized, prospective trial of antioxidant supplementation in critically ill surgical patients. Ann Surg 236.6 (2002): 814–822.

Norred CL. Complementary and alternative medicine use by surgical patients. AORN J 76.6 (2002): 1013–1021.

Norred CL et al. Use of complementary and alternative medicines by surgical patients. Am Assoc Nurse Anesth J 68.1 (2000): 13–118.

Pittler MH, Ernst E. Kava extract for treating anxiety. Cochrane Database Syst Rev 1 (2003): CD003383.

Rosenfeldt F et al. Coenzyme Q10 therapy before cardiac surgery improves mitochondrial function and in vitro contractility of myocardial tissue. J Thorac Cardiovasc Surg 129.1 (2005): 25–32.

Rosenfeldt FL et al. Coenzyme Q10 improves the tolerance of the senescent myocardium to aerobic and ischemic stress: studies in rats and in human atrial tissue. Biofactors 9.2–4 (1999): 291–299.

Rosenfeldt FL et al. The effects of ageing on the response to cardiac surgery: protective strategies for the ageing myocardium. Biogerontology 3.1–2 (2002): 37–40.

Ryan M. Many have a part to play. J Pharmacy Prac Res 33.1 (2003): 4.

Schneider C et al. [Spontaneous hyphema caused by Ginkgo biloba extract]. J Fr Ophtalmol 25.7 (2002): 731–732.

Sigurjonsdottir HA et al. Liquorice-induced rise in blood pressure: a linear dose-response relationship. J Hum Hypertens 15.8 (2001): 549–552.

Silverstein DD, Spiegel AD. Are physicians aware of the risks of alternative medicine? J Community Health 26.3 (2001): 159–174.

Smith PF et al. The neuroprotective properties of the Ginkgo biloba leaf: a review of the possible relationship to platelet-activating factor (PAF). J Ethnopharmacol 50.3 (1996): 131–139.

Taggart DP et al. Effects of short-term supplementation with coenzyme Q10 on myocardial protection during cardiac operations. Ann Thorac Surg 61.3 (1996): 829–833.

Tanaka J et al. Coenzyme Q10: the prophylactic effect on low cardiac output following cardiac valve replacement. Ann Thorac Surg 33.2 (1982): 145–151.

Tsen LC et al. Alternative medicine use in presurgical patients. Anesthesiology 93.1 (2000): 148–151.

Valli G et al. Benefits, adverse effects and drug interactions of herbal therapies with cardiovascular effects. J Am Coll Cardiol 39.7 (2002): 1083–1095.

Wolf HR. Does Ginkgo biloba special extract EGb 761 provide additional effects on coagulation and bleeding when added to acetylsalicylic acid 500 mg daily? Drugs R D 7.3 (2006): 163–172.

Yun KL et al. Time related quality of life after elective cardiac operation. Ann Thorac Surg 68.4 (1999): 1314–1320.

Zhou M et al. Effects of coenzyme Q10 on myocardial protection during cardiac valve replacement and scavenging free radical activity in vitro. Torino: J Cardiovasc Surg 40.3 (1999): 355–361.

Ziegler G et al. Efficacy and tolerability of valerian extract LI 156 compared with oxazepam in the treatment of non-organic insomnia: a randomized, double-blind, comparative clinical study. Eur J Med Res 7.11 (2002): 480–486.

CHAPTER 10

CANCER AND THE SAFETY OF COMPLEMENTARY MEDICINES

Complementary medicine (CM) is commonly used by oncology patients and therefore it is important for healthcare providers to become familiar with this use (Bernstein & Grasso 2001, Ernst & Cassileth 1998, Greenlee et al 2009, Richardson et al 2000). Typically, cancer patients use vitamins and herbal medicines, spiritual practices and psychosocial and physical therapies. Utilisation of CM therapies often increases after a diagnosis of cancer, with studies indicating that well over 50% of patients with cancer integrate CM into their treatment (Beatty et al 2012, Fox et al 2013, Vapiwala et al 2006). Unfortunately, relatively few cancer patients using CM receive information from their conventional healthcare providers and communication between patients and doctors about CM is virtually non-existent (Ernst 2003, Moran et al 2013). Oncologists surveyed in a recent study estimated CM use by their patients at around 30%, a significant underestimation of the current increased trend of CM integration (Fox et al 2013).

Patients with cancer want access to reliable and authoritative information about CM so that they can discuss benefits and limitations with their healthcare providers and make an informed decision about use. A study of children with cancer has revealed that parents also want information about CM, especially at the beginning of treatment and also in the hospital wards (Molassiotis & Cubbin 2004). Medical and CM practitioners, pharmacists and nurses can play an important role in this regard and do much to guide and support patients using or considering CM. However, in order to provide an informed and rational opinion, healthcare providers require a working knowledge of CM and an awareness of its benefits and potential to cause harm. They also need to keep an open mind, have access to reliable resources and develop collaborative partnerships across several disciplines.

Various types of CM are utilised in the oncology setting and can be divided into a number of broad categories (NCCAM 2009):

- Biologically-based CM: herbal therapies, vitamins and dietary supplements and whole-diet therapies such as the Paleolithic diet or Gerson diet.

- Energy medicine: biofield therapies such as Qigong, Reiki or therapeutic touch and bioelectromagnetic-based therapies such as pulsed and/or magnetic fields, therapeutic touch and crystal therapy.

- Manipulative and physical therapies: chiropractic, osteopathic and relaxation/lymphatic massage.

- Mind–body medicine and counselling: meditation, prayer, spiritual healing, art therapy, chanting and music therapy, dance, yoga, Qigong, tai chi, cognitive–behavioural therapy and patient support groups/cancer support centres (CRCs).

- Whole medical systems: homeopathic medicine, naturopathic medicine, traditional Chinese medicine and Ayurveda.

WHY DO PEOPLE WITH CANCER USE COMPLEMENTARY THERAPIES?

People with cancer choose CM as a means of addressing physical and psychosocial issues (Fox et al 2013).

For physical issues, CM is used to provide symptomatic relief from the disease and/or its treatments. This includes addressing symptoms such as pain, nausea and vomiting, fatigue, constipation, weight loss and cachexia and dyspnoea. It is sometimes used to minimise long-term adverse consequences of treatment, such as organ toxicity.

For psychosocial issues, CM offers an avenue for dealing with anxiety, depression, stress and fear. It also provides an opportunity for patient empowerment and can give a sense of control and improve wellbeing.

Patients with cancer utilise complementary treatment modalities such as herbs and supplements, functional diets, topical treatments, mind–body practices (e.g. yoga, meditation, imagery, music therapy), massage, acupuncture and techniques such as Reiki and healing touch. However, research indicates that the most frequently integrated CMs are biologically-based CMs, such as nutritional supplements and herbal therapies (Walshe et al 2012). Population-based studies indicate that females, and those with breast, head and neck, bowel and haematological cancers reported higher use of CM therapies; breast cancer patients being the most frequent users, with over 75% of patients using some form of CM (Wanchai et al 2010).

CM use typically decreases with advanced age and increases with education and socioeconomic status. Additionally, cancer survivors who have undergone chemotherapy, radiotherapy or other treatments (bone marrow/stem cell transplant, immunotherapy) report higher use of CM compared to survivors who had never had these treatments (Fox et al 2013, Tautz et al 2012, Walshe et al 2012). Perceived levels of satisfaction in CM users is also very high, with over 90% of patients indicating satisfaction in the therapies used, further increasing the likelihood that new patients will be encouraged to use CM by previous users or significant influencers, such as family and friends (Fox et al 2013, Öhlén et al 2006, Wanchai et al 2010).

Patients with cancer who use CM report various positive effects, such as reduced depression and anxiety, stress, nausea, pain and dyspnoea and improved physical energy, mood, concentration and optimism (Beatty et al 2012, Molassiotis & Cubbin 2004, Ponholzer et al 2003). According to research in children with cancer, CM use is associated with increased confidence, improved pain relief and relaxation (Molassiotis & Cubbin 2004). Importantly, most people with cancer do not expect CM to cure or slow their disease and generally use it as a supportive measure during conventional treatment, chiefly to relieve symptoms and emotional anguish and enhance recovery (Ponholzer et al 2003, Rees et al 2000, Richardson et al 2000, Wanchai et al 2010).

The use of CM is widespread and increasing, partly because of increased access to health information and the growth in research-based evidence supporting the effectiveness of complementary therapies. In addition, CM practitioners tend to have longer consultations than medical practitioners with patients and adopt a holistic approach that focuses on presenting symptoms, the patient's lifestyle and issues that encompass mind, body and spirit. The increased interest in health prevention strategies, such as diet and stress management, are also well catered for by complementary therapists, who see these approaches as essential to good clinical practice.

POOR DISCLOSURE

Although the use of CMs is popular among people with cancer, many do not inform their medical doctors that they are using it. Population-based studies show that at least 50% of cancer patients use some form of CM, with higher percentages of around 75% in some patient subgroups such as breast cancer patients (Fox et al 2013). However, relatively few patients discuss CM with their oncologists (Ge et al 2013). One of the main causes for non-disclosure is that doctors do not ask patients about CM use (Schiff et al 2011), and also because some patients anticipate disinterest or a negative response from their doctor, or think doctors are unable or unwilling to contribute meaningful information, or because it is perceived as irrelevant to the biomedical treatment course (Adler & Fosket 1999). If a patient does

---

CLINICAL NOTE — INTEGRATIVE ONCOLOGY

Integrative medicine may be described as 'practising medicine in a way that selectively incorporates elements of CM into comprehensive treatment plans alongside solidly orthodox methods of diagnosis and treatment' (Rees & Weil 2001). Integrative oncology (IO) is a subset of integrative medicine. It is a term being increasingly adopted to include CM, but integrated with conventional cancer treatment, as opposed to being considered a rival or true 'alternative' (Deng et al 2007, Smyth 2006). IO is an evolving evidence-based specialty that focuses on the roles of complementary therapies to increase the effectiveness of conventional cancer treatment programs by improving defined outcomes such as symptom control, quality of life, reduction of patients' distress, rehabilitation and prevention of recurrence (Sagar 2008). The core principles of IO include individualisation, holism, dynamism, synergism and collaboration (Leis et al 2008). CM therapies used in IO include natural medicines (botanicals, vitamins and minerals), nutrition, acupuncture, meditation and other mind–body approaches, music therapy, touch therapies, fitness therapies and others (Sagar 2006).

Integrative medicine in general has grown quickly in the United States and now virtually all major medical centres have departments devoted to integrative patient care, either as true stand-alone centres or departments with a research interest in this area (Ben-Arye et al 2012, Boyd 2007). This is particularly true of the major cancer centres, many of which — including Memorial Sloan Kettering Cancer Center, New York; M.D. Anderson Cancer Center, Houston, Texas; Johns Hopkins University, Baltimore, Maryland; Duke University, Durham, North Carolina; and the Dana Farber Cancer Institute, Boston, Massachusetts — have developed integrative cancer programs. In addition, programs such as the Cancer Treatment Centres of America have inpatient and outpatient programs with teams of practitioners, including medical oncologists, surgeons and radiation therapists, as well as credentialled naturopathic doctors, nutritionists, mind–body specialists and other integrative practitioners. Institutions are providing services to patients, exploring the effectiveness gap in their clinical services and are determining the efficacy of complementary therapies through randomised controlled trials and, increasingly, mixed method whole systems research (Sagar 2006).

For readers interested in keeping up to date with this evolving area, the journal *Integrative Cancer Therapies* is recommended, as it provides useful research and editorial information about CM in cancer care.

---

decide to inform their medical doctor, it is usually because they have a desire for their doctor to be fully informed, are concerned about interactions or want to be more informed about the therapy (Ge et al 2013). It is therefore not unusual for patients to be receiving treatment and advice from a variety of practitioners without a central healthcare provider coordinating and supervising care.

Lack of disclosure can give rise to serious problems such as drug interactions and failure to recognise CM-induced adverse effects and withdrawal effects. In oncology, this can have far-reaching consequences. Open and honest communication about CM should be the standard for both patients and clinicians in order to avoid or minimise adverse events and provide an opportunity for patients to express their personal preferences for treatment.

CM IN THE ONCOLOGY SETTING

Despite the increased interest in developing integrative approaches to cancer, many medical oncologists remain sceptical about the value of these modalities. A recent survey of paediatric oncologists indicates that the main concerns with patients using CM are about potential drug interactions, additional costs to the patient or that effective treatments may be ignored, prevented or delayed (Langler et al 2013). However, 65% of the respondents also indicated that they worry about a lack of competence on their own part to advise their patients about CM, and 85% expressed a desire for better education opportunities regarding CM interactions in oncology; these results are also noted in surveys of radiologists in oncology

(Bolderston et al 2008). There are several good reasons for oncologists and other staff to take such developments seriously and learn more about CM, instead of dismissing it as eccentric and unproven (Smyth 2006):

- **To enhance mutual respect between patient and doctor.** Oncology patients are using CM and yet all too often they are reluctant to discuss this or even to inform doctors that they are doing so. Mutual respect will help build communication pathways and provide the clinician with an opportunity to ensure that no harm is introduced unwittingly by patients themselves.

- **To encourage research into CM.** One of the major reasons for the medical profession's scepticism of CM is the poor evidence base for many of these treatments. Enquiry, instead of dismissal, will encourage further investigation and research into this area.

- **To increase doctors', pharmacists' and nurses' knowledge of CM.** With ever-increasing access to information and knowledge, patients will continue to challenge their professional advisers on every aspect of cancer management. CM approaches will continue to feature strongly in many patients' minds, placing demands on healthcare professionals in the years ahead. One way to help patients is to provide an informed, evidence-based opinion, while acknowledging that, in some cases, randomised studies may not be conducted for years, but that other forms of evidence may exist and provide guidance.

- **To help patients make safe choices and monitor their responses to treatment.** If a patient chooses to use CM, then helping them set appropriate goals and learn to self-monitor for safety issues or beneficial outcomes is both important and also helpful to the patient.

BENEFITS OF CM IN ONCOLOGY

A growing number of CM therapies are being subjected to clinical trials to determine their effectiveness and role in cancer treatment. In most instances, CM therapies are being investigated for symptom relief and improvements in quality of life.

A review in the *European Journal of Cancer* illustrated that the weight of evidence to support the use of some complementary approaches in cancer is clearly positive or showing a positive trend (Ernst 2003). According to the review, positive evidence exists for *Allium* spp vegetables (e.g. onions), detoxification, Sho-saiko-to, St John's wort, acupuncture and relaxation, while there is positive trend for green tea, phyto-oestrogens, Gerson diet, *Aloe vera*, melatonin, support group therapy, hypnotherapy, therapeutic touch and enzyme supplements.

Evidence is well-established for psychosocial therapies in cancer management, such as hypnosis, music therapy, meditation and stress management, and for acupuncture (Cassileth 1999). For example, there is evidence from randomised trials supporting the value of hypnosis for cancer pain and nausea; relaxation therapy, music therapy and massage for anxiety; and acupuncture for nausea (Vickers & Cassileth 2001). Studies involving people with cancer or cancer survivors report benefits of yoga for stress, anxiety, insomnia and cancer-related symptoms and show it increases quality of life (Bower et al 2005, Cohen et al 2004).

Results from clinical studies and/or experimental models indicate that several other therapies have the potential to reduce drug-induced side effects and toxicities. For example, a Cochrane systematic review that analysed the results of four trials using a Chinese decoction containing the herb astragalus (huang-qi) as an adjunct to chemotherapy concluded that co-administration of the herbal treatment with chemotherapy produced a significant reduction in nausea and vomiting and a decrease in the rate of leucopenia (Taixiang et al 2005). The review also stated that no evidence of harm was identified with use. The herbs ginger and baical skullcap have been found to reduce symptoms of cisplatin-induced nausea in experimental models (Aung et al 2003, Sharma & Gupta 1998, Sharma et al 1997), and animal and human studies suggest long-term carnitine administration may reduce cardiotoxic side effects of Adriamycin (Mijares & Lopez 2001, Waldner et al 2006). Additionally, preclinical and clinical studies suggest that anthracycline-induced cardiotoxicity can be prevented by administering coenzyme Q10 (CoQ10) during cancer chemotherapy which includes drugs such as doxorubicin and daunorubicin. Studies further suggest that CoQ10 does not interfere with the antineoplastic action of anthracyclines and might even enhance their anticancer effects (Conklin 2005). Many other natural substances, such as St Mary's thistle, grapeseed extract, St John's wort, parthenolide (from feverfew) and curcumin, show promise in preliminary studies in reducing chemotherapy-induced organ toxicity or other associated adverse effects and are discussed in individual monographs in this book. Research has also been conducted with individual antioxidant vitamins and minerals.

A comprehensive model of cancer care requires that patients take an active role in their healthcare and find partners to work with them during the process. Medical practitioners play a key role; however, many other healthcare providers can augment their work and help provide patients with holistic care. A number of complementary therapies have proven benefits and are considered safe. These should be made available to patients to increase their sense of wellbeing and improve their quality of life and experience of cancer, its treatments and recovery.

SUPPORTIVE MEASURES

Supportive care is that which helps patients and their families cope with cancer and its treatment, starting from prediagnosis, through the process of diagnosis and treatment, to cure, continuing illness or death, and into bereavement. It helps the patient to maximise the benefits of treatment and to live as well as possible with the effects of the disease.

A number of CM therapies and treatments can provide substantial support to people with cancer by providing symptomatic relief, enhanced quality of life and improved sense of wellbeing, without causing harm. CM use is an effective intervention for reducing stress and depression after a diagnosis of cancer, and a recent longitudinal study found that rates of post-cancer depression in patients who use CM are significantly lower than those who do not utilise CM therapies (Beatty et al 2012).

CM therapies also have important benefits in addition to those derived from their inherent therapeutic effect:
- They actively involve patients and provide a rare opportunity for them to exert control and tend to themselves or to have friends or family members assist them.

- Many CM therapies are time-honoured types of 'supportive care' that have been offered to patients for decades.
- Many are accessible.
- Some work by known mechanisms of action, whereas others may invoke a placebo response, an underutilised mechanism by which distress can be relieved and quality of life enhanced.

The information in Table 10.1 (pp 150) is a guide to some of the better-known and researched therapies and treatments that may provide supportive benefits for patients. To promote appropriate and safe use, each individual's characteristics, medication use, general health and overall situation needs to be assessed. Where herbal and nutritional medicines are mentioned, healthcare providers should check for potential interactions with drug therapy.

CM TO IMPROVE SURVIVAL

Although CM is most often used to treat symptoms and enhance wellbeing, to a lesser extent it is being used as a potential cure for cancer. Examples of some CM treatments that have been used by patients to prevent and cure cancer are listed in Table 10.2 (p 151) and 10.3 (p 151). Some of the listed treatments are currently under investigation and have been subject to in vitro and in vivo studies, whereas other treatments, such as Hoxsey therapy, the Di Bella regimen, shark cartilage and laetrile, are generally considered ineffective. A full review of the available evidence is beyond the scope of this chapter, but further information can be found in the relevant monographs. (Updated information is available at some of the websites listed in Table 10.5, pp 166.)

It is interesting to note that approximately two-thirds of commercially available anticancer drugs are derived from or related to natural products, including enzymes, hormones, plants and fungal extracts (Bryant et al 2003). For example, an extract of wild chervil was mentioned in an ancient medical text as a useful salve against tumours, and it is now known that podophyllotoxin, a cytotoxic agent, is present in the *Podophyllum* species of plants. The most recent anticancer products are the taxanes (paclitaxel and docetaxel), which are derived from the yew tree *Taxus baccata*, and the camptothecins (topotecan and irinotecan) from *Camptotheca accuminata*.

TABLE 10.1 CM THERAPIES USED TO SUPPORT CANCER PATIENTS	
CONDITION	**CM THERAPY**
Anxiety and stress	Acupressure: pressure with fingertips to key locations Aromatherapy: lavender, rosemary, chamomile and marjoram oils are popular; a few drops of oil in the bath, on a pillow, in an oil diffuser or in massage vehicle Meditation and other relaxation techniques: seated or lying down; class or DVD; visualisation and imagery Therapeutic massage: with a trained massage therapist Herbal medicines: brahmi, lemon balm, rhodiola, valerian, passionflower, kava kava, withania, Siberian ginseng; under professional supervision Nutritional supplements: vitamin B complex, SAMe Yoga: class or DVD; breathing exercises can be done by bedridden patients
Backache and muscle aches	Hydrotherapy: e.g. warm bath or spa Nutritional medicine: magnesium and/or calcium supplements, particularly if muscle cramping or muscle tension is a problem Therapeutic massage: with a trained massage therapist Herbal medicines: willowbark, devil's claw tea; or stronger forms under supervision
Depression	Herbal medicine: lemon balm, St John's wort, ginkgo, rhodiola Nutritional medicine: SAMe, fish oils, vitamin B complex Meditation and other relaxation techniques: seated or lying down; class or DVD Yoga: class or DVD; breathing exercises can be done by bedridden patients
Diarrhoea	Probiotics: recolonise bowel with beneficial bacteria Glutamine: symptom relief Herbal medicine: bilberry, chamomile, goldenseal, raspberry leaf tea; or stronger forms under supervision
Dyspepsia	Herbal medicine: dandelion, chamomile, peppermint, cinnamon, ginger, meadowsweet, fenugreek, raspberry leaf teas; or stronger forms under supervision Food supplements: probiotics, colostrum, glutamine
Headaches	Acupressure: pressure with fingertips to key locations Acupuncture Herbal medicine: willow bark, devil's claw Nutritional medicine: magnesium and calcium supplements; particularly if muscle tension is a problem
Nausea and vomiting	Acupuncture Possibly hypnosis Music therapy in combination with antiemetics for stronger effects Herbal medicine: ginger, cinnamon, peppermint tea; or stronger forms under supervision Lime juice taken in water
Pain	Acupuncture: may also increase mobility Biofeedback Herbal medicine: willowbark, ginger, devil's claw tea; or stronger forms under supervision Hypnosis Nutritional supplements: SAMe, fish oil supplements Therapeutic massage: with a trained massage therapist TENS daily for 6+ sessions; may improve fatigue and quality of life, provide acute pain relief and reduce analgesic requirements
Insomnia	Aromatherapy: lavender, rosemary, chamomile and marjoram oils are popular; a few drops of oil in the bath, on a pillow, in an oil diffuser or in massage vehicle Herbal medicine Lemon balm, passionflower, Siberian ginseng, valerian, chamomile tea; or stronger forms under supervision Therapeutic massage: with a trained massage therapist Meditation

TABLE 10.2 COMPLEMENTARY MEDICINES THAT HAVE BEEN USED TO IMPROVE CANCER CURE RATES	
COMPLEMENTARY MEDICINE	**COMMENTS**
Cat's claw (*Uncaria tormentosa*)	See monograph.
Chapparral	
Coenzyme Q10	There have been several positive case reports.
Curcumin	Attracting a lot of interest from researchers. See monograph.
Essiac tea	Herbal mixture originally formulated by an Ojibwa healer and popularised in the 1920s by a nurse, Rene Caisse. (Essiac is Caisse spelt backwards.) The four main herbs in Essiac tea are burdock root (*Arctium lappa*), Indian rhubarb (*Rheum palmatum*), sheep sorrel (*Rumex acetosella*) and the inner bark of slippery elm (*Ulmus fulva* or *U. rubra*).
Green tea	Attracting a lot of interest from researchers. See monograph.
Laetrile	A single compound isolated from a natural substance (apricot kernels and almonds); promoted as 'vitamin B17'.
MGN-3	This is a mushroom and rice bran extract.
Maitake mushroom extract (*Grifola frondosa*)	Maitake D-fraction is used.
Mistletoe extract	Has been subjected to clinical trials in Europe.
Pau d'arco	Used as a tea. Thought to be an old Inca remedy for many illnesses, including cancer. It is made from the bark of an indigenous South American evergreen tree, and its active ingredient, lapachol, has been isolated. See monograph for further information.
PC-SPES	Chinese formulation of eight herbs consisting of isatis (*Isatis indigotica*), either liquorice (*Glycyrrhiza glabra*) or Gan coa (*G. uralensis*), Chinese skullcap (*Scutellaria baicalensis*), reishi (Ganoderma lucidum), saw palmetto (*Serenoa repens* or *Sabal serrulata*), Asian ginseng (*Panax ginseng*), denodrantherm (*Denodrantherma morifolium*) and rabdosia (*Rabdosia rubescens*). It is no longer available, as it was also found to contain diethylstilboesterol and warfarin, which increase the risk of adverse effects.
714X	A liquid medicine made from camphor, nitrogen, ammonium salts, sodium chloride, and ethanol, generally given by injection.
Shark cartilage	Thought to have potential owing to antiangiogenic properties. See monograph for further information.

TABLE 10.3 CM THERAPIES THAT HAVE BEEN USED TO IMPROVE CANCER CURE RATES	
CM THERAPY	**COMMENTS**
Chelation therapy	The use of agents to chelate heavy metals.
The Di Bella regimen	Consists of melatonin, bromocriptine, retinoids, and either somatostatin or octreotide.
Electromagnetic therapy	
Fasting and juice therapies	
Hoxsey therapy	Consists of a caustic herbal paste for external cancers or a herbal mixture for 'internal' cancers, combined with laxatives, douches, vitamin supplements and dietary changes; one of oldest alternative cancer treatments in the United States, dating back to the 1920s.
Ozone therapy	

TABLE 10.4 CYTOCHROME ENZYMES INVOLVED IN THE METABOLISM OF CHEMOTHERAPEUTIC DRUGS	
CYTOCHROME ENZYME	**CHEMOTHERAPEUTIC DRUG**
CYP 1A1, 1A2	dacarbazine
CYP 2A6	cyclophosphamide, ifosfamide, tegafur
CYP 2B6	cyclophosphamide, ifosfamide
CYP 2C8	cyclophosphamide, ifosfamide, paclitaxel
CYP 2C9	cyclophosphamide, ifosfamide
CYP 2C19	teniposide
CYP 2D6	tamoxifen, doxorubicin, vinblastine
CYP 2E1	dacarbazine
CYP 3A4	teniposide, etoposide, epipodophyllotoxin, cyclophosphamide, ifosfamide, vindesine, vinblastine, vincristine, vinorelbine, paclitaxel, docetaxel, irinotecan, tamoxifen
CYP 3A5	etoposide, tipifarnib

RESEARCH APPROACHES AND CONSTRAINTS

The resurgence of medical pluralism has resulted in people with cancer developing their own combinations of biomedical, complementary and self-care strategies. Consequently, the need for a solid knowledge base for the non-surgical, non-radiotherapeutical and non-chemotherapeutical aspects of the treatment experience and their combinations is substantial and will only increase.

Until recently, research efforts in CM and cancer have concentrated mainly on testing a limited number of available treatments using the well-established pharmaceutical randomised controlled trial research model, with tumour size and/or survival as primary outcomes. This has already led to the publication of hundreds of randomised trials in the peer-reviewed literature. While this work is important and will continue, it does not reflect a patient's reasons for seeking CM treatments, which are not primarily tumour reduction, but improved well-being and symptom relief.

WHOLE SYSTEMS RESEARCH (WSR)

Cancer care is currently developing into a complicated network of interventions that are delivered at different times and places with different intentions. Some interventions are offered by healthcare professionals at an oncology centre; others are offered by CM practitioners; still others, such as special diets, meditation and OTC natural supplements, form part of a patient's individualised package of self-care. These treatment interventions are influenced by psychosocial factors such as the nature of the patient–provider relationship, varying levels of social support, and an individual patient's personality. Ultimately, a patient's outcomes are a result of all components of care, and it is likely that the effect of the whole is greater than the sum of its parts (Verhoef et al 2005). As a result, there is a need to consider whether the current research approaches in clinical cancer care adequately cover the ongoing treatment choices and combinations. One approach developed by CM researchers is whole systems research (WSR), which is proposed as an additional research method for modern systems of care, whether they include CM or not.

WSR is 'an emerging research framework specific for the investigation of the effectiveness of whole systems of healthcare' which focuses on the multidisciplinary approach taken by patients, rather than adopting a reductionist perspective where all variables remain constant except one that is altered. In WSR, issues are addressed, such as the ecological validity of the model, individualised patient-centred outcomes, patient–practitioner relationships, the context and environment of the intervention, and the interactions between the various components of the system (Kakai et al 2013). WSR focuses more on the individual patient and less on group-averaged results, under the assumption that there will be patient heterogeneity in response and that important information about the healing approach in that heterogeneity may otherwise be missed (Jonas et al 2006, Verhoef et al 2005). Integral to WSR is the belief that clinical research should reflect real-world practice and then be used to inform future clinical practice, hence the conclusion that WSR is the most appropriate form of research in integrative oncology (Sagar & Lawenda 2009). A mixed-methods approach that holds qualitative and quantitative research methods in equal esteem and captures information about different domains is advocated, because whole systems are complex and no single method can adequately capture the meaning, process and outcomes of these interventions (Verhoef et al 2005).

In summary, WSR is research that:

- encompasses the investigation of both the processes and the outcomes of complex interventions

- includes *all* aspects of any internally consistent approach to treatment (philosophical basis, patients, practitioners, setting of practice and methods/materials)

- acknowledges unique patient, family, community and environmental characteristics and perspectives.

OUTCOMES RESEARCH

Researchers in Canada determined nine outcome domains relevant to WSR (Fonnebo et al 2007) as follows: physical, psychological, social, spiritual, quality-of-life, holistic, individualised, process and context outcomes. At the same time, validated outcome instruments have been identified to measure these domains, as well as gaps where no adequate measures currently exist. Researchers in the UK and at the University of Arizona, United States, have led the way by conceptualising and developing these instruments, some examples of which are: Measure Yourself Medical Outcome Profile, Measure Yourself Concerns and Wellbeing, the Patient Enablement Questionnaire and the Consultation and Relational Empathy Measure (Fonnebo et al 2007).

EXPLORING EXCEPTIONAL PATIENTS

Becoming familiar with patients' individual experiences and collating information to find common themes is one method of identifying therapeutic approaches that show promising results and warrant further clinical research. In a way, this method of data collection is much like the practice of traditional healers of old, who were required to develop excellent observational and history-taking skills to learn more about the benefits and risks of treatments being applied.

This realisation has led to several international initiatives to collect and systematically categorise and review histories of patients who experience an unexpected benefit or spontaneous remission after CM treatments. Several research groups in different countries have initiated studies in this area, either collecting histories from the treatment providers or recruiting case histories mainly from patients themselves (Launso et al 2006). The US National Cancer Institute concentrates on a series of what they designate as 'best cases', whereas in Norway the National Research Centre in Complementary and Alternative Medicine (NAFKAM) includes both 'best' and 'worst' cases in its reviews.

LIMITED FUNDING

Despite the enormous popularity of CM, relatively little research has been conducted into the efficacy and safety of its use by people with cancer compared to similar research into conventional medicine. The literature on integrative medicine is expanding, but currently there is a lack of studies assessing the effectiveness of integrative programs. This scarcity of research is closely related to the difficulty in assessing relevant outcomes using validated measures due to the complex nature of CM. The role of therapeutic alliances in integrative medicine is often assumed to be crucial for patients' positive outcomes, but little research has focused on the entire integrative medicine program as a unit of analysis exploring the perspectives of patients/survivors, caregivers, CM providers and healthcare professionals. Examining the process and context by which healing occurs is crucial in CM research (Kakai et al 2013, Verhoef et al 2005). Currently, the majority of research into CM has been conducted in the United States, where a significant effort has been made, with government funding. In 1998

CLINICAL NOTE — SENATE ENQUIRY INTO SERVICES AND TREATMENTS OPTIONS FOR PERSONS WITH CANCER: KEY RECOMMENDATIONS

In June 2005 a report entitled 'The cancer journey: Informing choice' was released as a result of a Senate inquiry (Commonwealth of Australia 2005). The inquiry aimed to investigate the delivery of services and options for treatment for people diagnosed with cancer and to determine how less conventional and complementary cancer treatments can be assessed and judged. With regard to complementary medicine, several important recommendations were made, including a recommendation that the National Health and Medical Research Council provide a dedicated funding stream for research into complementary therapies and medicines and convene an expert working group to identify the research needs relating to complementary therapies, including issues around safety, efficacy and capacity building. The development of collaborative partnerships across disciplines was also advised. The Senate committee also recommended improved provision of authoritative information to patients and health professionals. Importantly, it recommended that where quality of life may be improved by complementary approaches, the means to make such therapies more accessible needs to be reviewed.

CLINICAL NOTE — NAFKAM: 'THE EXCEPTIONAL CASE HISTORY REGISTRY'

This registry is held at the National Research Centre in Complementary and Alternative Medicine (NAFKAM), University of Tromsø, Norway. It was initiated in 2002 and was the first international registry established for long-term collection of exceptional 'best' and 'worst' cases involving CM use. Its purpose was to establish a database that could contribute to the generation of knowledge about the factors influencing the development of exceptional disease courses after the use of complementary treatment. Researchers carry out a thorough medical evaluation of the case histories that patients send to NAFKAM. At the same time, NAFKAM is interested in collecting information about the experiences and the knowledge of people who themselves define their courses of illness as exceptional. The registry is seen as an important window to patient-based knowledge about disease and treatment courses.

Source: Galilei 2007

---

the Office of Cancer Complementary and Alternative Medicine (OCCAM) was established within the National Cancer Institute (NCI) in the United States to coordinate and enhance activities of the NCI in CM research as it relates to the prevention, diagnosis and treatment of cancer, cancer-related symptoms and side effects of conventional cancer treatments (see http://www.cancer.gov/). Since the establishment of OCCAM, the NCI's research expenditure for CM has more than quadrupled, from approximately US$28 million in 1998 to approximately US$105 million in 2011 (National Cancer Institute 2011).

In the UK, the National Cancer Research Institute has a complementary therapies clinical studies development group, which is looking at prioritising areas for study and methodological issues. In Australia and New Zealand there is still relatively little government funding for research in this area; however, the establishment of the National Institute of Complementary Medicine (NICM) in 2007 was an important step towards increasing awareness of this need and lobbying government and philanthropic organisations.

ADVERSE REACTIONS AND INTERACTIONS

One area of great concern is the potential for CMs to reduce the efficacy of oncology treatments or increase their adverse effects and toxicity beyond acceptable limits. In conventional drug therapy, interactions are an ongoing concern, although the clinical relevance of these interactions has not always been investigated. In the area of CM, the issue is even more complicated because much remains unknown about the mechanisms of action of many herbal and natural medicines, and relatively little drug interaction research has been conducted.

ADVERSE REACTIONS

Type A and type B adverse reactions are possible with all therapeutic agents, including complementary medicines (see Chapters 7 and 8). Type A effects are the most common and predictable because they are dose-related, generally of mild to moderate intensity, and reversible. Regarding vitamins, minerals and the cancer patient, toxicity concerns mainly relate to vitamin A and the minerals selenium and zinc.

Vitamin A

Cumulative toxicity is possible with daily doses exceeding 100,000 IU, although some adults can experience toxicity signs and symptoms at lower doses. Symptoms tend to resolve within days to weeks. Supplementation should be avoided in chronic renal failure and liver disease, and high-dose vitamin A should be avoided during radiochemotherapy.

Selenium

Cumulative toxicity is possible with daily doses exceeding 1000 micrograms/day. The organic form of selenium found in high-selenium yeast is less toxic and safer than other forms.

Zinc

Single doses of 225–450 mg can induce vomiting. Long-term daily use of 100–150 mg interferes with copper metabolism and can cause hypocuprinaemia, red blood cell microcytosis and neutropenia.

For further information about individual herbs, vitamins and minerals, refer to the relevant monographs.

INTERACTIONS

Cytotoxic anticancer drugs are among the strongest drugs available and tend to have a complex pharmacological profile, narrow therapeutic index, steep dose–toxicity curve and many pharmacokinetic and pharmacodynamic differences both within and between patients (Beijnen & Schellens 2004). Often combinations of medicines are used to address

the cancer itself, reduce the associated drug toxicities and provide palliation and symptom relief. As such, polypharmacy is standard practice. Additionally, many cancer patients are elderly and may be taking medicines for comorbid conditions such as cardiovascular disease, and as the number of concomitant medicines increases, so too does the risk of interactions (Blower et al 2005). Age-related changes to renal and hepatic functions and reduced homeostatic reserve are other complicating factors that make the prediction and avoidance of interactions difficult in this population.

As discussed in Chapter 8, there are two main categories of interaction, pharmacodynamic and pharmacokinetic, and a minor category known as physicochemical:

- **Pharmacodynamic** interactions occur when one substance alters the sensitivity or responsiveness of tissues to another. This type of interaction results in additive, synergistic or antagonistic drug effects and is frequently employed in clinical practice to improve patient outcomes. It is of particular concern when medicines used simultaneously have overlapping toxicities.

- **Pharmacokinetic** interactions occur when there is an alteration to the absorption, distribution, metabolism or excretion of a medicine. This interaction results in a change to the amount and persistence of available drug at receptor sites or target tissues. As a result, a change in magnitude of effect or duration of effect can occur, but no change to the type of effect is seen. This interaction is sometimes harnessed to increase serum levels of an expensive medicine without increasing the actual dose.

- **Physicochemical** interactions occur when two substances come into contact and are either physically or chemically incompatible. This type of interaction can take place during the manufacture or administration of medicines and result in the inactivation of one or both medicines.

Regardless of the mechanism involved, three possible outcomes can arise from an interaction: increased therapeutic or adverse effects; decreased therapeutic or adverse effects; or a unique response that does not occur when either agent is used alone.

Pharmacodynamic interactions
Antioxidants and chemotherapy

Chemotherapy-related toxicity is a major concern in oncology. The toxicity experienced with the use of chemotherapy agents can be sufficiently severe as to require dosage reduction, delays in treatment and even cessation of potentially effective treatments. Chemotherapy-induced toxicity is also a concern in those patients who are cured or achieve prolonged survival, but experience long-term side effects that reduce their quality of life (Weijl et al 2004). There is emerging evidence that malnourished cancer patients are at even higher risk for chemotherapy toxicity, and therefore nutritional support in the prevention of weight loss and hypoalbuminaemia are important considerations: specific nutrient support is indicated in all chemotherapy patients as a preventative (Bozzeti 2013).

Much debate has arisen about whether antioxidant supplementation alters the efficacy of cancer chemotherapy. Epidemiological studies show that a high intake of antioxidant-rich foods is inversely related to cancer risk, however, once cancer has occurred, there is a theoretical concern that high intake of substances with antioxidant activity will reduce patients' responsiveness to treatments that rely on inducing oxidative stress such as doxorubicin that is preferentially toxic to hypoxic cells (Borek 2004). Drugs with mechanisms of action which include free radical generation include, but are not limited to, alkylating agents (e.g. melphalan, cyclophosphamide), anthracyclines (e.g. doxorubicin, epirubicin), podophyllin derivatives (e.g. etoposide), platinum coordination complexes (e.g. cisplatin, carboplatin) and camptothecins (e.g. topotecan, irinotecan) (Labriola & Livingston 1999). Unfortunately, free radicals produced during the course of treatment are also a major source of serious side effects. For example, cisplatin and other platinum-induced toxicities include nephrotoxicity, ototoxicity and peripheral neuropathy, while doxorubicin and other anthracyclines often cause cardiotoxicity (Block et al 2007). There are other chemotherapy drugs that are thought to be less reliant on free radical production as a mechanism of action, such as plant-derived agents (e.g. vinca alkaloids and taxanes), antimetabolites (e.g. methotrexate, fluorouracil, cytarabine) and hormonal agents (Labriola & Livingston 1999).

Attempting to characterise chemotherapeutic compounds solely in this manner oversimplifies the issue, as most effective chemotherapeutic agents are multi-mechanistic and their relative ability to generate free radicals is not only dose-dependent but also dependent on the localisation and metabolism of the drug within specific tissues (Block et al 2007). Importantly, these cytotoxic drugs tend to have additional mechanisms of action that are not reliant on free radical generation, enabling them to target cells in a number of different ways.

Similarly, antioxidants have multiple mechanisms of action and, depending on their use and dosage, have the potential to serve as free radical molecules themselves.

Currently, clinical evidence is generally lacking to support concerns that antioxidant supplementation given concurrently with reactive-oxygen-species-(ROS)-generating chemotherapy will diminish the efficacy of treatment; however, the area remains underresearched and definitive evidence is still not available.

A historical perspective

The concept of administering antioxidant vitamins in cancer probably arose in the 1970s as a result of publications by Linus Pauling and Ewan Cameron. In one of their early papers entitled 'Orthomolecular treatment of cancer — the role of vitamin C in host defence', it was proposed that cancer treatment must be multidisciplinary and include all that medicine and surgery has to offer and also treatments that maximise the individual patient's resistance to cancer (Cameron & Pauling 1974). The phrase 'orthomolecular treatment' was described as a means of enhancing patients' responses, achieved by manipulating certain biochemical reactions. High-dose vitamin C supplementation was chosen as a good candidate to enhance host resistance, based on theoretical considerations, preliminary studies and the observation that many cancer patients had depleted vitamin C levels.

Cameron and Pauling went on to publish two controlled retrospective studies in 1976 and 1978 that showed the mean survival times were, respectively, more than four and three times as great for the ascorbate subjects as for the controls with the use of intravenously and orally administered high-dose vitamin C (Verrax & Buc Calderon 2008). Pauling and collaborators were convinced that high doses of ascorbate would increase the formation of collagen, leading to tumour encapsulation. Rapidly, several criticisms were raised about the design of the Pauling/Cameron studies since they were not randomised or placebo-controlled and had other methodological weaknesses. In an attempt to either duplicate or refute the amazing results obtained by Cameron and Pauling, the Mayo Clinic initiated different controlled double-blind studies, but these did not find that treatment was effective against advanced malignant disease.

In the last 30 years, our knowledge of the pharmacokinetics and pharmacodynamics of ascorbic acid has increased and provides the rationale to support its re-evaluation as adjuvant treatment for cancer patients. Indeed, ascorbic acid is cytotoxic against a wide variety of cancer cells, but presents a low toxicity towards normal cells, which could lead to the consideration of ascorbate as an interesting anticancer agent (Verrax & Buc Calderon 2008).

The evidence today

A number of comprehensive reviews in the peer-reviewed literature have assessed the effects of combined antioxidant and chemotherapy usage on different outcomes such as side-effect reduction, reduced toxicity and, to a lesser extent, survival. While there are some promising findings, particularly indicating that antioxidants reduce chemotherapy-induced toxicity, definitive conclusions about safety and efficacy cannot yet be drawn because of the variations in study design, intervention protocols, eligibility criteria, statistical power, timing of the observation or intervention, malignancy type and anticancer regimens (Borek 2004).

Block et al (2007) evaluated data from 19 randomised controlled trials ($n = 1554$ patients) in which studies measured survival and/or treatment-response levels of patients who were given antioxidants concurrently with chemotherapy in order to determine if the antioxidants enhanced or interfered with the efficacy of the chemotherapy. Reviewers found no evidence to support concerns that antioxidant supplementation diminished the efficacy of chemotherapy in study populations comprising mostly advanced or relapsed patients; overall,

studies showed a positive trend in the survival and response rates for the groups receiving the antioxidants. Although these results are certainly encouraging, only four studies provided adequate statistical data to support the positive conclusion made by Block et al.

Statistics were more robust to support the conclusion that antioxidant therapy reduced chemotherapy-induced toxicity. Seventeen studies reported on toxicity; 15 of these showed similar or reduced toxicities in the antioxidant group compared to controls; only one study reported significantly greater general toxicity, although the result was somewhat expected owing to the well-documented toxicities of high-dose vitamin A. One other study reported that two out of eight measured toxicities were non-significantly higher; however, the authors reported difficulty in interpretation because of poor patient compliance in the antioxidant group. More specifically, with regard to neurotoxicity, all 11 studies found antioxidant supplementation led to similar or less neurotoxicity compared to controls.

The comprehensive review looked at antioxidants with different mechanisms, such as free-radical scavengers that act as reducers or that break lipid chains (melatonin, N-acetylcysteine [NAC], vitamin E, glutathione [GSH], beta-carotene and vitamin C), metal chelators (vitamin C, epigallocatechin gallate from green tea [EGCG]), cellular protectors (vitamins A, C, E and melatonin), those that target and repair DNA aberrations (EGCG) and antioxidant enzymes created by combining with a protein to form selenoproteins (selenium, GSH). Only studies in which cancer patients were undergoing chemotherapy at the same time were included, as were all types of cancer and various chemotherapies that utilised the reactive oxygen species mechanism.

Some reviews have come to a similar conclusion (Simone & Simone 2008, Simone et al 2007). The authors evaluated 280 peer-reviewed in vitro and in vivo studies, including 50 human studies involving 8521 patients (5081 of whom were given nutrients) and concluded that studies have consistently shown that antioxidants do not interfere with therapeutic modalities for cancer. Furthermore, they contend that non-prescription antioxidants and other nutrients enhance the killing of therapeutic modalities for cancer, decrease their side effects and protect normal tissue. In 15 human studies, 3738 patients who took non-prescription antioxidants and other nutrients actually had increased survival rates.

By contrast, a 2008 review (Lawenda et al 2008) advises against the concurrent use of antioxidants during chemotherapy because of the possibility of tumour protection and reduced survival. The authors identified 16 randomised clinical trials that studied the concurrent use of antioxidant supplements and chemotherapy, six of which included a placebo control. Although no decrements in tumour response rates or survival rates were observed in the studies that reported response data, it was reported that none of the studies were sufficiently powered to evaluate these endpoints.

Theories explaining the observed improvement in survival and/or treatment response reported in some clinical studies with antioxidant supplementation have been offered (Conklin 2004, Block et al 2007). It is suggested that oxidative stress can slow the cell-cycle progression of cancer cells, which can interfere with the ability of anticancer agents to kill cells, and that the formation of reactive oxygen species (ROS), such as aldehydes, can inhibit drug-induced apoptosis and further diminish treatment effects. It is further proposed that the use of antioxidant agents during chemotherapy could enhance treatment effectiveness by decreasing this unwanted effect of ROS generation. In the 2007 review by Block et al, it was suggested that antioxidant therapy reduced free-radical-induced damage to normal tissues, leaving non-oxidative cytotoxic mechanisms unaffected. In this way, patients experienced fewer dose-limiting toxicities, so that more of them could successfully complete prescribed regimens.

Cisplatin and antioxidants

One of the most important drugs used for the treatment of a wide range of solid tumours is cisplatin, but it induces numerous toxicities that are mainly caused by the formation of free radicals, leading to oxidative organ damage. Long-term side effects of treatment include nephrotoxicity, loss of high-tone hearing and peripheral neuropathy. As a strategy to reduce oxidative damage and drug-induced toxicities, antioxidants (nutritional and herbal) have been investigated in both animals and humans, with

some studies showing amelioration or prevention of some side effects and possibly increased treatment effectiveness (Ali & Al Moundhri 2006, Lamson & Brignall 1999, Ohkawa et al 1988, Seifried et al 2003).

Neurotoxic protection

The neurotoxicity of chemotherapy depends not only on the anticancer agent used, the cumulative dose and the delivery method, but also on the capacity of the nerve to cope with the nerve-damaging process. The sensory and motor symptoms and signs of neurotoxicity are disabling, and have a significant impact on the quality of life for cancer patients. Moreover, the risk of cumulative toxicity may limit the use of highly effective chemotherapeutic agents. Therefore, prophylaxis and treatment of peripheral neurotoxicity secondary to chemotherapy are major clinical issues (De 2007).

Experimental and clinical studies have been conducted to investigate whether naturally-derived antioxidants prevent cisplatin-induced neurotoxicity, overall producing promising results. In a recent review of four trials, for example, the combination of vitamin E with cisplatin was shown in all trials to reduce the incidence of chemotherapy-induced peripheral neuropathy (Ben-Arye et al 2013, Wolf et al 2008). While no data was included on the long-term survival of the patients involved, numerous studies have been undertaken that failed to show a detrimental effect from combining vitamin E with chemotherapy. For instance, Argyriou et al (2005) conducted a randomised, open label trial with blind assessment to investigate whether vitamin E supplementation (600 mg/day) has a neuroprotective effect in chemotherapy-induced peripheral nerve damage. Thirty-one patients with cancer treated with six courses of cumulative cisplatin, paclitaxel or their combination regimens were randomly assigned to be controls receiving standard care, or to receive oral vitamin E at a daily dose of 600 mg/day during chemotherapy and for 3 months after its cessation. The incidence of neurotoxicity differed between the two groups, occurring in 25% patients taking vitamin E and 73% of controls ($P = 0.019$). A smaller trial found that a lower dose of only 300 mg/day vitamin E significantly reduced peripheral neurotoxicity in a group of 21 patients each receiving six cycles of cisplatin

($P < 0.01$). This supplementation was orally administered every day before treatment and continued for 3 months after cisplatin therapy and did not have any negative effects on cisplatin therapy (Pace et al 2003). More recently, the same group of researchers conducted a larger follow-up study of 108 cisplatin patients administered the same dose and frequency as previously described and noted that incidence of neurotoxicity was significantly lower in the vitamin E group at 5.9% compared to placebo 41.7% ($P < 0.01$). The severity of neuroxicity as measured by Total Neuotoxicity Score (TNS) was also significantly lower in the treatment group ($P < 0.01$) (Pace et al 2010).

In several experimental settings, the prophylactic administration of acetyl-L-carnitine (ALC), the acetyl ester of L-carnitine, prevented the occurrence of peripheral neurotoxicity commonly induced by chemotherapeutic agents and further promoted recovery of nerve function (De 2007). Later in vitro research suggested alpha-lipoic acid exerts neuroprotective effects against cisplatin-induced neurotoxicity in sensory neurons by protecting against mitochondrial toxicity, which is an early common event in cisplatin-induced neurotoxicity (Melli et al 2008).

Nephrotoxic protection

Many different agents have been shown to ameliorate experimental cisplatin-induced nephrotoxicity including antioxidants (e.g. melatonin, vitamin E, selenium, St John's wort, capsaicin, garlic powder, spirulina, tetramethyl-pyrazine, a major constituent of the Chinese herb *Ligusticum wallichii*, and many others) and modulators of nitric oxide (e.g. zinc histidine complex, L-arginine) (Ali & Al Moundhri 2006, Khan et al 2006, Mohan et al 2006, Razo-Rodriguez et al 2008, Saleh et al 2005, Shimeda et al 2005). Only a few of these agents have been tested in humans.

A randomised study using 4000 micrograms/day of selenium (as seleno-kappacarrageenan), given 4 days before to 4 days after treatment with cisplatin, found that it effectively reduced drug-induced nephrotoxicity and bone-marrow suppression (Hu et al 1997). Another randomised study that tested oral vitamin E (300 mg/day), given before treatment and continued for 3 months post-treatment, showed it significantly reduced the incidence and severity of neurotoxicity associated with cisplatin (Pace et al 2003).

Alternatively, combination therapy with vitamins C and E and selenium in 48 subjects failed to exert protective effects against cisplatin-induced nephrotoxicity and ototoxicity, according to a double-blind study (Weijl et al 2004). The doses used in that study were 1000 mg vitamin C (as L-ascorbic acid), 400 mg vitamin E (as DL-alpha-tocopherol-acetate) and 100 micrograms selenium (as sodium selenite), which was taken as a milky beverage 7 days before the onset of chemotherapy and continued until 3 weeks after cessation of therapy. Unfortunately, the interpretation of the results is difficult, as the study was hampered by very poor patient compliance, with only 36% of the intervention patients drinking the antioxidant-enhanced beverage for the duration of the test period. Additionally, the study has been criticised for using insufficient doses of antioxidants and, although supplementation led to a marked increase in plasma antioxidant levels before cisplatin treatment, enhanced levels were not maintained during chemotherapy. Clearly, further investigation is required.

Antioxidants and radiation therapy

Until recently, research attention has focused primarily on the interaction of antioxidants with chemotherapy, and relatively little attention has been paid to the interaction of antioxidants with radiotherapy. In general, oncologists take the view that antioxidants diminish the effectiveness of radiation therapy; however, there is great variation in the degree of concern over this issue. Considering that over 50% of radiotherapy patients are also utilising CM, more research, education and greater patient–practitioner communication is certainly warranted (Bolderston et al 2008, Moran et al 2013).

Reviews by Moss (2007) and Lawenda et al (2008) provide summaries of the available evidence to determine whether antioxidants interfere with radiation therapy. The different conclusions drawn by the two reviews clearly indicate that the issue of safety in this population is far from decided.

In the literature, published studies have reported on the use of alpha-tocopherol for the amelioration of radiation-induced mucositis; pentoxifylline and vitamin E to correct the adverse effects of radiotherapy; melatonin alongside radiotherapy in the treatment of brain cancer; retinol palmitate as a treatment for radiation-induced proctopathy; a combination of antioxidants and external beam radiation therapy as definitive treatment for prostate cancer; and the use of synthetic antioxidants, amifostine, dexrazoxane and mesna as radioprotectants. Moss (2007) concluded that, with few exceptions, most of the studies draw positive conclusions about the interaction of antioxidants and radiotherapy.

By contrast, Lawenda et al (2008) came to a different conclusion and advised against the concurrent use of antioxidant supplements. Five randomised clinical studies have been reported that investigated the use of high-dose vitamin E (400–600 mg/day or 400 IU/day), high-dose beta-carotene (30 mg/day) or melatonin (20 mg/night) in patients with head and neck cancers, non-small-cell lung cancer, brain metastases or glioblastoma multiforme, who were receiving radiotherapy. Two of these studies produced negative findings. The most concerning was that generated by Bairati et al (2005), who conducted a randomised, double-blind, placebo-controlled study involving 540 head and neck cancer patients treated with radiation therapy. Patients receiving supplementation with alpha-tocopherol (400 IU/day) and beta-carotene (30 mg/day) administered during radiation therapy and for 3 years thereafter tended to have less severe acute adverse effects during radiation therapy; however, the rate of local recurrence of the head and neck tumour tended to be higher in the supplement arm of the trial. Subgroup analysis published later found that interactions between antioxidant supplementation and cigarette smoking during radiation therapy were associated with an increase in both disease recurrence and cancer-specific mortality, whereas no increase in either of these outcome measures was observed for the non-smokers (Meyer et al 2008).

Lawenda et al (2008) point out that it is important to distinguish between high-dose and relatively low-dose antioxidant supplementation and the variations in antioxidant classes, because these differences may substantially define the efficacy and safety profiles of specific antioxidant supplements as therapy for cancer patients receiving selected chemotherapy agents or radiation therapy. Conklin, from the University of California, Los Angeles (UCLA) puts forward the theory that while radiation kills cells by generating high levels of free radicals, the effect is most successful in well-oxygenated tissues (Moss 2007). Tumours, particularly large ones, are often hypoxic at their core, thereby diminishing the effectiveness of radiation. He further suggests that the degree of free radical generation is proportional to the oxygen tension in the tissue, and with improved blood flow, resulting from relatively low-to-moderate doses of antioxidants, improved neoplastic activity may be seen. Conklin also makes the point that the dose of antioxidant supplementation must be sufficiently low to avoid the risk of diminishing treatment efficacy.

Increased risk of bruising and bleeding

A number of commonly used herbs and natural supplements demonstrate antiplatelet activity and have the potential to increase the incidence of bruising and/or bleeding when taken in sufficient dosage. This is of particular concern for patients undergoing major surgery who are taking anticoagulants or conventional antiplatelet agents. A list of these substances is given in Chapter 9.

Hormonally responsive tumours

Hormonal agents are used when a neoplasm is sensitive to hormonal growth controls in the body; for example, prostate cancer is stimulated by male androgens and breast cancer by oestrogen. Chemical treatment may consist of anti-androgens, anti-oestrogens and/or cytotoxic agents. Many constituents in herbs and everyday foodstuffs can theoretically stimulate or inhibit tumour growth or interact with hormonal treatments. The flavonoid group of naturally occurring chemicals provides a good example.

Flavonoids are polyphenolic compounds widely found in vegetables, nuts, fruits, beverages (e.g. coffee, tea and red wine) and medicinal herbs such as St Mary's thistle and St John's wort. They exert a wide range of biochemical and pharmacological actions and have been the focus of much interest, especially with regard to their cancer-protective activities, which are attributed to free-radical scavenging, modification of the enzymes that activate or detoxify carcinogens and inhibiting the induction of the transcription factor activator protein-1 activity by tumour promoters (Moon et al 2006).

Some of these compounds have been found to decrease oestrogen biosynthesis; for example, the flavones chrysin and baicalin, the flavonones (naringenin) and isoflavones (genistein, biochanin A) (Moon et al 2006). This is achieved by inhibiting the activity of aromatase (cytochrome P19) and could theoretically have a use in breast and prostate cancer (Kao et al 1998). Additionally, some flavonoids, such as soy isoflavones, can bind to oestrogen receptors and might slow down cell proliferation as a consequence (Wood et al 2006). Unfortunately, the bioavailability of many dietary flavonoids tends to be low, so effects seen in vitro do not necessarily reflect in vivo responses; however, this may not be true for herbal preparations or functional foods with concentrated flavonoid levels that may achieve much higher plasma concentrations.

Soy and isoflavones

Dietary soy isoflavones have attracted a lot of attention as potential cancer-protective agents, chiefly because of observations that high consumption in Asian diets has been correlated with lower incidence of prostate and breast cancers. Currently the data available is contradictory and it is still unclear under what conditions soy isoflavones have cancer protective effects, if at all.

The potential for soy isoflavones to either enhance or antagonise the effects of anticancer medicines such as tamoxifen has also been investigated in several experimental models. Most studies have focused on genistein, because of its relatively strong binding (in comparison to daidzein) to the alpha- and beta-oestrogen receptors and its oestrogenic/anti-oestrogenic activities, which are stronger than those of other isoflavones (Constantinou et al 2005). Some studies have raised the possibility that genistein could compete with tamoxifen for oestrogen receptors and thereby decrease the drug's efficacy, an observation seen in two experimental models (Constantinou et al 2005, Ju et al 2002). Alternatively, research conducted with daidzein has produced positive results and showed that it enhanced the effect of tamoxifen against mammary carcinogenesis in the rat model (Constantinou et al 2005). In fact, the combination of tamoxifen/daidzein was more effective than tamoxifen alone for reducing tumour burden, incidence and multiplicity, as well as increasing tumour latency. When these results are taken together, it appears that although the isoflavone genistein may have a deleterious effect when combined with tamoxifen, the use of soybeans in combination with tamoxifen is not necessarily dangerous and beneficial effects may even be possible.

Drug inactivation — chemical incompatibility

Predicting interactions between natural products and chemotherapeutic drugs is difficult and occasionally unexpected findings come up. The following case highlights the challenges in making interaction predictions in the area of IO and provides a good example of drug inactivation caused by a natural compound.

In recent years, chemopreventive and chemotherapeutic effects of green tea have been reported in different malignancies and have become well known. Epigallocatechin-3-gallate (EGCG), the most abundant and biologically active polyphenol in green tea, selectively inhibits cell growth and induces apoptosis in cancer cells without adversely affecting normal cells. The antitumour effects of EGCG include inhibition of angiogenesis, modulation of growth-factor-mediated proliferation, suppression of oxidative damage, induction of apoptosis and cell-cycle arrest. As a result, it has become a popular beverage among people with cancer or at risk of cancer.

Shammas et al (2006) reported that EGCG demonstrated potent and specific antimyeloma activity in experimental models, thereby suggesting it could have a role in chemoprevention and possibly treatment of multiple myeloma. As a result, a few years later EGCG was tested in vitro and in vivo to investigate whether combining it with the proteasome inhibitor bortezomib (BZM), commonly used in the treatment of multiple myeloma, would result in an increase in the drug's antitumour activity (Golden et al 2009). The results were surprising, as green tea extract almost completely blocked the effects of BZM both in vitro and in vivo.

Upon further investigation, it was found the interaction was due to a 1,2-benzene diol moiety contained in some of the green tea constituents, particularly the epigallocatechin-gallate (EGCG) which formed stable covalent bonds with the boronic acid moiety of BZM. The formation of the new boronate product resulted in little to none of the proteasome-blocking effect usually observed for BZM, thereby neutralising the cytotoxic activity of BZM. The pronounced antagonistic function of EGCG was evident only with boronic acid-based proteasome inhibitors (bortezomib, MG-262, PS-IX), but not with several non-boronic acid proteasome inhibitors (MG-132, PS-I, nelfinavir).

Although the in vivo component of this study was carried out in mice, the evidence is compelling and strongly suggests that in current practice the combination of BZM and green tea should be avoided until proven safe in clinical studies. It is important to note that this interaction was not based on an antioxidant/free radical mechanism and hence cannot be extrapolated to other antioxidants based solely on their free radical scavenging activity. Whether other agents containing the 1,2-benzene diol moiety also interact with boronic acid-based proteasome inhibitors in the same way is unknown, but it would be prudent to avoid concurrent use until safety is established. Some components containing the 1,2-benzene diol moiety found in the diet and as constituents in several herbal medicines include quercetin and myricetin, which have previously been shown to inhibit BZM in vitro (FT Liu et al 2008).

Pharmacokinetic interactions

Pharmacokinetic interactions often involve metabolising enzymes or drug transporters that have great significance in chemotherapy. Cytochrome enzymes (CYP) and drug transporters in the intestinal epithelium affect the bioavailability of many oral chemotherapy agents and can induce multidrug resistance.

P-glycoprotein

One mechanism responsible for multidrug resistance is overexpression of the adenosine-triphosphate (ATP)-binding cassette-containing family of proteins such as P-glycoprotein (P-gp), which has a counter-transport role and actively forces substrates out of cells. These proteins are expressed in both healthy cells, such as the blood–brain barrier, and resistant tumour cells, and act as a barrier. Of significance, they are highly expressed in the lumen of the gut and can substantially impede the oral uptake of several anticancer medicines (Beijnen & Schellens 2004). Examples of anticancer medicines that are P-gp substrates are:

- daunorubicin
- docetaxel
- doxorubicin
- paclitaxel
- taxol
- tacrolimus
- vinblastine
- vincristine.

An interaction will occur when a substrate is co-administered with another substance that alters the expression of the relevant counter-transport protein. With regard to P-gp, expression can be altered by a number of factors, such as common foods, herbs and pharmaceutical medicines. A promising strategy is to use P-gp inhibitors to increase drug bioavailability and reverse multidrug resistance in tumours; for example, the use of oral cyclosporin and paclitaxel has proved successful in a phase II study of people with advanced non-small-cell lung cancer (Kruijtzer et al 2002). Alternatively, P-gp inducers can have the opposite effect and reduce the bioavailability of P-gp substrates and increase drug resistance: they should be avoided when medicines that are P-gp substrates are administered.

Herbal and natural medicines affecting P-gp

The influence of herbal and natural medicines on P-gp expression has only recently been investigated, so much is still unknown and speculative. To date, most research has centred on St John's wort (*Hypericum perforatum*), which has significant P-gp induction effects, as demonstrated in clinical testing (Durr et al 2000). Studies have found that, after 16 days of continual use, P-gp expression can increase 4.2-fold. The hyperforin constituent is responsible for the induction effect, which is achieved by activation of the pregnane X receptor (Moore et al 2000). In Europe, some manufacturers have produced low-hyperforin-containing herbal products, which may not have the same effect. Besides St John's wort, the isoflavone genistein is reported in other studies to inhibit P-gp-mediated drug transport (Castro & Altenberg 1997).

Alternatively, rosemary extract acts as a P-gp inhibitor. According to an in vitro study, multidrug-resistant mammary tumour cells treated with rosemary extract produced an increase in intracellular concentrations of doxorubicin and vinblastine, both of which are P-gp substrates (Plouzek et al 1999), and the same effects were not seen in cells that lack P-gp expression. More recently, an in vitro study identified that bitter melon (*Momordica charantia*) leaf extract exhibited dose-dependent P-gp inhibition, which resulted in intracellular vinblastine accumulation (Limtrakul et al 2004). The effect was not seen for the fruit. Many other natural substances affect P-gp and have potential as useful adjuncts in the chemotherapeutic treatment of cancer.

Cytochromes and metabolism

Many drugs undergo two phases of metabolism: phase I, or functionalisation reactions, and phase II, or conjugation reactions. Many medicines, nutrients, environmental toxins and endogenous substances undergo metabolism by the CYP P450 system during phase I metabolism. As a result, an active substance can be converted into an inactive, less active, more active or toxic metabolite, or an inactive prodrug can be converted into an active one. Although there are over 50 enzymes in the CYP system, the most important for drug metabolism are CYP1A2, 2D6 and 3A4. In particular, CYP3A4 is involved in the metabolism of many anticancer medicines, some examples of which are the oxazaphosphorines (cyclophosphamide, ifosfamide) and the taxanes (paclitaxel, docetaxel) (Beijnen & Schellens 2004) (see also Table 10.4).

Interactions occur when CYP substrates and inducers or inhibitors are taken at the same time.

Herbal and natural supplements affecting CYP enzymes

Many factors can interfere with CYP activity, such as the ingestion of foreign compounds (e.g. environmental contaminants) or of certain constituents found in food, beverages, herbs or medicines. Of the herbal medicines commonly available, most research has been conducted with St John's wort, which significantly induces CYP enzymes, particularly CYP3A4 with long-term administration (Durr et al 2000, Roby et al 2000, Ruschitzka et al 2000). Once again, these effects are attributed to the interaction between hyperforin and the pregnane X receptor, which regulates expression of CYP3A4 mono-oxygenase. In this way, hyperforin increases the availability of CYP3A4, resulting in enzyme induction (Moore et al

2000). Clinically, this means that serum levels of those medicines that are CYP3A4 substrates will be reduced, which can reduce drug effectiveness and possibly induce therapeutic failure.

In recent years a growing number of other herbal medicines have been subjected to interaction studies and investigated for effects on CYP isoenzymes and transporter proteins, using new in vitro and in vivo techniques. The evidence from these tests suggests that several other herbal medicines have the potential to affect drug absorption and/or metabolism. However, readers are advised that translation of in vitro data to clinical practice is problematic and imperfect, and in vivo testing is required before an interaction prediction can be made.

For example, silymarin, the active constituent group from St Mary's thistle, significantly decreases CYP3A4 activity in primary cultures of human hepatocytes; however, four clinical studies have found no clinically significant effects in vivo (Gurley et al 2004, DiCenzo et al 2003, Leber & Knauff 1976, Piscitelli et al 2002). The daily doses of silymarin used in the clinical studies ranged from 210 mg to 480 mg.

ELIMINATION

Although most anticancer medicines are eliminated though metabolism, some, such as the platinum compounds and methotrexate, are eliminated mainly by the kidneys through glomerular filtration and active tubular secretion (Beijnen & Schellens 2004). Urinary excretion can be altered by substances that affect urinary pH, which will affect renal tubular reabsorption. One substance sometimes used by cancer patients is ascorbic acid. Although low-dose ascorbic acid is unlikely to cause detrimental effects, high doses that acidify the urine can affect the excretion of drug metabolites, which precipitate in the renal tubules at low pH. As a result, there has been a theoretical concern that high-dose vitamin C could precipitate methotrexate. A study by Sketris et al (1984) investigated the proposed interaction and found that it does not appear to be clinically significant; however, caution is still advised.

CLINICAL IMPLICATIONS OF INTEGRATIVE MEDICINE

People with cancer expect their healthcare providers to work with them to achieve adequate symptom relief, improved quality of life and a cure. In order for this to be achieved, a holistic approach that combines several different disciplines is best.

Although the role of some forms of CM in cancer is still unclear, there is evidence to support the use of several approaches as supportive therapies. When these are considered safe and provide benefits, either for symptom relief or improvements in wellbeing and quality of life, they should be made available and become a part of standard protocol. This requires access to reliable information and a collaborative partnership with a variety of healthcare providers, based on mutual respect and open communication.

SHARED DECISION MAKING
A wide range of patient- and doctor-related factors affect clinical decision making and subsequent use or disuse of CM.

1. General safety issues
Patient safety is paramount. Medicinal CM treatments (CMs) can pose a risk to patients via several mechanisms:
- Interference with blood clotting. Cancer patients often have low platelets at various points throughout their treatment, either as a direct result of the cancer itself, or as a temporary side effect from the chemotherapy or radiotherapy. CMs that significantly inhibit blood clotting may increase the risk of haemorrhage.
- Interactions with conventional chemotherapy drugs or radiation therapy resulting in diminished therapeutic effect.
- Interactions with conventional chemotherapy drugs or radiation therapy resulting in increased toxicity and/or other side effects.

Product quality is particularly important to assess in this population. For example, products contaminated with microorganisms can have serious consequences for immunosuppressed patients who have limited ability to mount an immune response.

Such concerns obviously do not relate to non-medicinal CM therapies such as massage and meditation, which may provide significant improvement to patients' wellbeing and quality of life during treatment. In this regard, finding an appropriately trained and credentialled practitioner with experience in treating cancer patients provides some safeguard against possible harm.

2. Availability of credible information sources
Credible, accurate and timely information is required for both patients and healthcare providers in order for evidence-based patient-centred care to occur.

CLINICAL INTEREST — THE COSA POSITION STATEMENT ON COMPLEMENTARY MEDICINE

During 2012–13, the Complementary and Integrative Therapies Interest Group within the Clinical Oncology Society of Australia (COSA) undertook a major initiative, which resulted in the COSA position statement regarding CM use by people with cancer (COSA 2013). After an in-depth search through the peer-reviewed literature, it was revealed that no clear guidelines existed that would help oncology healthcare professionals when their patients were using or considering using CM, either as adjunctive therapy or as an alternative to standard oncology practices. This meant oncologists and other doctors, pharmacists and allied health professionals could be easily confused as to their obligations ethically, professionally and legally and compromise patient safety and autonomy as a result.

The working party, chaired by Dr Lesley Braun, consisted of experts with a range of backgrounds in medicine, pharmacy, medical ethics, psychology, research, government regulation and integrative medicine, together with a consumer advocate. They were assisted by an advisory group which provided further expertise in legal matters, integrative oncology and general and community medicine.

The final document is the result of a true inter-disciplinary effort which aims to improve patient outcomes and help all involved in the therapeutic relationship to work more effectively together. It provides guidance for health professionals involved in the treatment of cancer patients.

See: https://www.cosa.org.au/media/1150/cosa_cam-position-statement_may-2013.pdf

Asking patients about their interest in and use of CM therapies is essential for good practice. Understanding their reasons for use and the information sources to which they have referred when making such decisions is also important. For many patients, family and friends are the main sources of information; others use CM practitioners, the internet, books and magazines.

When discussing the reliability of the information, some points to guide the patient may include:

- Was the internet site used an officially recognised and registered site? Is it frequently updated and what are the credentials of the authors providing content for the site?

- Was the internet site supporting a profit-driven enterprise? Was information in advertorial style, rather than independently written?

- If CM practitioners were consulted, are they registered or accredited with a professional association? What is their training and experience? Credentials?

- Healthcare providers should ensure that they:
  - have access to current, credible and relevant information sources
  - have effective information-seeking skills to locate information from databases and other resources
  - are able to critically evaluate the information retrieved
  - have a network of reliable CM practitioners who can provide additional information about treatments when necessary, as sometimes the peer-reviewed medical press has little useful information about some CM treatments.

3. Evidence of efficacy and safety

Evidence-based, patient-centred care means amassing and evaluating the best available evidence and involving patients in a shared decision-making process that takes into account their individual circumstances and wishes.

The emerging picture shows that the evidence base is greater for some CM therapies than others, and there is an urgent need for more research from a variety of perspectives and methodological approaches. Peer-reviewed journals provide a good starting point for gathering evidence, and frequently updated databases written by people expert in CM are also useful. It is important to note what evidence exists, but also what is missing and remains unknown. Importantly, keep in mind that *a lack of evidence is not necessarily evidence of a lack of effectiveness*. It is likely that some CM treatments being used by patients are effective, but have not yet been subjected to clinical trials. Table 10.5 gives a list of useful internet information sources.

When reviewing the evidence, look for:

- in vitro tests and studies with animal models that provide information about mechanisms, pharmacokinetic influences and the potential effects in humans, although they are not definitive

- clinical studies to provide more relevant information — consider the patient group involved, intent of treatment, interventions used (dose, form, time frames, administration method, type of extract), what other medications were also used (where relevant) and outcomes measured

- up-to-date, comprehensive reviews of the literature.

4. Intent behind using CM treatment

CM therapies are generally used as adjuncts to conventional treatments and, in the case of cancer, to improve quality of life, address symptoms and reduce toxic side effects. Far less common is their use as a potentially curative treatment. The decision to use CM therapies for symptom relief requires different consideration from using CM for curative purposes or as an alternative to conventional care.

5. Severity of disease

The use of CM by people with readily curable cancers is often viewed differently to its use by people with difficult-to-treat cancers or by palliative patients.

Highly curable cancers

When conventional treatments have a high cure rate, concomitant use of less proven treatments should be avoided unless there is clear evidence that it will not diminish outcomes. For example, testicular cancer currently has a 98% 5-year survival rate when treated aggressively with chemotherapy (Cancer Council

TABLE 10.5 USEFUL WEB-BASED INFORMATION SOURCES

Information source and URL	Description
National Cancer Institute (USA) http://cancer.gov	The National Cancer Institute (NCI) is a component of the National Institutes of Health (NIH), one of eight agencies that compose the Public Health Service (PHS) in the Department of Health and Human Services (DHHS). The NCI, established under the *National Cancer Act* 1937, is the Federal Government's principal agency for cancer research and training. The website includes cancer topics, clinical trials, cancer statistics, research and funding, and cancer-related news.
Office of Cancer Complementary and Alternative Medicine http://cam.cancer.gov/	The Office of Cancer Complementary and Alternative Medicine (OCCAM) was established in October 1998 to coordinate and enhance the activities of the National Cancer Institute (NCI) in the arena of complementary and alternative medicine (CAM). The website includes CAM information, research resources, the NCI Best Case Series, clinical trials, grant application information, and funding opportunities in cancer CAM.
PDQ Cancer Information Summaries: Complementary and Alternative Medicine http://www.cancer.gov/cancertopics/pdq/cam	Electronic resource containing summaries of complementary therapies.
PDQ Cancer Clinical Trials http://www.cancer.gov/clinicaltrials/search	The Physician Data Query (PDQ) holds many clinical trials in its international registry and is maintained by the NCI. Users can perform tailored searches focusing on type of cancer, trial type (treatment, supportive care, screening, prevention, genetics, diagnostic), location, status (active or closed), phase, sponsor and drug name.
Cancer Research Portfolio http://fundedresearch.cancer.gov/nciportfolio/	Electronic source for searching, organising and analysing NCI-supported research by organ/cancer site and/or by broad area of scientific interest, such as biology, cancer aetology, prevention, early detection, diagnosis, prognosis, treatment, cancer control, survivorship, outcomes research and scientific model systems.
National Center for Complementary and Alternative Medicine (USA) http://nccam.nih.gov/	The National Center for Complementary and Alternative Medicine (NCCAM) is one of the 27 institutes and centres that make up the National Institutes of Health (NIH). Congress established NCCAM in 1998 to explore complementary and alternative healing practices in the context of rigorous science, to train complementary and alternative medicine (CAM) researchers and to disseminate authoritative information to the public and professionals.
Office of Dietary Supplements (USA) http://ods.od.nih.gov/	The US Dietary Supplement Health and Education Act 1994 authorised the establishment of the Office of Dietary Supplements (ODS) at the NIH to promote scientific research in the area of dietary supplements. The website covers background information about claims and labelling for dietary supplements and botanicals, tips for supplement users, how to spot health fraud, and access to US Department of Agriculture and NIH databases.
American Cancer Society http://www.cancer.org/	The American Cancer Society (ACS) is a nationwide community-based voluntary health organisation. With headquarters in Atlanta, Georgia, the ACS has state divisions and more than 3400 local offices. The ACS journal *CAA Cancer Journal for Clinicians* archives numerous articles on CAM.
Consumer Labs http://www.consumerlab.com/	ConsumerLab.com, LLC (CL) provides independent test results and information to help consumers and healthcare professionals evaluate health, wellness and nutrition products. It publishes results of its tests on its site, including listings of brands that have passed testing. Products that pass CL's testing are eligible to bear the CL Seal of Approval.

(Continued)

TABLE 10.5 USEFUL WEB-BASED INFORMATION SOURCES *(continued)*	
Information source and URL	**Description**
UK information service chisuk.org.uk/	Complementary health information service, UK
NCI-SUPPORTED CANCER RESEARCH PROGRAMS AND CANCER PROGRAMS (USA)	
http://www.mskcc.org/cancer-care/integrative-medicine	Integrative Medicine at Memorial Sloan-Kettering Cancer Center
Cam-cancer	http://www.cam-cancer.org/
http://www.dana-farber.org/Adult-Care/Treatment-and-Support/Patient-And-Family-Support.aspx	Dana-Farber Cancer Institute Zakim Center for Integrated Therapies
http://www.dukecancerinstitute.org/	Duke Comprehensive Cancer Center
http://www.hopkinsmedicine.org/cam/	The Johns Hopkins Center for Complementary and Alternative Medicine
http://www.compmed.umm.edu/default.asp	The University of Maryland Center for Integrative Medicine
http://www.mdanderson.org/education-and-research/departments-programs-and-labs/programs-centers-institutes/integrative-medicine-program/index.html	The University of Texas M.D. Anderson Cancer Center Complementary/Integrative Medicine Education Resources
http://www.medicine.virginia.edu/research/research-centers/cancer-center	University of Virginia Cancer Centre Complementary Cancer Care Program
mdanderson.org/	University of Texas, complementary medicine information site

Sources: Lee 2005, Schmidt & Ernst 2004, Vickers & Cassileth 2001

Victoria 2012). The chemotherapy used for this type of cancer commonly involves cisplatin. Although some clinical studies indicate that concurrent use of antioxidants is likely to be safe, until definitive evidence becomes available it is prudent to avoid use during curative treatment.

If the patient understands the risks associated with the use of complementary medicinal agents during curative treatment, and voluntarily decides to use CM treatment, a compromise may sometimes be reached. It is reasonable to suggest the patient takes CM treatment in between treatment cycles, but abstains for a certain time period before, during and after curative treatment to minimise the risk of drug interactions. The washout period between treatments will depend on the pharmacokinetics of the agents being used. For chemotherapy, for example, St John's wort should be discontinued at least 7 days before any chemotherapy that is metabolised by the CYP3A4 enzymatic pathway or involves the P-gp transporter (see Chapter 8). Treatment may be

recommenced after five times the elimination half-life of the chemotherapy agent. Making an accurate determination of appropriate washout periods is difficult owing to interpatient variability of pharmacokinetics, and the difficulty in interpreting pharmacokinetic data. As a result, a conservative estimation of the half-life is recommended.

The Micromedex database states that the drug cyclophosphamide has an elimination half-life of 3–12 hours (Commonwealth of Australia 2005). This means that St John's wort should not be started until 3 days (12 × 5 = 60 hours) after cessation of the cyclophosphamide. However, this has not taken into account the fact that cyclophosphamide has active metabolites that contribute to its pharmacological effect. No specific data are available in popular drug databases concerning the half-life or the metabolic pathway of the primary active metabolite, but a case study of 12 people has been reported that identified 77% of the active metabolite present in serum 8 hours after administration. Assuming linear elimination kinetics, the elimination half-life of the active metabolite is extrapolated to be 17.3 hours; thus, the patient should wait for at least 86.5 hours before recommencing St John's wort. In such cases, if the cyclophosphamide is being given at regular intervals (often every 14 or 21 days), the most practical option is to abstain throughout treatment and recommence 4 days after the final treatment cycle has ended.

The use of CMs during active chemotherapy attracts a greater risk of drug interactions and is more problematic. It is essential to gather credible information about the known and unknown benefits and risks and to provide this to patients, so they can be involved in making an informed decision. If patients with a readily curable cancer experience drug-induced toxicities that jeopardise their ability to continue treatment or necessitates dose reduction, then concurrent use of antioxidants and other organ-protective treatments may be more acceptable and provide a useful option.

Difficult-to-cure cancers

When conventional treatments do not have a high cure rate, or a patient's response to treatments has been poor, a different situation arises. The combined use of CMs with conventional treatments is more acceptable in this setting, although thoughtful judgement still applies.

Numerous CM therapies have been shown to reduce a variety of chemotherapy-related side effects and/or pose no obvious risk to patients. In addition, CMs shown to have potential to increase the efficacy of chemotherapy can be further explored (with less ethical problems) in this patient group.

For example, ovarian cancers in the advanced stages are often treated with single-agent cisplatin or carboplatin. Treatment cessation or dose reductions are most often due to toxicities and/or renal impairment. Various antioxidants have been shown to reduce chemotherapy-induced peripheral neuropathy (Wolf et al 2008), renal toxicity and haematological toxicity (Block et al 2007) and may play an important role in reducing additional organ damage. Some clinical studies further suggest that co-administration may improve survival outcomes. As a result, combined use of antioxidants and other CMs with chemotherapy may present patients with a good option.

Prevention and enhancing quality of life in cancer survivors

Good knowledge and critical analysis of CM research is important for clinicians who counsel patients about preventing cancer recurrence and meeting survivorship needs. Considering that 64% of cancer patients survive more than 5 years beyond diagnosis, oncologists and CM practitioners are challenged to expand their focus from acute care to managing the long-term health consequences of cancer treatment and ensuring the integration of cancer prevention into their practices (Sagar & Lawenda 2009). When a patient has initiated CM integration during cancer therapy, it is reasonable to expect that they may want to continue utilising CM in some form, such as a specialised diet or supplementation, after treatment. Reasons for this include enhancing quality of life, reducing fatigue and improving energy levels, enhancing immune function and the interest in continuing positive lifestyle changes to prevent recurrence.

There are numerous dietary and lifestyle changes that survivors may wish to explore, with different levels of evidence to support their use. For example, a patient may reduce refined sugar intake in an ongoing manner due to research suggesting that excess dietary sugar increases cancer risk and promotes cancer cell growth via an increase in growth hormones, including insulin and insulin-like growth factor (Dixon 2012). Some food groups, such as dairy, are associated with increased risk of some types of cancer such as prostate cancer (Newmark & Heaney 2010), but may be protective in others such as breast cancer (Dong et al 2011). Lack of lifestyle modification plays a very significant role in the development of new cancers, and may be a factor in the relapse of previously treated disease. Preventive lifestyle changes such as increased physical activity are very important in bowel cancer prevention (Meyerhardt et al 2006a, 2006b) and in breast cancer (Larsson et al 2007). Weight loss was found to be a significant contributor to disease-free survival in the Women's Intervention and Nutrition Study, which focused on limiting dietary saturated fat in breast cancer survivors (Chlebowski et al 2006). A systematic review of publications on green tea research concludes that the tea may have beneficial effects on cancer prevention (Liu et al 2008); however, the constituents of green tea, including the polyphenolic catechins such as epigallocatechin-3-gallate may not be an appropriate CM during treatment with bortezomib, as discussed earlier in this chapter.

Guidance regarding evidence-based health promotion strategies are important for the promotion of disease-free survival, and oncologists are uniquely positioned to deliver this information: which may be as simple as the guidelines set forth by the World Cancer Research Fund that advocate maintaining a low glycaemic diet, decreasing red meat, salt and alcohol intakes, while increasing the intake of whole fruits, vegetables, legumes and grains (WCRF 2007).

Studies that focus on the effect of CM on quality of life (QoL) measures show varying levels of improvement with regard to physical QoL, but all show that the inclusion of CM during and after cancer treatment improved overall and mental QoL. Reviews by Schneerson et al (2013) and Wesa et al (2008) indicate that yoga and meditation/mindfulness during and after treatment improves QoL measures. However, even though the improvements are statistically significant, it is difficult to determine whether the true effect is due to the yoga/meditation itself or from difficulty in blinding and confounding factors, such as incidental social interaction. Further studies where the 'control' group is a social opportunity may clarify the difference between the 'intervention effect' and the 'trial effect' (Schneerson et al 2013).

Palliative care

The goal of palliative care is the achievement of the best quality of life for patients and their families. It involves the active holistic care of patients with advanced, progressive illness so they can live as actively as possible. It also involves assisting patients to die as they have lived, when the time arrives. Respecting a patient's choice during this period is of supreme importance. Providing relief from pain and other symptoms is paramount.

CM therapies are more accepted in the palliative care setting and can provide an important means of improving patients' quality of life, as the potential benefits of treatment tend to outweigh the potential risks. There is also a greater emphasis on patients' values and lifestyle habits in the delivery of quality care at the end of life, which allows more flexibility in patient care.

> It is important to remember that the ultimate decision to use or disuse CM treatments lies with the patient.

Besides providing physical benefits, the use of various CM therapies and medicinal treatments may provide significant psychological benefits for patients and their families if they have a strong need to feel they have tried everything possible that is available to them. The use of CM during this stage may assist them in coming to terms with the disease and subsequently help the family in the bereavement period.

Unfortunately, indiscriminate use of CM treatments during this period may also occur as patients and families search desperately for new treatments. Research on breast cancer patients indicates that the most common sources of information for use in decision making lie outside the medical system, including families and friends (49%), followed by the media (39%), whereas within the medical system, the GP played the major role (40%), followed by the outpatient oncologist with 20% (Tautz et al 2012). Although family and friends may be true advocates for the patient's wishes in some cases, inappropriate and unqualified advice in the use of some CMs may have detrimental effects and place an unwanted burden on the patient physically, psychologically and financially if they comply with family wishes while suffering added discomfort to do so (Öhlén et al 2006). In the UK, national guidelines for the use of complementary therapies in supportive palliative care provide a comprehensive overview of the key issues involved in CM provision and make recommendations for the safe and appropriate use of CM treatments in this population (Tavares 2003).

Communicating with patients

The patient–practitioner communication gap is a common phenomenon with regard to CM therapies in oncology. Failure to integrate information regarding health advice and therapies may interfere with provision of effective and safe care, whether complementary or conventional. In addition, communication barriers may cause safety issues, such as delayed or missed diagnoses, as well as adverse events from conventional–CM treatment interactions (Gulla

& Singer 2000). It is well documented that a lack of good communication and failure to include the patient's perspective is responsible for most formal complaints and litigation in health care malpractice, which involves lack of due care resulting in patient injury (Brophy 2014, Cohen & Kemper 2005). Because of the above issues of safety and efficacy, which could impact on patient care, doctors and CM providers are urged to inquire about concurrent therapies and monitor them for safety and efficacy in order to accurately estimate clinical risk (Deng et al 2007).

Various measures have been proposed in an attempt to close this gap. Schiff et al (2011) proposes a user-friendly framework for better communication between doctors, CM practitioners and patients in order to achieve better therapeutic outcomes. They propose more frequent use of the referral letter with the inclusion of four critical 'content elements', as represented by the mnemonic DIGS: conventional or CM diagnosis, with explanations of terminology when appropriate; possible CM–conventional treatment interactions; description of the treatment plan and goals and finally the quality of supplement/herb when prescribed (Schiff et al 2011). A communication-prompting list is suggested as a framework for clinicians, including reminders to: understand, respect, ask, explore, respond, discuss, advise, summarise, document and monitor CM therapies. Further to this, Ben-Arye et al (2013) provide a flow chart of a recommended stepwise approach to establishment of open non-judgemental oncologist–patient dialogue on CM use during adjuvant chemotherapy and radiotherapy, focusing on discussion, respect and trust.

Clearly, the need for doctors to assist patients in treatment decision making is considerable and requires more than just a basic knowledge of common CMs (Ben-Arye et al 2012). Doctors also need to have effective (and non-judgemental) communication skills to manage the discussion. They must also be prepared to provide information and advice about the benefits and likely outcomes of treatment, potential risks and complications, side effects and complementary treatment options. This information is needed to meet the traditional ethical principles of non-maleficence (do no harm), beneficence (offer a benefit), respect for autonomy and medical pluralism (Ben-Arye et al 2008, Schiff & Ben-Arye 2011, Schiff et al 2011, Verhoef et al 2006).

PRACTICE TIPS TO PROMOTE PATIENT SAFETY

1. **Ask all patients about the use of CMs.**
   According to the literature, many patients fail to disclose use of CMs to hospital staff; however, disclosure is more likely if they are asked directly (Tautz et al 2012). Some patients may not understand what is meant by the term 'complementary medicine', so consider using phrases such as 'vitamins, minerals or herbal medicines' or 'natural medicines'. If a patient is also seeing a CM practitioner who is prescribing CM treatments, it may be important to contact the practitioner and start an open dialogue to promote patient safety and continuity of care.

2. **Clearly communicate about risks and benefits, known and unknown.**
   If a patient is using a CM that has known or suspected potential to cause adverse outcomes, an honest discussion about what is known and unknown about the risks should ensue. If the patient still wishes to continue using the CM product against professional advice, the patient should be asked to sign a form listing the potential adverse effects to acknowledge that the attending doctor or pharmacist has recommended against continued use. This should also be documented in the patient's medication history and/or discharge summary.

3. **Suspend use of complementary medicines known or suspected to pose a safety risk.**
   Pharmacokinetic data about the drugs involved in treatment will help determine appropriate washout periods.

4. **If in doubt, refer to drug information centres, peer-reviewed literature or reputable resources for further information.**
   Evidence is accumulating about CM at a rapid rate and it would be unreasonable to expect all healthcare professionals to keep up to date with these changes. However, referring to reputable information sources when unsure about patient safety is essential for best practice.

5. **Document information and recommendations in the patient's chart.**
   A patient's CM use should be documented in the medication history and/or discharge summary as appropriate. The name, strength, brand and dose used should be recorded.

6. **Consider if and when a patient can resume taking the CM.**
   If use of an effective CM has been withdrawn, recommencement will be required to restore the patient's response. This should be discussed when taking the medication history.

7. **Recommend CMs with known safety and benefits.**
   If research indicates a CM has significant patient benefits and is low-risk, then evidence-based practice dictates it should be considered in the patient's management. Furthermore, if a patient is experiencing beneficial outcomes from the use of a CM product in the time prior to cancer treatment and the available evidence indicates efficacy and safety, continued use should be considered and carefully monitored.

8. **If an adverse event does occur, report this through the relevant channels.**
   Case reports provide useful clues that can guide future research to better determine factors affecting patients' safety.

REFERENCES

Adler SR, Fosket JR. Disclosing complementary and alternative medicine use in the medical encounter: a qualitative study in women with breast cancer. J Fam Pract 48.6 (1999): 453–458.

Ali BH, Al Moundhri MS. Agents ameliorating or augmenting the nephrotoxicity of cisplatin and other platinum compounds: A review of some recent research. Food Chem Toxicol 44.8 (2006): 1173–1183.

Argyriou AA et al. Vitamin E for prophylaxis against chemotherapy-induced neuropathy: a randomized controlled trial. Neurology 64.1 (2005): 26–31.

Aung HH et al. Scutellaria baicalensis extract decreases cisplatin-induced pica in rats. Cancer Chemother Pharmacol 52.6 (2003): 453–458.

Bairati I et al. Randomized trial of antioxidant vitamins to prevent acute adverse effects of radiation therapy in head and neck cancer patients. J Clin Oncol 23.24 (2005): 5805–5813.

Beatty LJ et al. Evaluating the impact of cancer on complementary and alternative medicine use, distress and health related QoL among Australian women: A prospective longitudinal investigation. Complementary Therapies in Medicine 20 (2012): 61–69.

Beijnen JH, Schellens JH. Drug interactions in oncology. Lancet Oncol 5.8 (2004): 489–496.

Ben-Arye E et al. Ethical issues in integrative oncology. Hematol Oncol Clin N Am 22 (2008): 737–753.

Ben-Arye E et al. The role of health care communication in the development of complementary and integrative medicine. Patient Education and Counseling 89 (2012): 363–367.

Ben-Arye E et al. Advising patients on the use of non-herbal nutritional supplements during cancer therapy: a need for doctor-patient communication. Journal of Pain and Symptom Management 46.6 (2013): 887–896.

Bernstein BJ, Grasso T. Prevalence of complementary and alternative medicine use in cancer patients. Oncology 15.10 (2001): 1267–1272.

Block KI et al. Impact of antioxidant supplementation on chemotherapeutic efficacy: A systematic review of the evidence from randomized controlled trials. Cancer Treat Rev 33.5 (2007): 407–418.

Blower P et al. Drug–drug interactions in oncology: why are they important and can they be minimized? Crit Rev Oncol Hematol 55.2 (2005): 117–142.

Bolderston A et al Radiation therapists' experiences with complementary alternative medicine use by their patients: a preliminary study. Journal of Medical Imaging and Radiation Sciences 39 (2008): 128–134.

Borek C. Dietary antioxidants and human cancer. Integrative Cancer Therapies 3.4 (2004): 333–341.

Bower JE et al. Yoga for cancer patients and survivors. Cancer Control 12.3 (2005): 165–171.

Boyd DB. Integrative oncology: the last ten years — a personal retrospective. Altern Ther Health Med 13.1 (2007): 56–64.

Bozzeti F. Nutritional support of the oncology patient. Crit Rev Oncol/Hematol 87 (2013): 172–200.

Brophy E. Health care decision-making, CM and the law. Advances in Integrative Medicine 1 (2014): 40–43.

Bryant B et al. Pharmacology for health professionals. Sydney: Elsevier, 2003.

Cameron E, Pauling L. The orthomolecular treatment of cancer. I. The role of ascorbic acid in host resistance. Chem Biol Interact 9.4 (1974): 273–283.

Cancer Council Victoria. Cancer Survival Victoria 2012 Available: http://www.cancervic.org.au/downloads/cec/cancer-survival-victoria-2012.pdf 29/7/2014.

Cassileth BR. Evaluating complementary and alternative therapies for cancer patients. CA Cancer J Clin 49.6 (1999): 362–375.

Castro AF, Altenberg GA. Inhibition of drug transport by genistein in multidrug-resistant cells expressing P-glycoprotein. Biochem Pharmacol 53.1 (1997): 89–93.

Chlebowski, RT et al. Dietary fat reduction and breast cancer outcome: interim efficacy results from the Women's Intervention Nutrition Study. J. Natl. Cancer Inst. 98.24 (2006): 1767–1776.

Cohen L et al. Psychological adjustment and sleep quality in a randomized trial of the effects of a Tibetan yoga intervention in patients with lymphoma. Cancer 100.10 (2004): 2253–2260.

Cohen MH, Kemper KJ. Complementary therapies in pediatrics: a legal perspective. Pediatrics 115 (2005): 774–780.

Commonwealth of Australia. The cancer journey: Informing choice. Report of the Senate Community Affairs References Committee on the inquiry into services and treatment options for persons with cancer, June 2005.

Conklin KA. Chemotherapy-associated oxidative stress: impact on chemotherapeutic effectiveness. Integr Cancer Ther 3.4 (2004): 294–300.

Conklin KA. Coenzyme q10 for prevention of anthracycline-induced cardiotoxicity. Integr Cancer Ther 4.2 (2005): 110–130.

Constantinou AI et al. The soy isoflavone daidzein improves the capacity of tamoxifen to prevent mammary tumours. Eur J Cancer 41.4 (2005): 647–654.

COSA. Position statement on the use of complementary and alternative medicine by cancer patients. Clinical Oncological Society of Australia, 2013.

De GD. Acetyl-L-carnitine for the treatment of chemotherapy-induced peripheral neuropathy: a short review. CNS Drugs 21 (Suppl 1) (2007): 39–43.

Deng GE et al. Integrative oncology practice guidelines. J Soc Int Oncology 5.2 (2007): 65–84.

DiCenzo R et al. Coadministration of milk thistle and indinavir in healthy subjects. Pharmacotherapy 23.7 (2003): 866–870.

Dixon S. Nutrition in complementary and alternative medicine. Seminars in Oncology Nursing, 28.1 (2012): 75–84.

Dong JY et al. Dairy consumption and risk of breast cancer: a meta-analysis of prospective cohort studies. Breast Cancer Res Treat 127 (2011): 23–31.

Durr D et al. St John's wort induces intestinal P-glycoprotein/MDR1 and intestinal and hepatic CYP3A4. Clin Pharmacol Ther 68 (2000): 598–604.

Ernst E. The current position of complementary/alternative medicine in cancer. Eur J Cancer 39.16 (2003): 2273–2277.

Ernst E, Cassileth BR. The prevalence of complementary/alternative medicine in cancer: a systematic review. Cancer 83.4 (1998): 777–782.

Fonnebo V et al. Cancer and complementary medicine: an international perspective. Support Care Cancer 15.8 (2007): 999–1002.

Fox P et al. Using a mixed methods research design to investigate complementary alternative medicine (CAM) use among women with breast cancer in Ireland. European Journal of Oncology Nursing 17 (2013): 490–497.

Galilei. 'The knowledgeable patients': announcement of the conference of National Research Centre in Complementary and Alternative Medicine, University of Tromso, Norway, 2007.

Ge J et al. Patient–physician communication about complementary and alternative medicine in a radiation oncology setting. Int J Radiation Oncol Biol Phys, 85.1 (2013): e1–e6.

Golden EB et al. Green tea polyphenols block the anticancer effects of bortezomib and other boronic acid-based proteasome inhibitors. Blood 113.23 (2009): 5927–5937.

Greenlee H et al. Complementary and alternative therapy use before and after breast cancer diagnosis: the pathways study. Breast Cancer Research and Treatment 117.3 (2009), 653–665.

Gulla J, Singer AJ. Use of alternative therapies among emergency department patients. Ann Emerg Med 35 (2000):226–228.

Gurley BJ et al. In vivo assessment of botanical supplementation on human cytochrome P450 phenotypes: Citrus aurantium, Echinacea purpurea, milk thistle, and saw palmetto. Clin Pharmacol Ther 76.5 (2004): 428–440.

Hu YJ et al. The protective role of selenium on the toxicity of cisplatin-contained chemotherapy regimen in cancer patients. Biol Trace Elem Res 56.3 (1997): 331–341.

Jonas WB et al. Proposal for an integrated evaluation model for the study of whole systems healthcare in cancer. Integr Cancer Ther. 5.4(2006): 315–319.

Ju YH et al. Dietary genistein negates the inhibitory effect of tamoxifen on growth of estrogen-dependent human breast cancer (MCF-7) cells implanted in athymic mice. Cancer Res 62.9 (2002): 2474–2477.

Kakai H. A Community of Healing: Psychosocial Functions of Integrative Medicine Perceived by Oncology Patients/Survivors, Healthcare Professionals, and CAM Providers. J Sci Heal. 9.6 (2013): 365–371.

Kao YC et al. Molecular basis of the inhibition of human aromatase (estrogen synthetase) by flavone and isoflavone phytoestrogens: A site-directed mutagenesis study. Environ Health Perspect 106.2 (1998): 85–92.

Khan M et al. Spirulina attenuates cyclosporine-induced nephrotoxicity in rats. J Appl Toxicol 26.5 (2006): 444–451.

Kruijtzer CM et al. Phase II and pharmacologic study of weekly oral paclitaxel plus cyclosporine in patients with advanced non-small-cell lung cancer. J Clin Oncol 20.23 (2002): 4508–4516.

Labriola D, Livingston R. Possible interactions between dietary antioxidants and chemotherapy. Oncology 13.7 (1999): 1003–1008.

Lamson DW, Brignall MS. Antioxidants in cancer therapy: their actions and interactions with oncologic therapies. Altern Med Rev 4.5 (1999): 304–329.

Langler A et al. Attitudes and beliefs of paediatric oncologists regarding complementary and alternative therapies. Complementary Therapies in Medicine 21S (2013): S10–S19.

Larsson SC et al Diabetes mellitus and risk of breast cancer: a meta-analysis. Int. J. Cancer 121.4 (2007): 856–862.

Launso L et al. Exceptional disease courses after the use of CAM: selection, registration, medical assessment, and research. an international perspective. J Altern Complement Med 12.7 (2006): 607–613.

Lawenda BD et al. Should supplemental antioxidant administration be avoided during chemotherapy and radiation therapy? J Natl Cancer Inst 100.11 (2008): 773–783.

Leber HW, Knauff S. Influence of silymarin on drug metabolizing enzymes in rat and man. Arzneimittel-Forsch 26.8 (1976): 1603–1605.

Lee CO. Communicating facts and knowledge in cancer complementary and alternative medicine. Semin Oncol Nurs 21.3 (2005): 201–214.

Leis AM, Weeks LC, Verhoef MJ. Principles to guide integrative oncology and the development of an evidence base. Curr Oncol 15 (Suppl 2) (2008): s83–s87.

Limtrakul P et al. Inhibition of P-glycoprotein activity and reversal of cancer multidrug resistance by Momordica charantia extract. Cancer Chemother Pharmacol 54.6 (2004): 525–530.

Liu FT et al. Dietary flavonols inhibit the anticancer effects of the proteasome inhibitor bortezomib. Blood 112.9 (2008): 3835–3846.

Liu J et al. Green tea (Camellia sinensis) and cancer prevention: a systematic review of randomized trials and epidemiological studies. Chinese Med. 3.12 (2008).

Melli G et al. Alpha-lipoic acid prevents mitochondrial damage and neurotoxicity in experimental chemotherapy neuropathy. Exp Neurol 214.2 (2008): 276–284.

Meyer F et al. Interaction between antioxidant vitamin supplementation and cigarette smoking during radiation therapy in relation to long-term effects on recurrence and mortality: A randomized trial among head and neck cancer patients. Int J Cancer 122.7 (2008): 1679–1683.

Meyerhardt, J et al. Physical activity and survival after colorectal cancer diagnosis. J. Clin. Oncol. 24.22 (2006a): 3527–3534.

Meyerhardt, J et al. Impact of physical activity on cancer recurrence and survival in patients with stage III colon cancer: findings from CALGB 89803. J. Clin. Oncol. 24.22 (2006b): 3535–3541.

Mijares A, Lopez JR. L-carnitine prevents increase in diastolic [Ca2+] induced by doxorubicin in cardiac cells. Eur J Pharmacol 425.2 (2001): 117–120.

Mohan IK et al. Protection against cisplatin-induced nephrotoxicity by Spirulina in rats. Cancer Chemother Pharmacol 58.6 (2006): 802–808.

Molassiotis A, Cubbin D. 'Thinking outside the box': complementary and alternative therapies' use in paediatric oncology patients. Eur J Oncol Nurs 8.1 (2004): 50–60.

Moon YJ et al. Dietary flavonoids: effects on xenobiotic and carcinogen metabolism. Toxicol In Vitro 20.2 (2006): 187–210.

Moore LB et al. St. John's wort induces hepatic drug metabolism through activation of the pregnane X receptor. Proc Natl Acad Sci USA 97 (2000): 7500–7502.

Moran MS et al. A prospective, multicenter study of complementary/alternative medicine (cam) utilization during definitive radiation for breast cancer. Int J Radiat Oncol Biol Phys 85 (2013): 40–46.

Moss RW. Do antioxidants interfere with radiation therapy for cancer? Integr Cancer Ther 6.3 (2007): 281–292.

National Cancer Institute. Annual Report of Complementary and Alternative Medicine. US Department of Health and Human Services/ National Institutes of Health. 2011. Available http://cam.cancer.gov/ cam_annual_report_fy11.pdf 8 October 2014.

NCCAM National Center for Complementary and Alternative Medicine. What is CAM? (2009).

Newmark HL, Heaney RP. Dairy products and prostate cancer risk. Nutr Cancer 62 (2010): 297–299.

Ohkawa K et al. The effects of co-administration of selenium and cis-platin (CDDP) on CDDP-induced toxicity and antitumour activity. Br J Cancer 58.1 (1988): 38–41.

Öhlén J et al. The influence of significant others in complementary and alternative medicine decisions by cancer patients. Social Science & Medicine 63 (2006): 1625–1636.

Pace A et al. Neuroprotective effect of vitamin E supplementation in patients treated with cisplatin chemotherapy. J Clin Oncol 21.5 (2003): 927–931.

Pace A et al Vitamin E neuroprotection for cisplatin neuropathy. Neurology 4.9 (2010): 762–766.

Piscitelli SC et al. Effect of milk thistle on the pharmacokinetics of indinavir in healthy volunteers. Pharmacotherapy 22.5 (2002): 551–556.

Plouzek CA et al. Inhibition of P-glycoprotein activity and reversal of multidrug resistance in vitro by rosemary extract. Eur J Cancer 35 (1999): 1541–1545.

Ponholzer A et al. Frequent use of complementary medicine by prostate cancer patients. Eur Urol 43.6 (2003): 604–608.

Razo-Rodriguez AC et al. Garlic powder ameliorates cisplatin-induced nephrotoxicity and oxidative stress. J Med Food 11.3 (2008): 582–586.

Rees RW et al. Prevalence of complementary therapy use by women with breast cancer: A population-based survey. Eur J Cancer 36.11 (2000): 1359–1364.

Rees L, Weil A. Integrated medicine. BMJ 322.7279 (2001): 119–120.

Richardson MA et al. Complementary/alternative medicine use in a comprehensive cancer centre and the implications for oncology. J Oncol 18 (2000): 2505–2514.

Roby CA et al. St John's Wort: effect on CYP3A4 activity. Clin Pharmacol Ther 67 (2000): 451–457.

Ruschitzka F et al. Acute heart transplant rejection due to Saint John's wort. Lancet 355 (2000): 548–549.

Sagar SM. Integrative oncology in North America. J Soc Integr Oncol 4.1 (2006): 27–39.

Sagar SM, Lawenda BD. The Role of Integrative Oncology in a Tertiary Prevention Survivorship Program. Prev Med. 49.2–3 (2009): 93–98.

Sagar SM. How do we evaluate outcome in an integrative oncology program? Curr Oncol 15 (Suppl 2) (2008): s78–s82.

Saleh S, et al. Protective effects of L-arginine against cisplatin-induced renal oxidative stress and toxicity: role of nitric oxide. Basic Clin Pharmacol Toxicol 97.2 (2005): 91–97.

Schiff E et al. Bridging the physician and CAM practitioner communication gap: Suggested framework for communication between physicians and CAM practitioners based on a cross professional survey from Israel. Patient Education and Counseling 85 (2011): 188–193.

Schiff E, Ben-Arye E. Complementary therapies for side effects of chemotherapy and radiotherapy in the upper gastrointestinal system. European Journal of Integrative Medicine 3 (2011): 11–16.

Schmidt K, Ernst E. Assessing websites on complementary and alternative medicine for cancer. Ann Oncol 15.5 (2004): 733–742.

Schneerson C et al. The effect of complementary and alternative medicine on the quality of life of cancer survivors: A systematic review and meta-analyses. Complementary Therapies in Medicine 21 (2013): 417–429.

Seifried HE et al. The antioxidant conundrum in cancer. Cancer Res 63.15 (2003): 4295–4298.

Shammas MA et al. Specific killing of multiple myeloma cells by (-)-epigallocatechin-3-gallate extracted from green tea: biologic activity and therapeutic implications. Blood 108.8 (2006): 2804–2810.

Sharma SS et al. Antiemetic efficacy of ginger (Zingiber officinale) against cisplatin-induced emesis in dogs. J Ethnopharmacol 57.2 (1997): 93–96.

Sharma SS, Gupta YK. Reversal of cisplatin-induced delay in gastric emptying in rats by ginger (Zingiber officinale). J Ethnopharmacol 62.1 (1998): 49–55.

Shimeda Y et al. Protective effects of capsaicin against cisplatin-induced nephrotoxicity in rats. Biol Pharm Bull 28.9 (2005): 1635–1638.

Simone CB et al. Antioxidants and other nutrients do not interfere with chemotherapy or radiation therapy and can increase kill and increase survival, Part 2. Altern Ther Health Med 13.2 (2007): 40–47.

Simone CB, Simone CB II. Re: Should supplemental antioxidant administration be avoided during chemotherapy and radiation therapy? J Natl Cancer Inst 100.21 (2008): 1558–1559.

Sketris IS et al. Effect of vitamin C on the excretion of methotrexate. Cancer Treat Rep 68.2 (1984): 446–447.

Smyth JF. Integrative oncology — what's in a name? Eur J Cancer 42.5 (2006): 572–573.

Taixiang W et al. Chinese medical herbs for chemotherapy side effects in colorectal cancer patients. Cochrane Database Syst Rev 1 (2005): CD004540.

Tautz E et al. Use of Complementary and Alternative Medicine in breast cancer patients and their experiences: A cross-sectional study. Euro J Cancer 48 (2012): 3133–3139.

Tavares M. National guidelines for the use of complementary therapies in supportive and palliative care. London: The Prince of Wales Foundation for Integrated Health/National Council for Hospice and Specialist Palliative Care Services, 2003.

Vapiwala, N. et al. Patient initiation of complementary and alternative medical therapies (CAM) following cancer diagnosis. Cancer J. 12 (2006) 467–474.

Verhoef MJ et al. Complementary and alternative medicine whole systems research: beyond identification of inadequacies of the RCT. Complement Ther Med 13.3 (2005): 206–212.

Verhoef M, Vanderheyden L. A whole systems research approach to cancer care: why do we need it and how do we get started? Integr Cancer Ther 5.4 (2006): 287–292.

Verrax J et al. The controversial place of vitamin C in cancer treatment. Biochem Pharmacol 76.12 (2008): 1644–1652.

Vickers AJ, Cassileth BR. Unconventional therapies for cancer and cancer-related symptoms. Lancet Oncol 2.4 (2001): 226–232.

Waldner R et al. Effects of doxorubicin-containing chemotherapy and a combination with L-carnitine on oxidative metabolism in patients with non-Hodgkin lymphoma. J Cancer Res Clin Oncol 132.2 (2006): 121–128.

Walshe R et al. Socio-demographic and medical correlates of the use of biologically based complementary and alternative medicines amongst recent Australian cancer survivors. Preventive Medicine 54 (2012) 23–26.

Wanchai A et al. Complementary and alternative medicine use among women with breast cancer: a systematic review. Clin J Onc Nurs 14.4 (2010) E45–E55.

WCRF (World Cancer Research Fund/American Institute for Cancer Research). Food, Nutrition, Physical Activity and the Prevention of Cancer: A Global Perspective. American Institute for Cancer Research, Washington DC. 2007.

Weijl NI et al. Supplementation with antioxidant micronutrients and chemotherapy-induced toxicity in cancer patients treated with cisplatin-based chemotherapy: a randomised, double-blind, placebo-controlled study. Eur J Cancer 40.11 (2004): 1713–1723.

Wesa K et al. Integrative Oncology: complementary therapies for cancer survivors. Hematol Oncol Clin N Am 22 (2008): 343–353.

Wolf S et al. Chemotherapy-induced peripheral neuropathy: Prevention and treatment strategies. European Journal of Cancer 44.11 (2008): 1507–1515.

Wood CE et al. Dietary soy isoflavones inhibit estrogen effects in the postmenopausal breast. Cancer Res 66.2 (2006): 1241–1249.

CHAPTER 11

HERBS AND NATURAL SUPPLEMENTS IN PREGNANCY

INTRODUCTION

Most women take over-the-counter (OTC) medicines at some point during their pregnancy. This may occur intentionally or inadvertently during the early stages of pregnancy. The advice on many product labels and package inserts is to 'consult your doctor' or 'consult your healthcare provider' before using a particular medicine, yet many healthcare providers are poorly equipped to weigh up the benefits of taking, or not taking, a particular medicine during pregnancy. The risk/benefit assessment is possibly even more complex when considering the safety and efficacy of complementary medicines (CMs).

Medical and complementary medicine practitioners, pharmacists and other healthcare providers face similar challenges when advising the pregnant patient about CMs. Despite their popularity, there is very little published evidence regarding the efficacy and safety of natural medicines during pregnancy and lactation. Modern and traditional texts may warn against use; however, little information is provided about the evidence used to come to such a recommendation. Information about the potential efficacy of CMs in pregnancy is also scarce.

This chapter aims to provide readers with an introduction to the fundamental concepts and concerns surrounding the use of CMs in pregnancy. Part 1 explores the use of herbs and natural supplements in pregnancy from a contemporary and traditional approach. Safety and

evidence issues are discussed in Part 2. Central to this section is a discussion about the methods of establishing the safety of any medicine in pregnancy. Part 3 provides a guide as to how the information presented in this chapter may be used to shape clinical practice.

PART 1 — HERBS AND NATURAL SUPPLEMENTS USED IN PREGNANCY

It is commonly known that CM is widely used throughout the world. In many countries traditional medicine continues to form the basis of primary healthcare (WHO 2002). There is an increasing trend in developed countries, including Australia, for the use of traditional and complementary medicines (MacLennan et al 2002, Thomas et al 2001, Tindle et al 2005, Xue et al 2007). The literature indicates that women frequently use CM during pregnancy; however, usage estimates vary considerably due to variations in the definition of CM used, geographical location, socioeconomic and cultural influences. For example, surveys conducted in Europe, the United States and Canada indicate the prevalence of CM usage in pregnancy to range from 7.1 to 96% (Forster et al 2006). Australian statistics estimate that between 10% (Henry & Crowther 2000) and 91% (Forster et al 2007) of all pregnant women will use CM at some stage during their pregnancy. Specifically in regards to herbal medicines, although the majority of women discontinue taking herbal medicines once they are aware of their pregnancies, some others may commence taking them on the advice of their maternity care providers (Ranzini et al 2001).

Surveys of Australian women have identified that nutritional supplements are frequently taken before and throughout pregnancy. During the preconception period, the most common supplements used are folate (29–33%), multivitamins (11–12%) and other supplements including vitamin C, calcium and iron (12–15%). During pregnancy, folate use increases to 70–79% of women (particularly in the first trimester), multivitamins 27–35%, iron 38–52% and other supplements including calcium, vitamin B_6 (predominantly in the first trimester) and zinc. The herbal medicine most often used in pregnancy is raspberry leaf (particularly in the last trimester) (Forster et al 2007, Maats & Crowther 2002).

Despite the widespread use of CM, pregnant women do not always disclose their use of CMs to their healthcare providers. In one study only 1% of participants' medical records listed their CM use (Maats & Crowther 2002), while another study reported 75% of women had informed their primary care provider (Tsui et al 2001). This is problematic as it is a missed opportunity for women to receive informed advice about the effectiveness and safety of the medicines they have chosen to use and prevent unsafe outcomes. Unsupervised use potentially increases the risk of drug interactions with prescribed medicines and contributes to the under-reporting of side effects and adverse outcomes.

Some pregnant women are motivated to take CMs in lieu of conventional medicine as they regard them as safer treatments (Hollyer et al 2002). Sometimes self-prescribed use is justified, such as using nutritional supplements to meet increased nutritional requirements or to treat a pregnancy-related health issue (e.g. nausea or general pregnancy preparation) or to treat non-pregnancy specific problems (e.g. the common cold) (Henry & Crowther 2000, Maats & Crowther 2002, Nordeng & Havnen 2004).

Pregnant women appear to use a variety of information sources to aid their selection of CMs including healthcare practitioners (Forster et al 2007, Tsui et al 2001), friends, family members (Hollyer et al 2002, Maats & Crowther 2002, Nordeng & Havnen 2004, Tsui et al 2001) and media sources (e.g. magazines and internet) (Tsui et al 2001).

NUTRITIONAL MEDICINE

Pregnant women choose to use nutritional medicines as symptomatic treatment to improve their own health in general and to optimise the healthy development of the growing child and its safe delivery.

Most clinicians will be aware of the changes in nutritional requirements that occur in pregnancy and the need for women to increase their dietary intake of certain nutrients such as iron, calcium, folate and others. Nutritional supplements are sometimes used to help women achieve these higher intake levels and correct preexisting deficiencies. The National Health and Medical Research Council (NHMRC) nutritional guidelines for the adequate intake of vitamins and minerals (Australian Government 2006) provides guidelines for nutritional requirements during pregnancy; however, they are only estimates based on extrapolated data from other populations and models, and do not take into account the individual's specific needs. In practice, a detailed diet and lifestyle history is necessary and sometimes additional pathology testing to enable clinicians to make more appropriate individual recommendations.

Besides enabling women to meet their basic nutritional needs, nutritional supplements are also used in larger doses to act as pharmacological agents to ameliorate symptoms and address a specific health complaint. For example, calcium and magnesium supplements have been used to reduce the severity of leg cramps, pyridoxine to alleviate nausea and folate to reduce the incidence of neural tube defects. Appendix 11.1 (p. 190) lists common nutritional supplements and their use in pregnancy. Appendix 11.2 (p. 198) lists dosage recommendations for the nutrients.

Long-term impact of maternal nutrition

The 'developmental origins of disease' hypothesis suggests that the benefits of a nutritional intervention may extend much further than those more immediate outcomes. Environmental factors during development, such as maternal nutrition, have been shown to influence the expression of our phenotype. The most sensitive time for this influence has been shown in-utero. Fetal nutrition can alter the body's structure, function and metabolism, subsequently affecting the risk of developing diseases later in life (Barker 2004). Longitudinal studies from around the world have found low birth weight (in relation to gestational age) is associated with increased risk of coronary heart disease, stroke, hypertension and type 2 diabetes in adulthood (Barker 2007). Furthermore, maternal vitamin D status during pregnancy appears to influence the bone-mineral density of offspring, even in late childhood (Javaid et al 2006). Similarly, there is some evidence suggesting that calcium supplementation during pregnancy can reduce the offspring's blood pressure during their childhood (Hatton et al 2003).

HERBAL MEDICINE

Herbal medicines are used in pregnancy as pharmacological agents. They are used as foods, such as ginger, in extract form (liquid and solid dose forms) and also as teas. In many developing countries, herbal medicines have been used as the dominant form of medicine and continue to play a major role in healthcare, reproductive health and midwifery (WHO 2002).

A traditional approach

Although conception is a problem for some women nowadays, a more common problem throughout the ages was contraception. Ethnobotanical studies conducted in many parts of the world reveal that herbal medicines have been used widely to prevent conception and induce miscarriage for generations, and in some parts of the world, their use continues despite the availability of pharmaceutical contraceptive pills and devices. Besides this, herbal medicines have been used to enhance fertility, regulate menstruation, facilitate childbirth, help with expulsion of the placenta and promote lactation.

In many cultures, herbal healers have special reverence for herbs thought to have abortifacient or emmenagogue properties. These concepts are foreign in Western medicine and deserve some discussion.

Abortifacients

Plants have been used as a source of both contraceptives and early-term abortifacients since the times of ancient Egypt (Riddle 1991) and in some parts of the world this practice still occurs. The abortifacient effects of herbs are attributed to their inherent toxicity or ability to induce uterine contractions (Noumi & Tchakonang 2001). It is also suspected that abortifacient activity may be immune-mediated, hormonal or due to non-specific actions such as the ability to reduce uterine blood flow. Examples of western herbs with abortifacient potential due to suspected toxicity include: wormwood (*Artemisia absinthium*), pennyroyal (*Mentha pulegium*), poke root (*Phytolacca decandra*), pau d'arco (*Tabebuia avellanedae*), rue (*Ruta graveolens*) and tansy (*Tanacetum vulgare*) (Mills & Bone 2005).

Emmenagogues

The term 'emmenagogue' is used to describe a herb that will stimulate menstrual flow. These herbs have been traditionally indicated for delayed menstruation and developed a reputation as being contraindicated in pregnancy for fear they may induce miscarriage. Herbalists consider emmenagogues as exerting oxytocic-like effects which cause uterine contractions; however, this mechanism is unlikely to explain how they promote menses in a non-pregnant woman. Changes to lymph or blood flow and hormonal effects are more likely mechanisms. Examples of herbs found on many traditional lists thought to act as emmenagogues include aloe (*Aloe vera*), juniper (*Juniperus communis*), pennyroyal (*Mentha pulegium*), goldenseal (*Hydrastis canadensis*), black cohosh (*Cimicifuga racemosa*), blue cohosh (*Caulophyllum thalictroides*), dong quai (*Angelica polymorpha*), rue (*Ruta graveolens*), tansy (*Tanacetum vulgare*), and thuja (*Thuja occidentalis*). Some herbs considered as emmenagogues are also thought of as potential abortifacients if used in sufficient quantities (e.g. oxytocin agonists); however, not all abortifacients may act as emmenagogues, e.g. potentially toxic herbs with no hormonal or uterine effects.

Historical perspectives

The use of medicinal plants has occurred in Mexico since pre-Hispanic times. Nearly 10,000,000 indigenous people speaking nearly 85 different languages inhabit the region and many still depend upon plants for primary therapy from the diverse flora (almost 5000 medicinal plants) (Andrade-Cetto 2009). An ethnobotanical study of the medicinal plants from Tlanchinol, Hidalgo, Mexico identified several plants used as abortifacients: *Galium mexicanum* var *mexicanum, Ruta chalepensis, Zaluzania triloba* and *Tanacetum parthenium*. The herb *Cinnamomum verum* is generally considered useful to induce childbirth and *Pedilanthus tithymaloides* is used for ovarian pain.

The Criollo people of Argentina use a vast plant pharmacopoeia. To date, 189 species with 754 different medicinal applications have been recorded (Martinez 2008). The absence of a normal menstrual cycle and amenorrhoea are matters of concern among these people and are treated with emmenagogue plants, the most common being *Anemia tomentosa, Tripodanthus flagellaris, Lippia turbinata* and *Trixis divaricata*. Contraceptive herbs used in the region include: *Zea mays, Anemia tomentosa* and abortifacient herbs include: *Artemisia absinthium; Cheilantes buchtienii; Chenopodium aff. hircinum; Cuphea glutinosa; Ligaria cuneifolia; Lippia turbinata* and *Pinus* spp. (Martinez 2008).

Rama midwives in eastern Nicaragua currently use a diverse group of plants in the practice of midwifery: 162 species from 125 genera and 62 families (Senes et al 2008). This extensive ethnopharmacopoeia is employed to treat the many health issues of pregnancy, parturition, postpartum care, neonatal care and primary healthcare of women and children. The 22 most popular midwifery species are medicinals that are widely used by practitioners other than midwives, not only in eastern Nicaragua, but elsewhere. Very few herbal species are used as contraceptives in this region, whereas abortifacients are well known and mostly made with bitter-tasting plants, probably due to alkaloids and other bitter-tasting compounds. The most widely used abortifacients are decoctions made from the leaves and seeds of soursap and the roots of guinea hen. Others are decoctions made with the leaves and/or flowers of barsley, broom weed, trompet, sorosi and wild rice and the root of ginja.

Interestingly, midwives in other parts of the world use many Rama midwifery species for the same purpose. For example, the two species sorosi and lime are both widely regarded as important in midwifery in many parts of the world. Sorosi is one of the most widely used medicinals in eastern Nicaragua and elsewhere where it is used as an abortifacient, with similar use in Africa, Australia, Brazil, India, Malaysia, Philippines and the West Indies (Senes et al 2008). Lime is a domesticated crop used by the Rama and other indigenous groups of eastern Nicaragua as an abortifacient and to accelerate labour. It is also used to induce abortion by tribal people in India, Honduran midwives and the Tikunas of northwestern Amazonia.

Europe has a rich history of herbal medicine use, which continues to be popular today. Plants here were also used for reproductive health, to prevent conception and induce abortion, with women and midwives as the main keepers of herbal knowledge. Savin (*Juniperus sabina*) was one abortifacient herb of choice in Europe and pennyroyal, sage, thyme and rosemary were considered powerful emmenagogues (Belew 1999). Unlike some other parts of the world, information exchange down the generations was interrupted during the 18th and 19th centuries as there was a major shift in management of the birthing process (Schiebinger 2008). During this period, female practitioners with knowledge of herbal lore lost ground to obstetricians (men trained primarily as surgeons) and the use of plant-based treatments was gradually replaced with surgical procedures (Schiebinger 2008). As a result, much knowledge about European use of herbal medicines in fertility and reproduction was lost.

The North American Indians used herbal medicines extensively thoughout the reproductive life cycle and had many remedies for improving fertility, preventing miscarriage, treating symptoms during pregnancy and facilitating the birthing process. A large number of these treatments came to the knowledge of European settlers in North America through careful study, observation and subsequent clinical use. If repeated use indicated the treatments were effective, the herbs were recorded and prescribed by the Eclectic physicians who flourished from the mid-1800s to around 1920 in the United States (Belew 1999). Many of the herbal medicines used by the North American Indians and described by the Eclectic physicians are still in use today as part of the Western herbalists and traditional midwives cache of treatments.

The Eclectics considered black cohosh a 'remedy par excellence to stimulate normal functional activity of the uterus and ovaries' throughout the reproductive life cycle (Belew 1999). They reported that when used regularly at the end of pregnancy 'it will render labor easier and quicker, and give a better getting up'. Black haw was highly regarded by the Eclectic physicians, who used it both before and during pregnancy to prevent miscarriage, prepare for labour and relieve false labour pains and afterpains. The Eclectic physicians preferred to use cotton root (*Gossypium*) as an oxytocin agonist rather than the newly available sublingual oxytocin preparation because the herb was considered to have a more gentle action and produce more predictable results. Squaw vine (*Mitchella repens*) was well considered when enhanced fertility was called for. It was extensively used to promote menstruation and alleviate physical discomfort in the latter months of pregnancy, and was thought to be a good preparative to labour, rendering the birth of a child easier.

Contemporary use by Western herbalists

In Western herbal practice today, much knowledge about herbal safety and efficacy in pregnancy is drawn from North American and European traditions and traditional applications are largely used as a basis for prescriptions. Herbal medicines may be prescribed to regulate menstruation before conception, alleviate morning sickness and other symptoms related to pregnancy. A growing number of gynaecologists and obstetricians are working with herbalists to enhance patients' chances of conception and reduce miscarriage, sometimes in combination with IVF procedures.

Requests for abortifacient herbs in Western countries are virtually unheard of; however, some women still seek herbalists to provide '*partus* (birth) *preparatus* (prepare)' mixtures to prepare for childbirth and facilitate delivery. Traditionally the Eclectic physicians called these preparations 'mother's cordial'. They tend to be recommended in very low doses starting at 36 weeks gestation, increasing in dose each week until delivery. Herbs that have been used in *partus preparatus* preparations include: *Mitchella repens* (squaw vine), *Viburnum prunifolium* (black haw), *Rubus idaeus* (raspberry), *Chamaelirium luteum* (false unicorn), *Caulophyllum thalictroides* (blue cohosh) and *Cimicifuga racemosa* (black cohosh).

Today, Western herbalists are also asked for treatment to address pre- and postnatal depression, alleviate symptoms of dyspepsia, nausea and lower back pain and sometimes topical applications to reduce perineal discomfort and stretch marks associated with pregnancy. In addition, herbalists may be providing support for conditions unrelated to pregnancy, such as urinary tract or upper respiratory tract infections.

Unlike medical practitioners, Western herbalists are less concerned about teratogenicity than inducing miscarriage. To minimise the risk of harming the mother or fetus, several general guidelines are followed. Most importantly, traditional sources dictate that if known toxic herbs are avoided, then toxic side effects are unlikely to occur. In addition, other classes of herbs avoided during pregnancy include the following (Hess et al 2007):

- emmenagogues and abortifacients (discussed above)

- large quantities of herbs containing a high volatile oil content, especially during the first trimester. It is suspected that volatile oils contain constituents that could induce uterine contractions. Many kitchen spices contain volatile oils, which are not believed to be a problem when used in dietary amounts but could pose problems when used in concentrated preparations, e.g. rosemary, peppermint, thyme, sage. This contraindication is likely to be derived from European tradition

- stimulant laxative herbs containing anthraquinones. These herbal medicines stimulate peristalsis and can induce loss of water and electrolytes, intestinal cramps, loose bowels and dependency with chronic use. It is believed these harsh irritant effects may exert a reflex stimulating effect on the uterus causing uterine contractions. Stimulant laxative herbs include buckthorn, cascara (*Rhamnus* species), rhubarb, castor, senna and aloe. Aloe gel is not a problem as it contains a part of the plant that does not contain significant levels of anthraquinones

- herbs with hormonal actions such as *Trifolium pratense* (red clover) and *Vitex agnuscastus* (chastetree) may adversely influence fetal development

- thujone-containing herbs, e.g. *Achillea millefolium* (yarrow), *Thuja occidentalis* (thuja) or *Artemisia absinthium* (wormwood) due to its inherent toxicity concerns

This approach is based on traditional evidence and theoretical concerns, usually without any scientific evidence to confirm lack of safety. As such, a herbalist's approach to these herbs may be overly cautious and not borne out if scientific testing takes place in the future. For example, senna is traditionally avoided during pregnancy as it is an anthraquinone-containing herb; however, it is widely recommended as a safe and effective short-term stimulant laxative for constipation by medical practitioners (Tytgat et al 2003). Some herbalists also recommend against the use of several aromatherapy oils during the first trimester; however, there is no scientific evidence to suggest external use of such oils poses any serious danger.

PART TWO — SAFETY IN PREGNANCY

All medicines have the potential to affect maternal health, cross the placenta and affect fetal development. The most serious risk associated with medicine use in pregnancy is the possibility of teratogenesis, which can manifest as a structural abnormality, dysfunctional growth in utero and/or long-term functional defects. Other risks include miscarriage and neonatal withdrawal.

Birth defects naturally occur in 2–4% of all newborns and in the vast majority of cases the cause is unknown. Medication use is not considered to be a major contributor to the incidence of birth defects as less than 1% of cases can be attributed to drug use (Webster & Freeman 2001). It is likely that the use of CMs in Western countries is a far less important factor.

CRITICAL PERIODS IN HUMAN DEVELOPMENT

The safe use of any medicine in pregnancy must take into account the safety of the treatment to be used, the seriousness of the patient's presenting problem and the timing of exposure.

In the first 2 weeks prior to implantation, an insult is thought to have an all or nothing effect. Assuming the embryo survives, the risk of structural malformations to the fetus is greatest 17–70 days post-conception, a critical stage of organ development (Freyer 2008). After this time, organs continue to mature, so later adverse effects tend to be functional rather than

structural and major birth defects are unlikely. Functional defects are less obvious than structural ones and may only become obvious once the child is older. The central nervous system, eyes, teeth and external genitalia are the last to fully develop and continue to mature until the baby reaches full term.

If practitioner and patient agree that medicinal treatment is warranted, then minimising exposure during critical developmental times is essential. This means using the lowest effective dose of the least toxic substance for the shortest period of time.

TERATOGENESIS

Teratogens are agents that result in structural or functional defects in the development of fetal organs (Shehata & Nelson-Piercy 2000). Sources of exposure to these agents include: contaminated air, water, soil, food, beverages, household items and medicines (including CMs). Teratogens can cause a variety of effects, including embryo/fetal death, intrauterine growth restriction and increased risk of malformations and carcinogenesis (Shehata & Nelson-Piercy 2000). The exact mechanisms responsible for teratogenicity are unknown, but theories include damage to DNA, membranes, protein and mitochondria, enzyme inhibition and hormonal interference. Despite the potential for teratogens to have devastating consequences, only a relatively small number of fetuses exposed to these agents experience adverse effects (Freyer 2008). This relates to factors such as the dose and duration of exposure, genetic susceptibility of the fetus/embryo, timing of exposure, specific mode of action of the teratogen (Miller et al 2007) and nutritional and disease status of the mother–baby unit (Shehata & Nelson-Piercy 2000).

Data on herbal teratogens is limited and largely based on animal studies, which are not completely reliable. Blue cohosh is an example of a herb that has some evidence to suggest a potential teratogenic effect based on animal studies (Keeler 1976, Keeler et al 1976, Kennelly et al 1999). Other herbs that may increase the risk of fetal malformations (predominantly based on limited animal data) include aloe, andrographis, cat's claw, Jamaica dogwood, pau d'arco, pennyroyal, poke root, tribulus and white horehound (Mills & Bone 2005). There is very little evidence of teratogenic activity or adverse pregnancy outcomes from the use of nutrititional supplements with the notable exception of high-dose vitamin A. Interestingly, nutrient *deficiencies* such as vitamin A, folate, vitamin B_{12}, vitamin D, iodine and zinc have been found to have adverse effects including teratogenesis emphasising the important role these nutrients play in normal embryonic and fetal development.

Neonatal withdrawal

While the fetus is in utero, the placenta supplies it with nutrients and other substances, as well as drugs. When the baby is born, placental supply ceases, which can lead to neonatal withdrawal syndromes for certain drugs such as beta-blockers, SSRIs and other antidepressants, opiates and alcohol (Freyer 2008, Sanz et al 2005). It is not known whether the use of CMs during the final trimester can also induce withdrawal syndromes.

HOW IS SAFETY EVALUATED IN PREGNANCY?

One of the hardest challenges a clinician faces is advising a pregnant patient about the safety of a treatment. A key factor to consider is the strength of evidence indicating the treatment is safe or, as so often happens in pregnancy, the lack of evidence indicating it is unsafe. More specific factors are the dose of medicine to be used, precise timing of exposure and duration of exposure.

When evaluating the effectiveness of a treatment, prospective randomised trials and meta-analyses are widely considered the gold standards. When evaluating safety in pregnancy, there is a paucity of such trials because pregnant women tend to be excluded, so other methods of information-gathering are required. Epidemiological studies, tests with animal models, post-marketing surveillance systems, case reports and traditional use provide the main inputs into establishing safety; however, each method has limitations and should not stand alone without corroborating evidence from another source.

Epidemiological studies

Epidemiological studies are also known as population studies. Due to their large participant numbers, epidemiological studies can detect large and small size effects and sometimes rare outcomes, if the study population is sufficiently large and follow-up is sufficiently complete. As such, they may provide useful information regarding safety in pregnancy.

Considering that the incidence of fetal malformations is already small (2–4%) extremely large participant numbers would be required to detect a slight increase above what might normally be expected. For example, a study would require 35,000 women in order to establish with 95% confidence level that a medicine changes the naturally-occurring frequency of a congenital malformation by 1% (Lee et al 2000). Unfortunately, most epidemiological studies have inadequate statistical power to detect this outcome as they lack sufficient patient numbers. As such, no medicine (pharmaceutical or complementary) has proven safety based on reliable epidemiological data involving sufficient numbers of women.

Animal studies

Animal studies of reproductive toxicity are required for all new drugs before they are licensed; however, they are not required for CMs. While they can provide some assurance of safety, animal tests have limited usefulness as results do not always extrapolate accurately to humans. For example, the drug thalidomide did not cause birth defects in animal models; however, it had a potent effect in humans (Webster & Freeman 2001). Far more common is the problem of false positives, whereby medicines that produce defects in animals are later found to be relatively safe in humans (e.g. corticosteroids) (Lee et al 2000). It is likely that the excessive doses used in testing increase the risk of producing a false positive as there is greater embryonic and maternal exposure to the medicine than would be expected in clinical practice. This should be kept in mind when interpreting the results of drug or herbal medicine testing in animal models.

Post-marketing surveillance systems

In many cases, more meaningful safety data only become available once a medicine is in widespread use and women knowingly or inadvertently take it during pregnancy. Those medicines with high effect rates will be detected more quickly than less potent teratogens. For example, the teratogenic effect of isotretinoin was detected about one year after it came onto the market whereas the anti-epileptic drug valproic acid was available in Europe in the 1960s, yet it took approximately 20 years of use by millions of women before its teratogenic potential was identified (Webster & Freeman 2001).

Post-marketing surveillance systems are set up to detect unfavourable outcomes and highlight adverse events rather than establishing safety, an inherently more difficult endpoint.

Adverse event case reports

Adverse event case reports are an account of an individual's suspected response to a treatment. Case reports are notoriously unreliable, as they tend to lack sufficient detail to clearly establish causality and fully eliminate the influence of confounding factors. Individual case reports become more convincing when a series of similar reports are collected.

Several factors should be considered when interpreting a case report; firstly, was the exposure to the medicine at the appropriate critical stage in pregnancy (usually first trimester) and was the dose used clinically relevant and similar for all cases? Additionally, if a complementary medicine is implicated, has the medicine been tested for contaminants and adulteration to exclude extrinsic factors and did the treatment involve a single entity or combination therapy (the norm in complementary medicine)? Finally, the traditional body of evidence that accompanies herbal medicines may provide further insights when interpreting cases.

The following three cases are presented as examples of the literature. They involve the herbs dong quai, Korean ginseng and blue cohosh. The reports indicate a probable link between herbal use and adverse outcome; however, none of the products implicated was tested for herbal authenticity or the presence of contaminants or adulterants, an essential step towards drawing a definitive conclusion.

Examples of case reports:

A 32-year-old woman, 3 weeks postpartum, developed acute headache, weakness, lightheadedness and vomiting with a blood pressure reading of 195/85 mmHg (Nambiar et al 1999). She reported using dong quai for postpartum weakness and had not been taking any other medicines. Her 3-week-old son's blood pressure was also raised at 115/69. Within 48 hours of stopping herbal treatment, blood pressure normalised for both the mother and the breastfed child.

In 1990, a case report published in *JAMA* described a 30-year-old mother who had taken *Panax ginseng* (650 mg twice a day) throughout pregnancy and during lactation of her 2-week-old baby (Koren et al 1990). The boy was noted to have signs of androgenisation, thick black pubic hair, hair over the entire forehead, swollen red nipples and enlarged testes. After 2 weeks, his pubic and forehead hair began to fall out and was scant by 7.5 weeks. Excessive androgen production was ruled out and the authors suspected the effects were producted by hormonal activity of the herbal product. Letters to the editor were subsequently exchanged suggesting the product contained Siberian ginseng and not *Panax ginseng* (Awang 1991). The story does not end here as Siberian ginseng has no significant androgenic activity in vivo which could account for the effects observed (Awang 1991, Waller et al 1992). It is now suspected that the herbal product was not substituted for Siberian ginseng but instead *Periploca sepium* (called Wu jia or silk vine), as American herb companies importing Siberian ginseng from China have been known to be supplied with two or three species of *Periploca* (Awang 1991).

A newborn infant presented with acute myocardial infarction associated with profound congestive heart failure and shock (Jones & Lawson 1998). The mother had been ingesting blue cohosh (*Caulophyllum thalictroides*) in the month prior to delivery to facilitate the birthing process. She had been instructed to take one tablet daily but elected to take three times the recommended dose in the 3 weeks prior to delivery. During this time she noticed an increase in uterine contractions and a decrease in fetal activity. The infant eventually recovered after being critically ill for several weeks. Attending doctors excluded other causes of myocardial infarction and indicated blue cohosh was responsible for the adverse event. On late follow-up at 2 years of age the child was doing well with good exercise tolerance and normal growth and development. However, cardiomegaly persisted, left ventricular function remained mildly reduced and he was still receiving digoxin therapy.

Clinical studies

While prospective clinical studies of herbal safety in pregnancy are problematic, retrospective studies are easier to conduct. Establishing cause–effect relationships beyond reasonable doubt are rare due to the myriad of confounding factors present; however, they may identify common or palpable problems that could be investigated in appropriate models.

Example: echinacea

A Canadian study involving 412 pregnant women investigated the safety of echinacea in pregnancy (Gallo et al 2000). These women had contacted a teratogen information service (Motherisk Program) between 1996 and 1998 with concerns about the safety of ingesting echinacea during pregnancy. Half the group had already taken the herb, whereas the others decided against use, so were enrolled as a control group. Of the 206 women in the echinacea group, 112 (54%) used the herb in the first trimester and 17 (8%) used it throughout their pregnancies. No significant differences were seen between the groups for rates of major and minor malformations or any pregnancy outcome including delivery method, maternal weight gain, gestational age, infant birth weight or fetal distress.

Long-term use

Long-term use of a medicine by large populations of women without apparent increase in adverse events is considered to contribute towards evidence of safety. For example, the Australian Drug Evaluation Committee (ADEC) has classified the drug metoclopramide as relatively low risk because the 'drug has already been taken by large numbers of pregnant women and women of child-bearing age without proven increase in fetal harm' (Bryant et al 2003).

The term 'long-term use' in relation to herbal medicine may actually refer to hundreds or even thousands of years of use, not just decades, as is the case with pharmaceutical medicines. In fact, many herbal medicines, such as ginger and garlic, have been used as both foods and medicines since antiquity. This has allowed a large body of longitudinal and retrospective evidence to accumulate which gives herbalists an extra dimension to consider.

Like all forms of evidence, traditional evidence has its limitations and must be interpreted carefully. It is likely that traditional healers would have found it easier to identify poisonous herbs and herbs that induce acute or obvious adverse effects than those which induce insidious, rare or delayed-onset adverse outcomes. There may also be significant differences in the way a herbal medicine is grown, prepared and used today compared with older times, thereby allowing larger doses to be taken and different herbal constituents to be absorbed (Tannis 2003).

WEIGHING UP THE EVIDENCE

For both pharmaceutical and complementary medicines, the evidence base is incomplete and insufficient to state with certainty that any medicine is safe in pregnancy. To build a case for safety, evidence from multiple sources must be considered to fill in as many gaps in knowledge as possible.

In regards to complementary medicines, any evidence supporting or contraindicating use during pregnancy must be based on the totality, quality and relevance of the evidence. In general, the greater the consistency of evidence from different sources, the stronger the evidence is overall.

In Australia, the Australian Drug Evaluation Committee (ADEC) has classified drugs on their potential to cause harm during pregnancy. Eight categories are listed and each describes the evidence used to indicate safety or lack of safety (see Table 11.1). They rely on evidence gathered from animal models and postmarketing surveillance systems and also consider the proven, suspected or expected potential of a drug to cause adverse outcomes (e.g. cytotoxic drugs).

Proposing a different system for complementary medicines

A similar grading system is required for CMs, which builds a case for safety or harm based on considering multiple forms of evidence. Ideally the new system should take into account the availability of a traditional body of evidence and the relative lack of data available from animal studies. It should also take into account the relative safety of OTC CMs in comparison to scheduled pharmaceutical drugs and whether the association between exposure and proposed adverse outcome is biologically plausible.

Table 11.2 (p. 174) is a safety matrix that synthesises different forms of evidence, including taking note of what is known and what

TABLE 11.1 ADEC PREGNANCY CATEGORIES (AUSTRALIA)	
CATEGORY A	Drugs which have been taken by a large number of pregnant women and women of childbearing age without any proven increase in the frequency of malformations or other direct or indirect harmful effects on the fetus having been observed.
CATEGORY B1	Drugs which have been taken by only a limited number of pregnant women and women of childbearing age, without an increase in the frequency of malformation or other direct or indirect harmful effects on the human fetus having been observed. Studies in animals have not shown evidence of an increased occurrence of fetal damage.
CATEGORY B2	Drugs which have been taken by only a limited number of pregnant women and women of childbearing age, without an increase in the frequency of malformation or other direct or indirect harmful effects on the human fetus having been observed. Studies in animals are inadequate or may be lacking, but available data show no evidence of an increased occurrence of fetal damage.
CATEGORY B3	Drugs which have been taken by only a limited number of pregnant women and women of childbearing age, without an increase in the frequency of malformation or other direct or indirect harmful effects on the human fetus having been observed. Studies in animals have shown evidence of an increased occurrence of fetal damage, the significance of which is considered uncertain in humans.
CATEGORY C	Drugs which, owing to their pharmacological effects, have caused or may be suspected of causing harmful effects on the human fetus or neonate without causing malformations. These effects may be reversible. Accompanying texts should be consulted for further details.
CATEGORY D	Drugs which have caused, are suspected to have caused or may be expected to cause, an increased incidence of human fetal malformations or irreversible damage. These drugs may also have adverse pharmacological effects. Accompanying texts should be consulted for further details.
CATEGORY X	Drugs which have such a high risk of causing permanent damage to the fetus that they should not be used in pregnancy or when there is a possibility of pregnancy.

Note: For drugs in the B1, B2 and B3 categories, human data are lacking or inadequate and subcategorisation is therefore based on available animal data. The allocation of a B category does NOT imply greater safety than the C category. Drugs in category D are NOT absolutely contraindicated in pregnancy. Moreover, in some cases the D category has been assigned on the basis of suspicion.
Based on: Medicines in Pregnancy Working Party of the Australian Drug Evaluation Committee. *Prescribing medicines in pregnancy. An Australian categorisation of risk of drug use in pregnancy.* 4th edn. Canberra: Commonwealth of Australia, 1999. *http://www.tga.gov.au/hp/medicines-pregnancy.htm*

remains unknown. Traditional and scientific evidence from various sources are compared and theoretical reasoning is considered. The matrix has been weighted so scientific evidence is given greater credence than traditional evidence; however, it must be acknowledged that, in many cases, scientific evidence to support safety will be unavailable.

USING THE SAFETY MATRIX

Clinicians are recommended to use information in the monographs of this text as a starting point for gathering information about evidence of safety in pregnancy. Supplementary information will be required from frequently updated databases and traditional monograph pharmacopeias. Five common herbs are reviewed here as examples of how the matrix may be used:

echinacea, ginger, raspberry leaf, black cohosh and chaste tree.

Echinacea spp. (Echinacea)
Classification: Likely safe
- Traditional evidence: available? Y
  - Traditional evidence: cautions or contraindicates? NA
  - Traditional evidence: if cautions: biologically plausible? NA
- Scientific evidence: available? Y
  - Scientific evidence: human or animal studies find NO known pharmacological effects of concern in pregnancy? Y
  - Scientific evidence: toxicological or pharmacological profile studies find NO known

TABLE 11.2 COMPLEMENTARY MEDICINE SAFETY MATRIX				
TRADITIONAL EVIDENCE → / SCIENTIFIC EVIDENCE ↓	WELL-DOCUMENTED TRADITIONAL EVIDENCE UNAVAILABLE	TRADITIONAL EVIDENCE DOES NOT CONTRAINDICATE AGAINST USE	TRADITIONAL EVIDENCE CAUTIONS OR CONTRAINDICATES USE DUE TO POSTULATED NON-SPECIFIC MECHANISMS THAT ARE NOT BIOLOGICALLY PLAUSIBLE	TRADITIONAL EVIDENCE CONTRAINDICATES USE BASED ON DESCRIPTIONS OF SPECIFIC ADVERSE EFFECTS OR IS USED AS AN ABORTIFACIENT
There are *no animal or human studies* available to support safety	Consider as unsafe because safety remains unknown	Likely to be safe but safety cannot be confirmed Scientific evidence unavailable to support or refute traditional safety claim	Likely to be safe but best used under professional guidance Scientific evidence unavailable to support or refute traditional contraindication	Unsafe Scientific evidence unavailable to support or refute traditional contraindication
Human and animal studies demonstrate there are *no known pharmacological activities* of the substance or its components relevant to therapeutic use in humans known to be associated with fetal damage, abortifacient activity or any other adverse reproductive effects	Safe	Safe Scientific evidence supports traditional safety claim	Likely to be safe but best used under professional guidance Scientific evidence does not support traditional contraindication	Likely to be safe but best used under professional guidance Scientific evidence does not support traditional contraindication
The toxicological or pharmacological profile of the substance indicates that there are *no known pharmacological actions* of the substance or its components relevant to therapeutic use in humans which could cause fetal damage, abortifacient activity or any other adverse reproductive effects	Safe	Safe Scientific evidence supports traditional safety claim	Likely to be safe but best used under professional guidance Scientific evidence does not support traditional contraindication	Likely to be safe but best used under professional guidance Scientific evidence does not support traditional contraindication
Human or animal studies *have shown* evidence of pharmacological activity for the substance or its components relevant to therapeutic use in humans which could cause fetal damage, abortifacient effects or any other adverse reproductive effects	Unsafe	Unsafe Scientific evidence refutes traditional safety claim	Unsafe Scientific evidence supports traditional contraindication	Unsafe Scientific evidence supports traditional contraindication

pharmacological effects of concern in pregnancy? NA
- Scientific evidence: human and/or animal studies find evidence of pharmacological effects adverse to pregnancy, e.g. abortifacient? Y

One animal study highlighted concerns about use during the first trimester demonstrating the risk of spontaneous abortions, with pregnant mice fed *Echinacea purpurea* daily, increased as 50% of fetuses were lost by mid-pregnancy (Chow et al 2006). Human studies, however, indicate it is generally considered safe in pregnancy when used in recommended doses (Mills & Bone 2005). A recent study of a prospective cohort study found that oral consumption during the first trimester did not increase the risk of malformations and was recommended as safe for use during pregnancy (Perri et al 2006). Additional evidence from a prospective cohort study suggests it is safe during pregnancy with no increase in the risk for major malformations; however, large-scale controlled trials are unavailable (Gallo et al 2000). This particular study involved 206 women who used echinacea during their pregnancy (54% in the first trimester and 8% in all trimesters). Fifty-eight per cent of participants used capsules or tablets (doses ranging from 250 to 1000 mg/day) and 38% used tinctures (dose varied from 5 to 10 to a maximum of 30 drops per day). Most used the echinacea for only a short period of time compared with a control group matched by disease (upper respiratory tract ailments), maternal age, alcohol and cigarette use. There was no statistical differences between the groups for any of the end points analysed — major and minor malformations, miscarriages and neonatal complications.

Zingiber officinalis (Ginger)

Classification: Likely to be safe, but safety cannot be confirmed for high-dose supplements (concentrated extracts), safe for usual dietary intake
- Traditional evidence: available? Y
  - Traditional evidence: cautions or contra-indicates? Y
  - Traditional evidence: if cautions: biologically plausible? N
- Scientific evidence: available? Y

- Scientific evidence: human or animal studies find NO known pharmacological effects of concern in pregnancy? Y
- Scientific evidence: toxicological or pharmacological profile studies find NO known pharmacological effects of concern in pregnancy? NA
- Scientific evidence: human and/or animal studies find evidence of pharmacological effects adverse to pregnancy e.g. abortifacient? Y

Traditionally used as an anti-emetic, ginger has encouraging research to support its use during pregnancy for nausea and vomiting (Borrelli et al 2005) and no adverse effects have been reported in several studies examining ginger in treatment of nausea and vomiting in pregnancy. Ginger's anti-nausea and anti-emetic mechanism of action has not been fully elucidated, although several hypotheses have been proposed. It has been reported that symptoms of nausea and vomiting during pregnancy improve in a manner directly correlated to improvements in pregnancy-induced gastric dysrhythmias. Therefore, ginger's actions in pregnancy may be due to a direct effect of the medicine on the gastrointestinal tract (Chaiyakunapruk et al 2006, Matthews et al 2010).

A recent systematic review assessed 10 RCTs that investigated ginger in pregnancy. Five trials reported ginger to be more effective than placebo, four trials found ginger to be equally effective in the management of nausea and vomiting compared to vitamin B_6 and dimethhydrinate. Compared with dimenhydrate, ginger caused fewer side effects and none of the studies raised any concerns about safety in pregnant women (Dante et al 2013). The Cochrane Collaboration reached the conclusion that the efficacy of ginger was equal to that of either vitamin B6 or dimenhydrinate (Matthews et al 2010).

Another systematic review of 4 double-blind RCTs ($n = 449$) and one prospective observational cohort study ($n = 187$) evaluated the effects of ginger on pregnancy outcomes. The preparation used in the trials was a ginger root powder or extract, taken 3–4 times daily (total dose ranging from 1.0–1.5 g) from 8 to 20 weeks' gestation. No dose was provided in the prospective study. No difference in the occurrence of spontaneous abortions, stillbirth, term delivery and caesarean deliveries, neonatal death, gestational age and congenital abnormalities were found between those women who took ginger compared to those taking vitamin B$_6$ or placebo, or the general population (Borrelli et al 2005).

Unfortunately, there is a lack of consensus regarding its safety during pregnancy. Soudamini et al (1995) suggest ginger contains possible mutagenic properties; however, this effect appears to be counteracted by zingerone, another constituent present in the whole rhizome (Nakamura & Yamamoto 1982). Traditionally, ginger has been contraindicated in labour due to the possibility of increased postpartum haemorrhage and in large doses it is traditionally thought to act as emmenagogue (Grieve 1971). German Commission E suggest that ginger is contraindicated in pregnancy, while more recent research suggests that doses up to 2 g/day of dried ginger root have been used safely. When considered in a comparison of recent research, the proposed notion of haemorrhage is unlikely. Teratogenicity studies in rats show that even at very large doses (ginger tea up to 50 g/L) it had no impact on maternal toxicity or fetal malformations; however, embryo losses were double compared to the controls. No evidence of maternal toxicity was found for a patented extract of ginger (EV.EXT 33) given in doses of up to 1000 mg/kg/body weight daily to pregnant rats during the period of organogenesis (Weidner & Sigwart 2001).

Rubus idaeus (raspberry leaf)

Classification: Likely to be safe, but safety cannot be confirmed (first trimester), likely to be safe (second and third trimester)
- Traditional evidence: available? Y
  - Traditional evidence: cautions or contraindicates? N
  - Traditional evidence: if cautions: biologically plausible? NA
- Scientific evidence: available? Y
  - Scientific evidence: human or animal studies find NO known pharmacological effects of concern in pregnancy? Y
  - Scientific evidence: toxicological or pharmacological profile studies find NO known pharmacological effects of concern in pregnancy? Y
  - Scientific evidence: human and/or animal studies find evidence of pharmacological effects adverse to pregnancy, e.g. abortifacient? Y

Raspberry leaves appear to have a dual effect on the uterus, acting as both a stimulant and a relaxant to the uterine musculature (Bamford et al 1970). The use of this herb in concentrated form is traditionally recommended only in the second and third trimesters due to its possible effects on the uterus. Traditional evidence and the select pharmacological studies highlight that this herbal medicine has an effect on uterine contractions (Bamford et al 1970). Unfortunately, there is limited research on both the efficacy and the safety of raspberry leaf. In one retrospective trial, raspberry leaf was associated with some shortening of labour and a decreased need for mechanical assistance (forceps or vacuum), although the difference was not statistically significant (Parsons et al 1999). In another study, raspberry did not shorten the first stage of labour. The only clinically significant findings were shortening of the second stage of labour (mean difference = 9.59 minutes) and lower rate of forceps deliveries between the treatment group and the control group (19.3% vs 30.4%) (Simpson et al 2001).

Two clinical studies evaluating the safety of raspberry leaf in pregnancy have reported no evidence of toxicity in either mother or child (Parsons et al 1999, Simpson et al 2001) although evidence from older animal studies is less clear (Burn & Withell 1941, Whitehouse 1941). In one systematic review, no adverse effects were described in the mothers (increase in blood pressure, increase in blood loss at birth, preterm or post-term labour), and no significant relationships were found between raspberry consumption and neonatal outcomes (Apgar score, birth weight) (Dante et al 2013).

Although raspberry leaf has been in traditional use for a very long time, the evidence regarding safety, efficacy and active constituents is weak. The chemical constituents responsible for the effect on uterus or other smooth muscle are not clearly determined. Some of the constituents, such as flavonoids, have repeatedly been shown to have a relaxing effect on smooth muscle (Mullen et al 2002); however, more research is required.

Cimicifuga racemosa (Black cohosh)

Classification: Unsafe (first and second trimester). Likely to be safe but cannot be confirmed (labour)

- Traditional evidence: available? Y
  - Traditional evidence: cautions or contra-indicates? Y
  - Traditional evidence: if cautions: biologically plausible? Y
- Scientific evidence: available? Y
  - Scientific evidence: human or animal studies find NO known pharmacological effects of concern in pregnancy? N
  - Scientific evidence: toxicological or pharmacological profile studies find NO known pharmacological effects of concern in pregnancy? N
  - Scientific evidence: human and/or animal studies find evidence of pharmacological effects adverse to pregnancy, e.g. abortifacient? Y

Black cohosh was traditionally used by the Native Americans for a variety of ailments including arthritis, menopausal symptoms and respiratory symptoms, and was commonly used to induce labour. It was widely used by the Eclectics in traditional Western Herbal Medicine as a partum preparatory if taken in the last few weeks of pregnancy (Felter & Lloyd 1905, 1983). Black cohosh has a variety of actions such as selective oestrogen–receptor modulator activity, anti-inflammatory and dopaminergic effects. Traditionally it is avoided during early pregnancy, but could be used to assist birth under professional supervision.

Vitex agnus castus (Chaste tree)

Classification: Likely to be safe, but cannot be confirmed

- Traditional evidence: available? Y
  - Traditional evidence: cautions or contra-indicates? N
  - Traditional evidence: if cautions — biologically plausible? NA
- Scientific evidence: available? Y
  - Scientific evidence: human or animal studies find NO known pharmacological effects of concern in pregnancy? Y
  - Scientific evidence: toxicological or pharmacological profile studies find NO known

pharmacological effects of concern in pregnancy? Y

  - Scientific evidence: human and/or animal studies find evidence of pharmacological effects adverse to pregnancy, e.g. abortifacient? N

Chaste tree has been traditionally used for a variety of gynaecological conditions such as aiding the expulsion of the placenta after birth and promoting menstruation. In the first trimester it is sometimes used to promote conception and/or support the growth and development of the fetus. North American herbalists traditionally recommended vitex to improve fertility and after pregnancy as a galactagogue (Felter & Lloyd 1905, 1983). As it is most commonly used by women of childbearing age, it is likely that some women may consume it unknowingly when in the early stages of pregnancy (Dougoua et al 2008). Vitex is believed to act on dopamine receptors to decrease prolactin levels, (Mills & Bone 2005). According to in vitro studies, it may bind to alpha and beta oestrogen-receptors.

PART THREE — ADVISING PATIENTS IN CLINICAL PRACTICE

At some stage of practice most clinicians have to consider the question 'Is this treatment safe in pregnancy?' The answer to such a question is never straightforward, as establishing safety in pregnancy with any degree of certainty is difficult.

Over the years medical practitioners and pharmacists have generally held the view that all medicines should be avoided during pregnancy, where possible. This has referred to the use of pharmaceutical medicines and is wise counsel. With the increasing popularity and accessibility of CMs, many have extended this caution to include herbal medicines under the assumption that the same safety issues apply. Indeed, the safety issues are similar and prudence is still required.

Naturopaths and herbal medicine practitioners hold a more targeted view and recommend a small number of herbal and nutritional medicines during different stages of pregnancy, while being mindful of many others which are considered contraindicated for various reasons.

It is easy for clinicians to adopt the conservative view that all herbal medicines are to be avoided throughout pregnancy; however, this is not useful in practice, especially as women will continue to take them in the belief that they are safe. In fact, it could be argued that best practice means considering all treatment options for safety and efficacy in pregnancy, including herbs and natural supplements.

When medicinal treatments present unacceptable risks or are ineffective, CM as a treatment domain offers a broad range of non-medicinal treatment options which can be considered by clinicians. For example, lifestyle prescriptions, dietary manipulation, massage, acupuncture and aromatherapy provided by appropriately trained practitioners can address a range of symptoms during this sensitive time.

FACTORS TO CONSIDER IN PRACTICE
Individual prescribing
The decision to prescribe or withdraw a CM must be made on an individual case-by-case basis. The safe use of any medicine in pregnancy must take into account the safety of the treatment being considered, the seriousness of the patient's presenting problem, maternal age and gestational age of the fetus and timing of exposure. This includes a consideration of the dose to be used, dosing interval and timing in respect to other medicines and food. Additionally, the patient's presenting health and nutritional status, comorbidities, kidney and liver function and personal attitude to treatment are important factors.

If practitioner and patient agree that a medicine is to be used, steps should be taken to reduce harm, such as recommending the lowest effective dose for the shortest period possible.

While special cautions exist for the first trimester, care must be taken at all stages of pregnancy as fetal growth and development continues.

Timing of the intervention
In practice, choosing the correct dose and administration form is essential and in pregnancy there is the additional consideration of correct timing, which is important for achieving a desired clinical result with a minimum of risk. For example, folate supplementation has been shown to prevent neural tube defects when administered in the preconception period and continued during the first trimester (Berry et al 1999, De-Reigil et al 2010). Similarly, antioxidant supplements appear to be ineffective in reducing preeclampsia when started later in pregnancy (Rumbold et al 2008); however, positive results in preeclampsia were reported in a study which commenced treatment in the first trimester with a broad spectrum antioxidant supplement (including vitamin A 1000 IU, vitamin C 200 mg, vitamin E 400 IU, folic acid 400 mcg, selenium 100 mcg, zinc 15 mg, copper 2 mg, N-acetyl cysteine 200 mg, iron 30 mg) (Rumiris et al 2006).

Informed consent
Evidence-based, patient-centred care means all clinicians are required to present risk/benefit information to their patient, who can then make an informed choice. This means an honest discussion between patient and practitioner about what is known and what remains unknown about the safety and efficacy of a treatment. Patients will no doubt vary in their interest and ability to comprehend and recall the necessary information, so written information and assurance that the woman understands the issues during the time of consultation is useful.

PRACTICE POINTS: GENERAL RULES FOR USING COMPLEMENTARY MEDICINES IN PREGNANCY

- Use CM within the Quality Use of Medicines (QUM) Framework.
- Consider the patient's presenting health status and comorbidities.
- Consider non-medicinal treatment options where appropriate, especially during the first trimester.
- Is such a treatment available and likely to be successful?

Risk–benefit analysis:
- If a CM is under consideration, what are the potential risks and benefits to the mother and fetus?
- What are the risks and benefits (for each) of not prescribing?

Timing of intervention:
- Avoid all medicinal agents where possible, especially in the first trimester.
- Carefully consider the timing of the intervention in regards to gestational age of the fetus: a fetus' susceptibility to toxic effects changes throughout gestation.
- Consider appropriate dose, dose frequency and duration of treatment.

Pharmacotherapy compared with complementary medicine:
- If the patient's condition is sufficiently severe that pharmacotherapy is being considered, clinicians should consider whether an appropriate CM treatment exists with a lower risk of harm.
- If clinician and patient decide a CM is to be used, the lowest possible dose should be used for the shortest period of time.
- CM is best prescribed by a qualified and appropriately trained health professional.

Counselling:
- Counsel pregnant women to avoid exposure to unnecessary medicines and chemicals.

Education and communication:
- If use of a CM is being considered, an open discussion about the potential benefits and potential risks must ensue, so patients can make an informed decision. This includes providing information about what is known about the safety of the treatment and what remains unknown.
- Communication is essential among all health professionals involved in obstetric patient management and the patient.
- Encourage patients to disclose CM use to all their obstetric team of health professionals.
- Special caution should be considered by women due to have elective caesarean section or other surgery. Presurgery cautions and recommendations should be considered.

Additional rules relating to the specific use of herbal medicines in pregnancy
- Avoid all known toxic and poisonous plants at all times, e.g. aconite, pennyroyal, tansy.
- Avoid all thujone-containing herbal medicines, e.g. *Achillea millefolium* (yarrow), *Thuja occidentalis* (thuja) or *Artemisia absinthium* (wormwood).
- Avoid internal use of pure volatile oils from herbal medicines throughout pregnancy. Herbal teas and small concentrations of oils used as flavouring are the exception, e.g. peppermint oil or food quantities of essential oil containing herbal medicines.
- Avoid emmenagogue herbal medicines throughout pregnancy.
- Herbs used to assist delivery should only be used under close professional supervision in the final 6 weeks of pregnancy.

APPENDIX 11.1: NUTRIENTS DURING PREGNANCY

NUTRIENT	THERAPEUTIC FUNCTION/JUSTIFICATION	DOSAGE RECOMMENDATIONS AND ISSUES
Vitamin A	Required for gene expression and cellular differentiation in organogenesis and embryonic development of the spinal cord and vertebrae, limbs, eyes and ears, and heart (Morriss-Kay & Sokolova 1996). Poor maternal status will result in risk of infant deficiency (Ortega et al 1997) associated with poor immune function and increased risk of infection morbidity and mortality in infants and children (Grubesic 2004, Huiming et al 2005) Maternal deficiency increases the risk of mortality (West et al 1999), premature rupture of membranes (Westney et al 1994), preterm delivery (Radhika et al 2002), reduced haemoglobin levels and anaemia (Bondevik et al 2000, Suharno et al 1993), night blindness (Livingstone et al 2003) and immune suppression (Cox et al 2006). A Cochrane review in 2011 (van den Broek et al 2010) pooled results of two large trials in Nepal and Ghana (95,000 women). These results indicated that there was no role for antenatal vitamin A supplementation to reduce maternal or perinatal mortality. However, the populations studied were probably different with regard to baseline vitamin A status and there were problems with follow-up. There is good evidence for antenatal vitamin A supplementation to reduce maternal anaemia for women who live in areas where vitamin A deficiency is common or who are HIV positive. There is also possibly some benefit to reduce maternal infection; however, these data sources are not high quality so further studies are required.	Excessive supplementation shown to be associated with adverse pregnancy outcomes particularly in the first trimester No association with moderate intake (<10,000 IU) and fetal malformations (Botto et al 1996, Johansen et al 2008, Martinez-Frias & Salvador 1990, Mastroiacovo et al 1999, Mills et al 1997, Shaw et al 1997, Werler et al 1990) Supplement labels must carry the warning – when taken in excess of 3000 mcg retinol equivalents (10,000 IU), vitamin A may cause birth defects
Vitamin B_6 (pyridoxine)	Beneficial in the treatment of nausea of pregnancy (Jamigorn & Phupong 2007, Jewell & Young 2003, Sripramote & Lekhyananda 2003). Poor vitamin B_6 status may decrease the possibility of conception (Ronnenberg et al 2007) and increase the risk of early pregnancy loss (Goddijn-Wessel et al 1996, Ronnenberg et al 2007, Wouters et al 1993). Unfortunately vitamin B_6 is insufficiently studied. A Cochrane review established that there were few trials reporting clinical outcomes and mostly had unclear trial methodology and inadequate follow-up. There was not enough evidence to detect clinical benefits of vitamin B_6 supplementation in pregnancy and/or labour, other than one trial suggesting protection against dental decay. It is recommended that future trials assessing this and other outcomes such as orofacial clefts, cardiovascular malformations, neurological development, preterm birth, preeclampsia and adverse events are required (Thaver et al 2006).	RDI during pregnancy is increased slightly to 1.9 mg, and upper recommended level is 50 mg with no evidence of teratogenicity. High dose supplementation (mean 132 mg/day) for 9 weeks during the first trimester appears to be safe with no associated increase in risk for major malformations (Shrim et al 2006). Doses used in studies for nausea are 30–75 mg/day.

NUTRIENT	THERAPEUTIC FUNCTION/JUSTIFICATION	DOSAGE RECOMMENDATIONS AND ISSUES
Vitamin B_9 (folic acid)	Deficiency can lead to homocysteine accumulation, possibly associated with abnormalities of the placental vasculature and increased risk of miscarriage and preeclampsia (Dodds et al 2008, Napolitano et al 2008, Makedos et al 2007) and are associated with a two-fold increased risk of adult schizophrenia (Brown et al 2007). Intake of folic acid preconceptually and in the first 4–6 weeks of pregnancy reduces the risk of neural tube defects (NTD) by more than 50% (Berry et al 1999, Czeizel & Dudas 1992), and may also decrease risk of other congenital malformations including urinary tract and cardiovascular defects, limb deficiencies and hypertrophic pyloric stenosis (Czeizel 1998). The protective effects of higher folic acid intake was also demonstrated in a study from Chile, whereby fortification of flour with folic acid has led to a 55% reduction in NTD prevalence between 1999 and 2009. Individuals with polymorphisms in folate metabolism (methylenetetrahydrofolate reductase [MTHFR] gene) may be at greater risk of deficiency and subsequent adverse effects (Biselli et al 2008, Boyles et al 2008, Candito et al 2008, Coppede et al 2007, Steer et al 2008). In this instance, 5-methyl-tetrahydrofolate preparations are more advisable. A recent Cochrane review found a benefit for folic acid in improving mean birth weight (Lassi & Salam 2013).	Supplementation with folate has been linked with increased risk of multiple pregnancies (Czeizel 1998, Czeizel & Vargha 2004) although disputed by others (Li et al 2003). RDI in pregnancy is 600 mcg/day (200 mcg above non pregnancy state). Upper limit recommended in pregnancy is 1000 mcg due to the possibility of masking a vitamin B_{12} deficiency.
Vitamin B_{12} (cyanocobalamin)	Inadequate cobalamin status in pregnancy has been associated with several adverse outcomes such as preterm birth (Ronnenberg et al 2002), intrauterine growth-retardation (Muthayya et al 2006), increased risk for NTDs (Groenen et al 2004, Gaber et al 2007, Kirke et al 1993, Steen et al 1998, Suarez et al 2003, Wright 1995) and increased risk of miscarriage (Hubner et al 2008). It is also required for homocysteine metabolism, whereby increased levels have been associated with numerous conditions including preeclampsia (Napolitano et al 2008) and recurrent pregnancy loss (Hubner et al 2008). Inadequate maternal status may result in an infant with poor stores, and this may be further exacerbated by low stores in breast milk (Allen 1994).	The RDI is slightly increased to 2.6 mcg/day in pregnancy. There is no upper level of intake as there is no evidence of adverse effects. Deficiency (indicated by macrocytic changes) may be masked by high dose folic acid supplementation.
Vitamin C	Vitamin C deficiency has been suggested to play a role in several adverse pregnancy outcomes such as preeclampsia, intrauterine growth restriction and pre-labour rupture of fetal membranes (PROM). A Cochrane review reported no difference between women supplemented with vitamin C (alone or combined with other supplements) compared with placebo for the risk of stillbirth, miscarriage, birth weight, placental abruption or intrauterine growth restriction (Rumbold & Crowther 2005, Rumbold et al 2005). Required for healthy immune function and significantly reduces the risk of urinary tract infections during pregnancy (Ochoa-Brust et al 2007).	The recommended intake of vitamin C is slightly increased in pregnancy to 60 mg/day. Early reports of high-dose maternal supplementation causing 'conditioned or rebound scurvy' in infants (Cochrane 1965, Rhead & Schrauzer 1971) have not been replicated in subsequent studies (Diplock et al 1998).

(Continued)

NUTRIENT	THERAPEUTIC FUNCTION/JUSTIFICATION	DOSAGE RECOMMENDATIONS AND ISSUES
Vitamin D	Vitamin D supplementation in a single or continued dose during pregnancy increases serum vitamin D concentrations. A recent Cochrane review analysing results from three trials involving 463 women suggest that women who receive vitamin D supplements during pregnancy were less likely to have a low birth weight baby below 2500 grams compared to women receiving no treatment or a placebo (De-Regil et al 2012). High prevalence of vitamin D deficiency in pregnancy and lactation has been reported (Ainy et al 2006, Hollis & Wagner 2004, Judkins & Eagleton 2006, Sachan et al 2005, van der Meer et al 2006). Maternal status also affects the infant's vitamin D status (Hollis & Wagner 2004) and intrauterine growth of long bones (Morley et al 2006), poor infant skeletal growth and mineralisation (Zeghoud et al 1997). In severe maternal deficiency, there is an increased risk of rickets in the infant (Specker 1994). Glucose intolerance (Maghbooli et al 2008), bone health and risk of osteoporotic fracture risk later in life may also be influenced (Javaid et al 2006). It is important for normal brain development (Cui et al 2007, Eyles et al 2003) with fetal deficiency leading to alterations in brain structure and function (Almeras et al 2007, Feron et al 2005). Supplementation may protect against multiple sclerosis (Munger et al 2004, 2006) and reduce the risk of later preeclampsia in the infant (Hypponen et al 2007). Conversely, maternal concentrations of > 75 nmol/L of 25 (OH)-vitamin D in pregnancy may increase the risk of eczema in infants and asthma in children, but did not negatively influence the child's intelligence, psychological health or cardiovascular system (Gale et al 2008).	The amount of vitamin D required during pregnancy and lactation to avoid deficiency may be higher than the recommended amount (RDI 5.0 mcg) (Hollis 2005, 2007, Vieth et al 2001). The recommended upper limit is 80 mcg (Australian Government 2006). Vieth et al (2001), however, found no adverse effects even at doses of 100 mcg (4000 IU) per day. Toxicity is rare, but may occur with excessive supplementation (Koutkia et al 2001). Breast milk is a poor source of vitamin D, with infants requiring an exogenous source within a few months (Challa et al 2005, Daaboul et al 1997, Hatun et al 2005, Sills et al 1994).
Vitamin E	Antioxidant activity is valuable in protecting the embryo (in vitro) and fetus from damage due to oxidative stress (Cederberg et al 2001, Jishage et al 2001, Wang et al 2002). Although oxidative stress plays an important role in the pathogenesis of preeclampsia (Gupta et al 2005), there is little evidence for the role of vitamin E in its prevention (Polyzos et al 2007). Some evidence suggests it was beneficial in women with poor antioxidant status (Rumiris et al 2006). Low maternal levels contribute to increased risk of wheezing and asthma in childhood (Devereux et al 2006) and supplementation was useful in reducing pregnancy-related leg cramps (Shahraki 2006) and increasing birth weight for gestation (Scholl et al 2006, Valsecchi et al 1999).	The recommended intake for vitamin E (7 mg) is not increased for pregnancy. High dose supplementation of vitamin E (400–1200 IU) appears to be safe and does not increase risk for major malformations, preterm deliveries, miscarriages or stillbirths (Boskovic et al 2005). The recommended upper limit in pregnancy is 300 mg/day (Australian Government 2006)

NUTRIENT	THERAPEUTIC FUNCTION/JUSTIFICATION	DOSAGE RECOMMENDATIONS AND ISSUES
Vitamin K	Poor maternal vitamin K levels can result in relative deficiency in newborn infants (Shearer 1992). Low intake combined with the reduced gastrointestinal bacterial synthesis puts infants at risk of Vitamin K deficiency bleeding (VKDB) due to the lack of activity of vitamin K-dependent clotting factors (II, VII, IX and X) (von Kries et al 1993). This is compounded in breastfed infants as breast milk contains lower levels compared to formula, although this may be increased with maternal supplementation during lactation (Greer et al 1997).	The recommended intake of vitamin K during pregnancy and lactation is the same as for a non-pregnant woman (60 mcg/day). To prevent infant health risks, prophylactic treatment of one intramuscular injection of 1 mg (0.1 mL) at birth, or 3 × 2 mg (0.2 mL) oral doses at birth, 3–5 days of age and at 4 weeks are recommended (Australian Government 2006).
Calcium	The newborn infant skeleton holds approximately 20–30 g calcium (Prentice 2003), 80% of which is acquired during the third trimester when the fetal skeleton is rapidly mineralising (Trotter & Hixon 1974). This increased demand for calcium during pregnancy is met by alterations to maternal calcium metabolism, particularly a two-fold increase in calcium absorption mediated by increases in 1,25-dihydroxyvitamin D and other mechanisms (Kovacs & Kronenberg 1997, Prentice 2003). A possible inverse relationship between calcium intake during pregnancy and risk of hypertension and preeclampsia has been suggested from epidemiological and clinical studies (Repke & Villar 1991, Villar & Belizan 2000, Villar et al 1983, 1987, 2003). Supplementation (1.0–2.0 g/day) is recommended to reduce the risk of preeclampsia, gestational hypertension (Hofmeyr et al 2006, 2007), and may also reduce the blood pressure of the offspring (Belizan et al 1997, Hatton et al 2003). Calcium supplementation during pregnancy has been shown to reduce maternal blood lead concentrations by an average of 11% by inhibiting the mobilisation of lead from bone and inhibiting intestinal absorption (Téllez-Rojo et al 2006). Supplementation (1200 mg) during lactation also reduces the risk of infant lead exposure by decreasing the concentration in breast milk by 5–10% (Ettinger et al 2006). A recent Cochrane review identified that calcium supplementation is associated with a significant protective benefit in the prevention of preeclampsia (Buppasiri et al 2011). Another Cochrane review determined that calcium supplementation halved the risk of preeclampsia, reduced the risk of preterm birth and reduced the occurrence of the composite outcome 'death or serious morbidity' (Hofmeyr et al 2010).	Although pregnancy is a time of high calcium requirement, there is no increase in the recommended daily intake for pregnancy (1000 mg). If supplementation is required, it appears to be safe to use (Hofmeyr et al 2006).

(Continued)

NUTRIENT	THERAPEUTIC FUNCTION/JUSTIFICATION	DOSAGE RECOMMENDATIONS AND ISSUES
Chromium	Deficiency is believed to have an effect on glucose intolerance (Jovanovic-Peterson & Peterson 1996, Jovanovic & Peterson 1999). Chromium may protect against maternal insulin resistance and gestational diabetes (Morris & Samaniego 2000); however, studies are contradictory (Aharoni et al 1992, Gunton et al 2001, Woods et al 2008).	Recommended daily intake during pregnancy is slightly increased to 30 mcg/day. Supplementation in gestational diabetes is likely to be safe (Jovanovic & Peterson 1999).
Iodine	Iodine deficiency occurs in both developing and developed countries (Becker et al 2006, Donnay et al 2013). Deficiency during pregnancy (defined as urinary iodine concentrations <150 mcg/L) has been found, even in areas considered to have generally adequate intake. In a study conducted in Rome where a salt iodination program has been introduced, only 4% of non-pregnant women were found to be iodine deficient (<100–199 mcg/L) compared to 92% of pregnant women, suggesting it may be necessary to monitor pregnant women even in regions where iodine deficiency is not common (Marchioni et al 2008). It enables the manufacture of maternal thyroid hormones, is protective against cretinism (Delange 2000) and development of fetal brain, protects against neurological damage (Perez-Lopez 2007), and is also supplied to the breastfed infant via breastmilk (Berbel et al 2007). Maternal hypothyroidism during early pregnancy is associated with other adverse outcomes including premature birth, preeclampsia, breech delivery and increased fetal mortality (Casey et al 2005, Haddow et al 1999, Pop 2004). It protects the mother from thyroid dysfunction which in turn protects the neonate's thyroid function and supports neurocognitive development in children (Ersino et al 2013). High-risk women (personal or family history of thyroid disorders or a personal history of other autoimmune diseases) have more than a six-fold increased risk of hypothyroidism during early pregnancy (Vaidya et al 2007)	Mild iodine deficiency (median UIE < 100 mcg/L) has been found in several areas in Australia including NSW and Victoria (Li et al 2006). To prevent iodine deficiency disorders, WHO, United Nations Children's Fund and International Council for the Control of Iodine Deficiency Disorders established that for a given population median urinary iodine concentrations (UIC) must be 150–249 mcg/L in clinically healthy pregnant women (Marchioni et al 2008). Iodine requirement increases during pregnancy and recommended intakes are 250–300 mcg/day (Delange 2007). To monitor iodine status, WHO suggest that a median urinary iodine concentration 250–500 mcg/day indicates adequate iodine intake in pregnancy (Zimmermann 2007).

NUTRIENT	THERAPEUTIC FUNCTION/JUSTIFICATION	DOSAGE RECOMMENDATIONS AND ISSUES
Iron	Iron requirements increase significantly in pregnancy to support expansion of maternal red blood cell mass and fetal growth (Bothwell 2000). Accurate assessment of iron status during pregnancy is more challenging due to the physiological changes occurring at this time (Milman et al 1991). Haemodilution affects iron parameters, such as haemoglobin concentration, haematocrit, serum iron, ferritin and total-iron binding capacity. Serum ferritin is regarded as the most reliable indicator of iron stores (Byg et al 2000), while haemoglobin levels are used as an inexpensive marker to diagnose anaemia (Reveiz et al 2007). The evaluation of iron status and the future risk of anaemia developing during pregnancy may be more accurate when done early in pregnancy before the maternal plasma volume expands (Scholl 2005). Demands are partly met by a progressive increase in iron absorption as the pregnancy advances (Bothwell 2000); however, depending on initial iron reserves this may not be sufficient to prevent deficiency (Casanueva et al 2003). The risk of iron deficiency increases with parity (Looker et al 1997). Maternal iron stores at conception appear to be a strong predictor of the risk of anaemia in later pregnancy (Bothwell 2000, Casanueva et al 2003). WHO estimates indicate that iron deficiency anaemia affects 22% of women during pregnancy in industrialised countries and 52% in non-industrialised countries (WHO 1992). Supplementation raised haemoglobin levels by 7.5 g/dL and reduced the risk of iron deficiency and iron-deficiency anaemia at term (Casanueva et al 2006, Pena-Rosas & Viteri 2006). Numerous studies have showed an association between adverse outcomes and iron deficiency anaemia, including increased risk of maternal mortality, infection, low birth weight and premature delivery. Fetal and infant iron deficiency may adversely impact on brain development, function and neurocognition (Grantham-McGregor & Ani 2001). Poor maternal iron status may contribute to reduced fetal stores (de Pee et al 2002, Emamghorashi & Heidari 2004, Preziosi et al 1997). However, in a recent cross-sectional study, pregnant women with iron deficiency or mild anaemia were not found to produce offspring with significantly altered iron levels (Paiva Ade et al 2007). Similarly, iron supplementation during the second half of pregnancy was not found to influence the iron status of the children at 6 months or 4 years of age (Zhou et al 2007). On a cautionary note, excessive iron supplementation resulting in high haemoglobin and increased iron stores may be associated with increased adverse pregnancy outcomes (Scholl 2005), including low birth weight and premature delivery (Casanueva & Viteri 2003). A recent Cochrane review involving more than 27,402 women concluded that prenatal supplementation with daily iron is effective in reducing the risk of low birth weight babies, and prevents maternal anaemia and iron deficiency in pregnancy (Peña-Rosas et al 2012).	The daily recommended intake of iron during pregnancy is increased to 27 mg/day. Upper limit is 45 mg based on the risk for side effects and potential systemic toxicity. A daily supplement of 40 mg ferrous iron from 18 weeks of gestation appears adequate to prevent iron deficiency in 90% of women (Milman et al 2005). However, individual assessment of iron status in early pregnancy may be useful to tailor the appropriate prophylaxis to prevent iron deficiency and iron deficiency anaemia: Ferritin ≤ 30 mcg/L — 80–100 mg ferrous iron/day; ferritin 31–70 mcg/L — 40 mg ferrous iron/day; those with ferritin > 70 mcg/L do not require supplementation (Milman et al 2006). High dose supplementation may reduce the absorption of zinc (Hambidge et al 1987, O'Brien et al 2000) and other divalent cations (copper, chromium, molybdenum, manganese, magnesium) (Rossander-Hulten et al 1991). Side effects of high dose supplementation typically include gastrointestinal disturbances — most commonly constipation and nausea (Melamed et al 2007).

(Continued)

NUTRIENT	THERAPEUTIC FUNCTION/JUSTIFICATION	DOSAGE RECOMMENDATIONS AND ISSUES
Magnesium	Magnesium is involved as a cofactor in more than 300 enzyme pathways (Wacker & Parisi 1968) and acts as a neuromuscular relaxant. The infant will contain 750 mg at birth (Prentice 2003). Positive trials highlight benefits of magnesium supplementation for leg cramps (Dahle et al 1995) and possibly pre-ecclampsia although evidence is inconsistent for this last indication (Adam et al 2001, Ahmed 2004, Dawson et al 2000, Duley et al 2003a, 2003b, 2003c, Handwerker et al 1995, Kisters et al 2000, Makrides & Crowther 2001, Omu et al 2008, Sanders et al 1999, Seydoux et al 1992, Shamsuddin et al 2005).	The recommended daily intake for magnesium during pregnancy is increased slightly to 350 mg (19–30 years) and 360 mg (31–50 years). The upper level of intake from non-food sources is 350 mg/day.
Zinc	Deficiency has been associated with adverse outcomes in pregnancy. Numerous animal models demonstrate an association between zinc deficiency and increased developmental abnormalities and fetal losses. Deficiency has also been associated with reduced interuterine growth, preterm delivery, labour and delivery complications, poor immunological development (Caulfield et al 1998) and congenital malformations (Hambidge et al 1977). A Cochrane review analysing results from studies assessed over 15,000 women and their babies concluded that zinc supplementation resulted in a small but significant reduction in preterm birth (Mori et al 2012). In humans acrodermatitis enteropathica, a genetic disease which produces severe zinc deficiency, has been found to increase fetal losses and malformations, most probably due to its key role in protein synthesis and cellular growth (King 2000). The usefulness of zinc supplementation during pregnancy is unclear. Supplementation has been shown to reduce preterm birth (Mahomed et al 2007), assist the accumulation of lean tissue in the infant during the first year of growth (Iannotti et al 2008) and reduce the risk of delivering via caesarean section (Mahomed et al 2007). While women with preeclampsia have significantly lower zinc and SOD levels compared to healthy pregnant women (Ilhan et al 2002), zinc supplementation had no significant effect in pregnancy hypertension or preeclampsia (Mahomed et al 2007), and no significant differences were seen for several other maternal or infant outcomes including pre-labour rupture of membranes, antepartum haemorrhage, post-term birth, prolonged labour, retention of placenta, meconium in liquor, smell or taste dysfunction, maternal infections, gestational age at birth or birth weight (Mahomed et al 2007).	Recommended daily intake during pregnancy is increased to 11 mg/day and recommended upper level of intake is the same as for adults at 40 mg/day. Vegans and vegetarians may need an additional 50%. The teratogenic effects of alcohol may be exacerbated by a concurrent zinc deficiency (Keppen et al 1985).

NUTRIENT	THERAPEUTIC FUNCTION/JUSTIFICATION	DOSAGE RECOMMENDATIONS AND ISSUES
Omega-3 (DHA/ EPA)	High fetal demands for omega-3 fatty acids result in maternal stores progressively decreasing throughout pregnancy (Al et al 1995, Bonham et al 2008). Important for optimal fetal and infant neurodevelopment and may be associated with benefits for other pregnancy and infant health outcomes including growth and development of the fetal and infant brain (Horrocks & Yeo 1999, Rogers et al 2013), improvements to children's eye–hand coordination (Dunstan et al 2008) and higher infant cognitive function (Hibbeln et al 2007, Oken et al 2005). Lower maternal intake was associated with increased risk of infants with poorer outcomes for prosocial behaviour, fine motor, communication and social development scores (Hibbeln et al 2007), increase risk of infant asthma (Olsen et al 2008), increased risk of postnatal depression (Levant et al 2006, 2008) and increased depressive symptoms in postpartum women (Hibbeln 2002). However, more recent studies have found no association (Browne et al 2006, Freeman et al 2008, Rees et al 2008, Sontrop et al 2008) or mixed outcomes (Su et al 2008). Lower dietary intake of fish (Oken et al 2007) and biochemical markers of omega-3 fatty acid intake (Mehendale et al 2008, Qiu et al 2006, Velzing-Aarts et al 1999) have been reported in women who develop preeclampsia. However, intervention studies with fish oil supplementation generally have not found a protective effect. In a Cochrane review there was no significant difference in risk of gestational hypertension (five trials) or preeclampsia (four trials) in those taking the fish oil (133 mg/day to 3 g/day) compared with control groups (Makrides et al 2006).	Fish oil supplementation during pregnancy appears to be safe. Mild side effects such as belching and unpleasant taste are reported (Freeman & Sinha 2007, Makrides et al 2006). Recommendations for dietary intake of EPA/ DHA (adequate intake) for pregnancy is 115 mg/day. Upper level of intake is recommended at 3 g for adults (no pregnancy specifications). Maternal dietary docosahexaenoic acid intake of at least 200 mg/day is associated with positive infant neurodevelopmental outcomes (Cetin & Koletzko 2008).
Probiotics	Prenatal and postnatal supplementation with probiotics may play a role in immune regulation and the prevention of allergies developing in the infant. Numerous positive studies in the prevention of allergies including eczema in the child have involved the following strains: *Lactobacillus reuteri* ATCC 55730 (Abrahamsson et al 2007) *Lactobacillus rhamnosus* strain GG (ATCC 53103) (Kalliomaki et al 2001, 2003, Rautava et al 2002) *Lactobacillus rhamnosus* GG (ATCC 53103); *L. rhamnosus* LC705 (DSM 7061); *Bifidobacterium breve* Bb99 (DSM 13692); and *Propionibacterium freudenreichii* ssp. *shermanii* JS (DSM 7076) (Kukkonen et al 2007) *Lactobacillus rhamnosus* strain GG and *Bifidobacterium lactis* Bb12 (Huurre et al 2008) Prophylactic enteral supplementation reduces the occurrence of necrotising enterocolitis and death in premature infants born less than 1500 g (Alfaleh & Bassler 2008), which may be due to normalisation of gut flora and stimulation of natural host defences (Hammerman & Kaplan 2006). Vaginal application reduces the risk of vaginal infections in pregnancy (Othman et al 2007).	Based on review of literature, prescription appears to be safe for internal and vaginal application.
Choline	Choline status in pregnancy influences the development of the memory centre (hippocampus) in the fetal brain, and may have a lifelong impact on memory (Zeisel 2004). It has been shown to improve cognitive function in the neonate and benefit extends into childhood (Boeke et al 2013).	The recommended daily intake is slightly increased at 440 mg/ day, with an upper level of 3000 mg.

APPENDIX 11.2: NHMRC DOSAGE RECOMMENDATIONS FOR PREGNANCY

NUTRIENT	RDI (NHMRC)	NUTRIENT	RDI (NHMRC)
Vitamin A	2600 IU	PABA	No guidelines available
Vitamin B$_1$ (thiamine)	1.4 mg	Coenzyme Q10	No guidelines available
Vitamin B$_2$ (riboflavin)	1.4 mg	Alpha lipoic acid	No guidelines available
Vitamin B$_3$ (niacin)	18 mg	Calcium	1000–1300 mg
Vitamin B$_5$ (pantothenic acid)	5 mg	Chromium	30 mcg
		Copper	1.3 mg
Vitamin B6 (pyridoxine)	1.9 mg	Iodine	220 mcg
Pyridoxal 5 phosphate (P5P)	No guidelines available	Iron	27 mg
Vitamin B$_9$ (folic acid)	600 mcg	Magnesium	350 mg
Folinic acid	No guidelines available	Manganese	5 mg
L-5-MTHF	No guidelines available	Potassium	2800 mg
Vitamin B$_{12}$ (cyanocobalamin)	2.6 mcg	Selenium	65 mcg
		Silica	No guidelines available
Vitamin C	60 mg	Zinc	11 mcg
Vitamin D	200 IU/5 mcg	Total omega-3 essential fatty acids	No guidelines available
Vitamin E	10 IU/7 mg		
Vitamin K	60 mcg	Total omega-6 essential fatty acids	No guidelines available
Betacarotene	800 mcg	DHA	220 mg
Bioflavonoids	No guidelines available	EPA	220 mg
Biotin	30 mcg	Evening primrose oil	No guidelines available
Choline	440 mg	Probiotics (mixed strains)	No guidelines available
Inositol	No guidelines available		

REFERENCES

Abrahamsson TR et al. Probiotics in prevention of IgE-associated eczema: a double-blind, randomized, placebo-controlled trial. J Allergy Clin Immunol 119.5 (2007): 1174–1180.

Adam B et al. Magnesium, zinc and iron levels in pre-eclampsia. J Matern Fetal Med 10.4 (2001): 246–250.

Aharoni A et al. Hair chromium content of women with gestational diabetes compared with nondiabetic pregnant women. Am J Clin Nutr 55.1 (1992): 104–107.

Ahmed R. Magnesium sulphate as an anticonvulsant in the management of eclampsia. J Coll Physicians Surg Pak 14.10 (2004): 605–607.

Ainy E et al. Changes in calcium, 25(OH) vitamin D3 and other biochemical factors during pregnancy. J Endocrinol Invest 29.4 (2006): 303–307.

Al MD et al. Maternal essential fatty acid patterns during normal pregnancy and their relationship to the neonatal essential fatty acid status. Br J Nutr 74.1 (1995): 55–68.

Alfaleh K, Bassler D. Probiotics for prevention of necrotizing enterocolitis in preterm infants. Cochrane Database Syst Rev 1 (2008): CD005496.

Allen LH. Vitamin B12 metabolism and status during pregnancy, lactation and infancy. Adv Exp Med Biol 352 (1994): 173–186.

Almeras L et al. Developmental vitamin D deficiency alters brain protein expression in the adult rat: implications for neuropsychiatric disorders. Proteomics 7.5 (2007): 769–780.

Andrade-Cetto A. Ethnobotanical study of the medicinal plants from Tlanchinol, Hidalgo, Mexico. Journal of Ethnopharmacology 122.1 (2009):163–171.

Australian Government, Department of Health and Ageing. National Health and Medical Research Council (NHMRC) and the New Zealand Ministry of Health (MoH). Nutrient Reference Values for Australia and New Zealand. Commonwealth of Australia, 2006. Available: https://www.nhmrc.gov.au/_files_nhmrc/publications/attachments/n35.pdf 5/8/2014.

Awang DV. Maternal use of ginseng and neonatal androgenization. JAMA 265.14 (1991): 1828.

Bamford DS et al. Br J Pharmacol 40 (1970): 161P

Barker DJ. The developmental origins of adult disease. J Am Coll Nutr 23.(6 Suppl) (2004): 588S–595S.

Barker DJ. The origins of the developmental origins theory. J Intern Med 261.5 (2007): 412–417.

Becker DV et al. Iodine supplementation for pregnancy and lactation — United States and Canada: Recommendations of the American Thyroid Association. Thyroid 16.10 (2006): 949–951.

Belew C. Herbs and the childbearing woman: Guidelines for midwives. Journal of Nurse-Midwifery 44(3) (1999): 231–252.

Belizan JM et al. Long-term effect of calcium supplementation during pregnancy on the blood pressure of offspring: follow up of a randomised controlled trial. BMJ 315(7103) (1997): 281–285.

Berbel P et al. Iodine supplementation during pregnancy: a public health challenge. Trends Endocrinol Metab 18.9 (2007): 338–343.

Berry RJ et al Prevention of neural-tube defects with folic acid in China. China–U.S. Collaborative Project for Neural Tube Defect Prevention. N Engl J Med 341.20 (1999): 1485–1490.

Biselli JM et al. Genetic polymorphisms involved in folate metabolism and elevated plasma concentrations of homocysteine: maternal risk factors for Down syndrome in Brazil. Genet Mol Res 7.1 (2008): 33–42.

Boeke CE et al. Choline intake during pregnancy and child cognition at age 7 years. Am J Epidemiol 177.12 (2013): 1338–1347.

Bondevik GT et al. Anaemia in pregnancy: possible causes and risk factors in Nepali women. Eur J Clin Nutr 54.1 (2000): 3–8.

Bonham MP et al. Habitual fish consumption does not prevent a decrease in LCPUFA status in pregnant women (the Seychelles Child Development Nutrition Study). Prostaglandins Leukotrienes and Essential Fatty Acids 78.6 (2008): 343–350.

Borrelli F et al. Effectiveness and safety of ginger in the treatment of pregnancy-induced nausea and vomiting. Obstet Gynecol 105.4 (2005): 849–856.

Boskovic R et al Pregnancy outcome following high doses of Vitamin E supplementation. Reprod Toxicol 20.1 (2005): 85–88.

Bothwell TH. Iron requirements in pregnancy and strategies to meet them. Am J Clin Nutr 72.(1 Suppl) (2000): 257S–264S.

Botto LD et al. Periconceptional multivitamin use and the occurrence of conotruncal heart defects: results from a population-based, case-control study. Pediatrics 98.5 (1996): 911–917.

Boyles AL et al. Folate and one-carbon metabolism gene polymorphisms and their associations with oral facial clefts. Am J Med Genet A 146A.4 (2008): 440–449.

Brown AS et al. Elevated prenatal homocysteine levels as a risk factor for schizophrenia. Arch Gen Psychiatry 64.1 (2007): 31–39.

Browne JC et al. Fish consumption in pregnancy and omega-3 status after birth are not associated with postnatal depression. Journal of Affective Disorders 90.2–3 (2006): 131–139.

Bryant B et al. Drugs in Pregnancy. Pharmacology for Health Professionals. Sydney: Mosby, 2003.

Buppasiri P et al. Calcium supplementation (other than for preventing or treating hypertension) for improving pregnancy and infant outcomes. Cochrane Database of Systematic Reviews 10 (2011).

Burn J, Withell E. A principle in raspberry leaves which relaxes uterine muscle. Lancet 5 (1941): 1–3.

Byg KE et al. Erythropoiesis: Correlations between iron status markers during normal pregnancy in women with and without iron supplementation. Hematology 4(6) (2000): 529–539.

Candito M et al. Nutritional and genetic determinants of vitamin B and homocysteine metabolisms in neural tube defects: a multicenter case-control study. Am J Med Genet A 146A.9 (2008): 1128–1133.

Casanueva E, Viteri FE. Iron and oxidative stress in pregnancy. J Nutr 133.(5 Suppl 2) (2003): 1700S–1708S.

Casanueva E et al. Iron and folate status before pregnancy and anemia during pregnancy. Ann Nutr Metab 47.2 (2003): 60–63.

Casanueva E et al. Weekly iron as a safe alternative to daily supplementation for nonanemic pregnant women. Arch Med Res 37(5) (2006): 674–682.

Casey BM et al. Subclinical Hypothyroidism and Pregnancy Outcomes. Obstet Gynecol 105(2) (2005): 239–245.

Caulfield LE et al. Potential contribution of maternal zinc supplementation during pregnancy to maternal and child survival. Am J Clin Nutr 68 (2 Suppl) (1998): 499S–508S.

Cederberg J et al. Combined treatment with vitamin E and vitamin C decreases oxidative stress and improves fetal outcome in experimental diabetic pregnancy. Pediatr Res 49.6 (2001): 755–762.

Cetin I, Koletzko B. Long-chain omega-3 fatty acid supply in pregnancy and lactation. Curr Opin Clin Nutr Metab Care 11.3 (2008): 297–302.

Chaiyakunapruk N et al. The efficacy of ginger for the prevention of postoperative nausea and vomiting: a meta-analysis. Am J Obstet Gynecol 194 (2006): 95–99.

Challa A et al. Breastfeeding and vitamin D status in Greece during the first 6 months of life. Eur J Pediatr 164(12) (2005): 724–729.

Chow G et al. Dietary Echinacea purpurea during murine pregnancy: effect on maternal hemopoiesis and fetal growth. Biol Neonate 89.2 (2006): 133–138.

Cochrane WA. Overnutrition in prenatal and neonatal life: a problem? Can Med Assoc J 93.17 (1965): 893–899.

Coppede F et al. Polymorphisms in folate and homocysteine metabolizing genes and chromosome damage in mothers of Down syndrome children. Am J Med Genet A 143A.17 (2007): 2006–2015.

Cox SE et al. Vitamin A supplementation increases ratios of proinflammatory to anti-inflammatory cytokine responses in pregnancy and lactation. Clin Exp Immunol 144.3 (2006): 392–400.

Cui X et al. Maternal vitamin D depletion alters neurogenesis in the developing rat brain. International Journal of Developmental Neuroscience 25(4) (2007): 227–232.

Czeizel AE. Periconceptional folic acid containing multivitamin supplementation. Eur J Obstet Gynecol Reprod Biol 78.2 (1998): 151–161.

Czeizel AE, Dudas I. Prevention of the first occurrence of neural-tube defects by periconceptional vitamin supplementation. N Engl J Med 327.26 (1992): 1832–1835.

Czeizel AE, Vargha P. Periconceptional folic acid/multivitamin supplementation and twin pregnancy. Am J Obstet Gynecol 191 3 (2004): 790–794.

Daaboul J et al. Vitamin D deficiency in pregnant and breast-feeding women and their infants. J Perinatol 17.1 (1997): 10–14.

Dahle LO et al (1995). The effect of oral magnesium substitution on pregnancy-induced leg cramps. Am J Obstet Gynecol 173(1): 175–180.

Dante, G et al. Herb remedies during pregnancy: a systematic review of controlled clinical trials, J. Mat-Fet and Neo Med 26.3 (2013): 306–312.

Dawson EB et al. Blood cell lead, calcium, and magnesium levels associated with pregnancy-induced hypertension and preeclampsia. Biol Trace Elem Res 74.2 (2000): 107–116.

de Pee S et al. The High Prevalence of Low Hemoglobin Concentration among Indonesian Infants Aged 3–5 Months Is Related to Maternal Anemia. J. Nutr. 132.8 (2002): 2215–2221.

De-Regil LM et al. Effects and safety of periconceptional folate supplementation for preventing birth defects. Cochrane Database of Systematic Reviews 10 (2010): CD007950.

De-Regil LM et al. Vitamin D supplementation for women during pregnancy. Cochrane Database of Systematic Reviews 2 (2012): CD008873.

Delange F. The role of iodine in brain development. Proc Nutr Soc 59.1 (2000): 75–79.

Delange, F. Iodine requirements during pregnancy, lactation and the neonatal period and indicators of optimal iodine nutrition. Public Health Nutr 10.12A (2007): 1571–1583.

Devereux G et al. Low maternal vitamin E intake during pregnancy is associated with asthma in 5-year-old children. Am J Respir Crit Care Med 174.5 (2006): 499–507.

Diplock AT et al. Functional food science and defence against reactive oxidative species. Br J Nutr 80 Suppl 1 (1998): S77–112.

Dodds L et al. Effect of homocysteine concentration in early pregnancy on gestational hypertensive disorders and other pregnancy outcomes. Clin Chem 54.2 (2008): 326–334.

Donnay S et al. Position statement of the working group on disorders related to iodine deficiency and thyroid dysfunction of the Spanish Society of Endocrinology and Nutrition. Endocrinología y Nutrición (2013): S1575–0922.

Dougoua JJ et al. Safety and efficacy of chastetree (Vitex agnus castus) during pregnancy and lactation, Can J Clin Pharmacol 15.1 (2008):e74–e79.

Duley L, Henderson-Smart D (2003). Magnesium sulphate versus diazepam for eclampsia. Cochrane Database Syst Rev(4): CD000127.

Duley L, Henderson-Smart D (2003). Magnesium sulphate versus phenytoin for eclampsia. Cochrane Database Syst Rev(4): CD000128.

Duley L et al. Magnesium sulphate and other anticonvulsants for women with pre-eclampsia. Cochrane Database Syst Rev(2) (2003): CD000025.

Dunstan JA et al. Cognitive assessment of children at age 2(1/2) years after maternal fish oil supplementation in pregnancy: a randomised controlled trial. Arch Dis Child Fetal Neonatal Ed 93.1 (2008): F45–50.

Emamghorashi F, Heidari T. Iron status of babies born to iron-deficient anaemic mothers in an Iranian hospital. East Mediterr Health J 10.6 (2004): 808–814.

Ersino G et al. Clinical assessment of goiter and low urinary iodine concentration depict presence of severe iodine deficiency in pregnant Ethiopian women: a cross-sectional study in rural Sidama, southern Ethiopia. Ethiop Med J. 51.2 (2013): 133–141.

Ettinger AS et al. Influence of maternal bone lead burden and calcium intake on levels of lead in breast milk over the course of lactation. Am J Epidemiol 163.1 (2006): 48–56.

Eyles D et al. Vitamin d3 and brain development. Neuroscience 118.3 (2003): 641–653.

Felter HW, Lloyd JU. King's American dispensatory, 18th edn, 3rd rev. vol 1, Eclectic Medical Publications, USA, 1905, reprinted 1983.

Feron F et al Developmental Vitamin D3 deficiency alters the adult rat brain. Brain Res Bull 65.2 (2005): 141–148.

Forster D et al. Herbal medicine use during pregnancy in a group of Australian women. BMC Pregnancy and Childbirth 6.1 (2006): 21.

Forster DA et al. The use of folic acid and other vitamins before and during pregnancy in a group of women in Melbourne, Australia. Midwifery 2007.

Freeman MP, Sinha P. Tolerability of omega-3 fatty acid supplements in perinatal women. Prostaglandins, Leukotrienes and Essential Fatty Acids 77.3–4 (2007): 203–208.

Freeman MP et al. Omega-3 fatty acids and supportive psychotherapy for perinatal depression: A randomized placebo-controlled study. J Affect Disord 110.1–2 (2008): 142–148.

Freyer AM Drug-prescribing challenges during pregnancy Obstetr, Gynaecol Repr Med, Review 18.7 (2008): 180–186.

Gaber KR et al. Maternal vitamin B12 and the risk of fetal neural tube defects in Egyptian patients. Clin Lab 53.1–2 (2007): 69–75.

Gale CR et al. Maternal vitamin D status during pregnancy and child outcomes. Eur J Clin Nutr 62.1 (2008): 68–77.

Gallo M et al. Pregnancy outcome following gestational exposure to echinacea: a prospective controlled study. Arch Intern Med 160.20 (2000): 3141–3143.

Goddijn-Wessel TA et al. Hyperhomocysteinemia: a risk factor for placental abruption or infarction. Eur J Obstet Gynecol Reprod Biol 66.1 (1996): 23–29.

Grantham-McGregor S, Ani C. A review of studies on the effect of iron deficiency on cognitive development in children. J Nutr 131.2S-2 (2001): 649S–668S.

Greer FR et al. Improving the vitamin K status of breastfeeding infants with maternal vitamin K supplements. Pediatrics 99.1 (1997): 88–92.

Grieve M. A modern herbal. New York, Dover, 1971.

Groenen P M et al. Marginal maternal vitamin B12 status increases the risk of offspring with spina bifida. Am J Obstet Gynecol 191.1 (2004): 11–17.

Grubesic RB. Children aged 6 to 60 months in Nepal may require a vitamin A supplement regardless of dietary intake from plant an animal food sources. Food Nutr Bull 25.3 (2004): 248–255.

Gunton JE et al. Serum chromium does not predict glucose tolerance in late pregnancy. Am J Clin Nutr 73.1 (2001): 99–104.

Gupta S et al. The role of placental oxidative stress and lipid peroxidation in preeclampsia. Obstet Gynecol Surv 60(12) (2005): 807–816.

Haddow JE et al. Maternal Thyroid Deficiency during Pregnancy and Subsequent Neuropsychological Development of the Child. N Engl J Med 341.8 (1999): 549–555.

Hambidge KM et al. The role of zinc in the pathogenesis and treatment of acrodermatitis enteropathica. Prog Clin Biol Res 14 (1977): 329–342.

Hambidge KM et al. Acute effects of iron therapy on zinc status during pregnancy. Obstet Gynecol 70.4 (1987): 593–596.

Hammerman C, Kaplan M. Probiotics and neonatal intestinal infection. Curr Opin Infect Dis 19.3 (2006): 277–282.

Handwerker SM et al. Ionized serum magnesium and potassium levels in pregnant women with preeclampsia and eclampsia. J Reprod Med 40.3 (1995): 201–208.

Hatton DC et al. Gestational calcium supplementation and blood pressure in the offspring. Am J Hypertens 16.10 (2003): 801–805.

Hatun S et al (2005). Vitamin D deficiency in early infancy. J. Nutr. 135(2): 279–282.

Henry A, Crowther C. Patterns of medication use during and prior to pregnancy: the MAP study. Aust N Z J Obstet Gynaecol 40.2 (2000): 165–172.

Hess H M et al. Herbs during pregnancy. Drugs during pregnancy and lactation, 2nd edn. Oxford: Academic Press, 2007, pp 485–501.

Hibbeln JR. Seafood consumption, the DHA content of mothers' milk and prevalence rates of postpartum depression: a cross-national, ecological analysis. J Affect Disord 69.1–3 (2002): 15–29.

Hibbeln JR et al. Maternal seafood consumption in pregnancy and neurodevelopmental outcomes in childhood (ALSPAC study): an observational cohort study. Lancet 369.9561 (2007): 578–585.

Hofmeyr GJ, Atallah, AN et al. Calcium supplementation during pregnancy for preventing hypertensive disorders and related problems. Cochrane Database Syst Rev 3 (2006): CD001059.

Hofmeyr GJ, Lawrie TA et al. Calcium supplementation during pregnancy for preventing hypertensive disorders and related problems. Cochrane Database of Syst Rev 8 (2010): CD001059.

Hofmeyr GJ et al. Dietary calcium supplementation for prevention of pre-eclampsia and related problems: a systematic review and commentary. Bjog 114.8 (2007): 933–943.

Hollis BW. Circulating 25-Hydroxyvitamin D Levels Indicative of Vitamin D Sufficiency: Implications for Establishing a New Effective Dietary Intake Recommendation for Vitamin D. J. Nutr. 135.2 (2005): 317–322.

Hollis BW. Vitamin D requirement during pregnancy and lactation. J Bone Miner Res 22 Suppl 2 (2007): V39–44.

Hollis BW, Wagner CL. Assessment of dietary vitamin D requirements during pregnancy and lactation. Am J Clin Nutr 79(5) (2004): 717–726.

Hollyer T et al. The use of CAM by women suffering from nausea and vomiting during pregnancy. BMC Complement Altern Med 2 (2002): 5.

Horrocks LA, Yeo YK. Health benefits of docosahexaenoic acid (DHA). Pharmacol Res 40.3 (1999): 211–225.

Hubner U et al. Low serum vitamin B12 is associated with recurrent pregnancy loss in Syrian women. Clin Chem Lab Med (2008).

Huiming Y et al. Vitamin A for treating measles in children. Cochrane Database Syst Rev 4 (2005): CD001479.

Huurre A et al. Impact of maternal atopy and probiotic supplementation during pregnancy on infant sensitization: a double-blind placebo-controlled study. Clin Exp Allergy (2008).

Hypponen E et al. Does vitamin D supplementation in infancy reduce the risk of pre-eclampsia? Eur J Clin Nutr 61.9 (2007): 1136–1139.

Iannotti LL et al. Maternal zinc supplementation and growth in Peruvian infants. Am J Clin Nutr 8.1 (2008): 154–160.

Ilhan N et al. The changes of trace elements, malondialdehyde levels and superoxide dismutase activities in pregnancy with or without preeclampsia. Clin Biochem 35.5 (2002): 393–397.

Jamigorn, M, Phupong V. Acupressure and vitamin B6 to relieve nausea and vomiting in pregnancy: a randomized study. Arch Gynecol Obstet 276.3 (2007): 245–249.

Javaid MK et al. Maternal vitamin D status during pregnancy and childhood bone mass at age 9 years: a longitudinal study. Lancet 367.9504 (2006): 36–43.

Jewell D, Young G. Interventions for nausea and vomiting in early pregnancy. Cochrane Database Syst Rev. 4 (2003): CD000145.

Jishage K-i et al. alpha-Tocopherol Transfer Protein Is Important for the Normal Development of Placental Labyrinthine Trophoblasts in Mice. J. Biol. Chem. 276.3 (2001): 1669–1672.

Johansen AM et al. Maternal dietary intake of vitamin A and risk of orofacial clefts: a population-based case-control study in Norway. Am J Epidemiol 167.10 (2008): 1164–1170.

Jones TK, Lawson BM. Profound neonatal congestive heart failure caused by maternal consumption of blue cohosh herbal medication. J Pediatr 132.3–1 (1998): 550–552.

Jovanovic L, Peterson M. Chromium supplementation for women with gestational diabetes mellitus. The Journal of Trace Elements in Experimental Medicine 12.2 (1999): 91–97.

Jovanovic-Peterson L, Peterson CM. Vitamin and mineral deficiencies which may predispose to glucose intolerance of pregnancy. J Am Coll Nutr 15(1) (1996): 14–20.

Judkins A, Eagleton C. Vitamin D deficiency in pregnant New Zealand women. N Z Med J 119.1241 (2006): U2144.

Kalliomaki M et al. Probiotics in primary prevention of atopic disease: a randomised placebo-controlled trial. Lancet 357.9262 (2001): 1076–1079.

Kalliomaki M et al. Probiotics and prevention of atopic disease: 4-year follow-up of a randomised placebo-controlled trial. Lancet 361.9372 (2003): 1869–1871.

Keeler RF. Lupin alkaloids from teratogenic and nonteratogenic lupins. III. Identification of anagyrine as the probable teratogen by feeding trials. J Toxicol Environ Health 1.6 (1976): 887–898.

Keeler RF et al. Lupin alkaloids from teratogenic and nonteratogenic lupins. IV. Concentration of total alkaloids, individual major alkaloids, and the teratogen anagyrine as a function of plant part and stage of growth and their relationship to crooked calf disease. J Toxicol Environ Health 1(6) (1976): 899–908.

Kennelly EJ et al. Detecting potential teratogenic alkaloids from blue cohosh rhizomes using an in vitro rat embryo culture. J Nat Prod 62.10 (1999): 1385–1389.

Keppen LD et al. Zinc deficiency acts as a co-teratogen with alcohol in fetal alcohol syndrome. Pediatr Res 19.9 (1985): 944–947.

King JC. Determinants of maternal zinc status during pregnancy. Am J Clin Nutr 71.(5 Suppl) (2000): 1334S–1343S.

Kirke PN et al. Maternal plasma folate and vitamin B12 are independent risk factors for neural tube defects. Q J Med 86.11 (1993): 703–708.

Kisters K et al. Membrane, intracellular, and plasma magnesium and calcium concentrations in preeclampsia. Am J Hypertens 13.7 (2000): 765–769.

Koren G et al. Maternal ginseng use associated with neonatal androgenisation. JAMA 264.22 (1990): 2866.

Koutkia P et al. Vitamin D intoxication associated with an over-the-counter supplement. N Engl J Med 345.1 (2001): 66–67.

Kovacs CS, Kronenberg HM. Maternal-fetal calcium and bone metabolism during pregnancy, puerperium, and lactation. Endocr Rev 18(6) (1997): 832–872.

Kukkonen K et al. Probiotics and prebiotic galacto-oligosaccharides in the prevention of allergic diseases: a randomized, double-blind, placebo-controlled trial. J Allergy Clin Immunol 119.1 (2007): 192–198.

Lassi ZS et al. Folic acid supplementation during pregnancy formaternal health and pregnancy outcomes. Cochrane Database Syst Rev 3 (2013): CD006896.

Lee A et al. Therapeutics in pregnancy and lactation. Oxford: Radcliffe Medical Press, 2000.

Levant B et al. Reduced brain DHA Content After a Single Reproductive Cycle in Female Rats Fed a Diet Deficient in N-3 polyunsaturated fatty acids. Biological Psychiatry 60.9 (2006): 987–990.

Levant B et al. Decreased brain docosahexaenoic acid content produces neurobiological effects associated with depression: Interactions with reproductive status in female rats. Psychoneuroendocrinol 33.9 (2008): 1279–1292.

Li Z et al. Folic acid supplements during early pregnancy and likelihood of multiple births: a population-based cohort study. Lancet 361.9355 (2003): 380–384.

Li M et al Are Australian children iodine deficient? Results of the Australian National Iodine Nutrition Study. Med J Aust 184.4 (2006): 165–169.

Livingstone C et al. Vitamin A deficiency presenting as night blindness during pregnancy. Ann Clin Biochem 40.Pt 3 (2003): 292–294.

Looker AC et al. Prevalence of iron deficiency in the United States. JAMA 277.12 (1997): 973–976.

Maats FH, Crowther CA. Patterns of vitamin, mineral and herbal supplement use prior to and during pregnancy. Aust N Z J Obstet Gynaecol 42.5 (2002): 494–496.

MacLennan AH et al. The escalating cost and prevalence of alternative medicine. Prev Med 35.2 (2002): 166–173.

Maghbooli Z et al. Correlation between vitamin D3 deficiency and insulin resistance in pregnancy. Diabetes Metab Res Rev 24.1 (2008): 27–32.

Mahomed K et al. Zinc supplementation for improving pregnancy and infant outcome. Cochrane Database Syst Rev. 2 (2007): CD000230.

Makedos G et al. Homocysteine, folic acid and B12 serum levels in pregnancy complicated with preeclampsia. Arch Gynecol Obstet 275.2 (2007): 121–124.

Makrides M, Crowther CA. Magnesium supplementation in pregnancy. Cochrane Database Syst Rev 4 (2001): CD000937.

Makrides M et al. Marine oil, and other prostaglandin precursor, supplementation for pregnancy uncomplicated by pre-eclampsia or intrauterine growth restriction. Cochrane Database Syst Rev 3 (2006): CD003402.

Marchioni E et al. Iodine deficiency in pregnant women residing in an area with adequate iodine intake. Nutrition 24(5) (2008): 458–461.

Martinez GJ. Traditional practices, beliefs and uses of medicinal plants in relation to maternal–baby health of Criollo women in central Argentina. Midwifery 24.4 (2008): 490–502.

Martinez-Frias ML, Salvador J. Epidemiological aspects of prenatal exposure to high doses of vitamin A in Spain. Eur J Epidemiol 6.2 (1990): 118–123.

Mastroiacovo P et al. High vitamin A intake in early pregnancy and major malformations: a multicenter prospective controlled study. Teratology 59.1 (1999): 7–11.

Matthews A et al. Interventions for nausea and vomiting in early pregnancy. Cochrane Database Syst Rev 9 (2010): CD007575.

Mehendale S et al. Fatty acids, antioxidants, and oxidative stress in pre-eclampsia. International Journal of Gynecology and Obstetrics 100.3 (2008): 234–238.

Melamed N et al. Iron supplementation in pregnancy — does the preparation matter? Arch Gynecol Obstet 276.6 (2007): 601–604.

Miller RK et al. General commentary on drug therapy and drug risks in pregnancy. Drugs during pregnancy and lactation, 2nd edn. Oxford: Academic Press, 2007, pp. 1–26.

Mills JL et al. Vitamin A and birth defects. American Journal of Obstetrics and Gynecology 177.1 (1997): 31–36.

Mills S, Bone K. The Essential Guide to Herbal Safety, Elsevier Churchill Livingstone, USA, 2005.

Milman N et al. Iron supplementation during pregnancy. Effect on iron status markers, serum erythropoietin and human placental lactogen. A placebo controlled study in 207 Danish women. Dan Med Bull 38.6 (1991): 471–476.

Milman N et al. Iron prophylaxis during pregnancy — how much iron is needed? A randomized dose–response study of 20–80 mg ferrous iron daily in pregnant women. Acta Obstet Gynecol Scand 84.3 (2005): 238–247.

Milman N et al. Body iron and individual iron prophylaxis in pregnancy — should the iron dose be adjusted according to serum ferritin? Ann Hematol 85.9 (2006): 567–573.

Mori R et al. Zinc supplementation for improving pregnancy and infant outcome. Cochrane Database Syst Rev 7 (2012): CD000230.

Morley R et al. Maternal 25-hydroxyvitamin D and parathyroid hormone concentrations and offspring birth size. J Clin Endocrinol Metab 91.3 (2006): 906–912.

Morris B et al. Increased chromium excretion in pregnancy is associated with insulin resistance. J Trace Elem Exper Med 13 (2000): 389–396.

Morriss-Kay GM, Sokolova N. Embryonic development and pattern formation. Faseb J 10.9 (1996): 961–968.

Mullen W et al Ellagitannins, flavonoids, and other phenolics in red raspberries and their contribution to antioxidant capacity and vasorelaxation properties. J Agric Food Chem 50 (2002): 5191–5196.

Munger KL et al. Vitamin D intake and incidence of multiple sclerosis. Neurology 62.1 (2004): 60–65.

Munger KL et al. Serum 25-hydroxyvitamin D levels and risk of multiple sclerosis. Jama 296.23 (2006): 2832–2838.

Muthayya S et al. Low maternal vitamin B12 status is associated with intrauterine growth retardation in urban South Indians. Eur J Clin Nutr 60.6 (2006): 791–801.

Nakamura H, Yamamoto T. Mutagen and anti-mutagen in ginger, Zingiber officinale. Mutat Res 103(2) (1982): 119–126.

Nambiar S et al. Hypertension in mother and baby linked to ingestion of Chinese herbal medicine [letter]. West J Med 171 (1999): 152.

Napolitano PG et al. Umbilical cord plasma homocysteine concentrations at delivery in pregnancies complicated by pre-eclampsia. Aust N Z J Obstet Gynaecol 48.3 (2008): 261–265.

Nordeng H, Havnen GC. Use of herbal drugs in pregnancy: a survey among 400 Norwegian women. Pharmacoepidemiol Drug Saf 13(6) (2004): 371–380.

Noumi E, Tchakonang NYC. Plants used as abortifacients in the Sangmelima region of Southern Cameroon. J Ethnopharmacology 76.3 (2001): 263–268.

O'Brien KO et al. Prenatal Iron Supplements Impair Zinc Absorption in Pregnant Peruvian Women. J. Nutr. 130.9 (2000): 2251–2255.

Ochoa-Brust GJ et al. Daily intake of 100 mg ascorbic acid as urinary tract infection prophylactic agent during pregnancy. Acta Obstet Gynecol Scand 86.7 (2007): 783–787.

Oken E et al. Maternal fish consumption, hair mercury, and infant cognition in a U.S. cohort. Environmental Health Perspectives 113.10 (2005): 1376–1380.

Oken E et al. Diet during pregnancy and risk of preeclampsia or gestational hypertension. Ann Epidemiol 17.9 (2007): 663–668.

Olsen SF et al. Fish oil intake compared with olive oil intake in late pregnancy and asthma in the offspring: 16 y of registry-based follow-up from a randomized controlled trial. Am J Clin Nutr 88.1 (2008): 167–175.

Omu AE et al. Magnesium sulphate therapy in women with pre-eclampsia and eclampsia in Kuwait. Med Princ Pract 17.3 (2008): 227–232.

Ortega RM et al. Vitamin A status during the third trimester of pregnancy in Spanish women: influence on concentrations of vitamin A in breast milk. Am J Clin Nutr 66.3 (1997): 564–568.

Othman M et al. Probiotics for preventing preterm labour. Cochrane Database Syst Rev 1 (2007): CD005941.

Paiva Ade A et al. Relationship between the iron status of pregnant women and their newborns. Rev Saude Publica 41.3 (2007): 321–327.

Parsons M et al. Raspberry leaf and its effect on labour: safety and efficacy. Aust Coll Midwives Inc J 12.3 (1999): 20–25.

Pena-Rosas JP, Viteri FE. Effects of routine oral iron supplementation with or without folic acid for women during pregnancy. Cochrane Database Syst Rev 3 (2006): CD004736.

Peña-Rosas JP et al. Daily oral iron supplementation during pregnancy. Cochrane Database Syst Rev 12 (2012): CD004736.

Perez-Lopez FR. Iodine and thyroid hormones during pregnancy and postpartum. Gynecol Endocrinol 23.7 (2007): 414–428.

Perri D et al. Safety and efficacy of echinacea (Echinacea angustifolia, E. purpurea, E. pallida) during pregnancy and lactation. Can J Clin Pharmacol 13.3 (2006): e262–267.

Polyzos NP et al. Combined vitamin C and E supplementation during pregnancy for preeclampsia prevention: a systematic review. Obstet Gynecol Surv 62.3 (2007): 202–206.

Pop VJ. Low concentrations of maternal thyroxin during early gestation: a risk factor of breech presentation? BJOG: Int J Obstetric Gynaecolo 111.9 (2004): 925–930.

Prentice A. Micronutrients and the bone mineral content of the mother, fetus and newborn. J Nutr 133.(5 Suppl 2) (2003): 1693S–1699S.

Preziosi P et al. Effect of iron supplementation on the iron status of pregnant women: consequences for newborns. Am J Clin Nutr 66.5 (1997): 1178–1182.

Qiu C et al. Erythrocyte omega-3 and omega-6 polyunsaturated fatty acids and preeclampsia risk in Peruvian women. Archives of Gynecology and Obstetrics 274.2 (2006): 97–103.

Radhika MS et al. Effects of vitamin A deficiency during pregnancy on maternal and child health. Bjog 109.6 (2002): 689–693.

Ranzini A et al. Use of complementary medicines and alternative therapies among obstetric patients. Obstet Gynecol 97.(4 Suppl 1) (2001): 546.

Rautava S et al. Probiotics during pregnancy and breast-feeding might confer immunomodulatory protection against atopic disease in the infant. J Allergy Clin Immunol 109.1 (2002): 119–121.

Rees AM et al. Omega-3 fatty acids as a treatment for perinatal depression: Randomized double-blind placebo-controlled trial. Australian and New Zealand Journal of Psychiatry 42.3 (2008): 199–205.

Repke JT, Villar J. Pregnancy-induced hypertension and low birth weight: the role of calcium. Am J Clin Nutr 54(1 Suppl) (1991): 237S–241S.

Reveiz L et al. Treatments for iron-deficiency anaemia in pregnancy. Cochrane Database Syst Rev(2) (2007): CD003094.

Rhead WJ, Schrauzer GN. Risks of long-term ascorbic acid overdosage. Nutr Rev 29.11 (1971): 262–263.

Riddle JM. Oral contraceptives and early-term abortifacients during classical antiquity and the middle ages. Past & Present 132.1 (1991): 3–32.

Rogers LK et al. DHA supplementation: current implications in pregnancy and childhood. Pharmacol Res 70.1. (2013):13–19.

Ronnenberg AG et al. Preconception homocysteine and B vitamin status and birth outcomes in Chinese women. Am J Clin Nutr 76.6 (2002): 1385–1391.

Ronnenberg AG et al. Preconception B-vitamin and homocysteine status, conception, and early pregnancy loss. Am J Epidemiol 166.3 (2007): 304–312.

Rossanber-Hulten L et al. Competitive inhibition of iron absorption by manganese and zinc in humans. Am J Clin Nutr 54.1 (1991): 152–156.

Rumbold A, Crowther CA. Vitamin C supplementation in pregnancy. Cochrane Database Syst Rev(2) (2005): CD004072.

Rumbold A, Crowther CA. Vitamin E supplementation in pregnancy. Cochrane Database Syst Rev(2) (2005): CD004069.

Rumbold A et al. Vitamin supplementation for preventing miscarriage. Cochrane Database Syst Rev(2) (2005): CD004073.

Rumbold A et al. Antioxidants for preventing pre-eclampsia. Cochrane Database Syst Rev(1) (2008): CD004227.

Rumiris D et al. Lower rate of preeclampsia after antioxidant supplementation in pregnant women with low antioxidant status. Hypertens Pregnancy 25. 3 (2006): 241–253.

Sachan A et al. High prevalence of vitamin D deficiency among pregnant women and their newborns in northern India. Am J Clin Nutr 81.5 (2005): 1060–1064.

Sanders R et al. Intracellular and extracellular, ionized and total magnesium in pre-eclampsia and uncomplicated pregnancy. Clin Chem Lab Med 37.1 (1999): 55–59.

Sanz EJ et al. Selective serotonin reuptake inhibitors in pregnant women and neonatal withdrawal syndrome: a database analysis. Lancet 365.9458 (2005): 482–517.

Schiebinger L. Exotic abortifacients and lost knowledge. The Lancet 371 (2008):718–719.

Scholl TO. Iron status during pregnancy: setting the stage for mother and infant. Am J Clin Nutr 81.5 (2005): 1218S–1222.

Scholl TO et al. Vitamin E: maternal concentrations are associated with fetal growth. Am J Clin Nutr 84.6 (2006): 1442–1448.

Senes M et al. Coenzyme Q10 and high-sensitivity C-reactive protein in ischemic and idiopathic dilated cardiomyopathy. Clin Chem Lab Med 46.3 (2008): 382–386.

Seydoux J et al. Serum and intracellular magnesium during normal pregnancy and in patients with pre-eclampsia. Br J Obstet Gynaecol 99.3 (1992): 207–211.

Shahraki AD. Effects of vitamin E, calcium carbonate and milk of magnesium on muscular cramps in pregnant women. J Med Sci 6.6 (2006): 979–983.

Shamsuddin L et al. Use of parenteral magnesium sulphate in eclampsia and severe pre-eclampsia cases in a rural set up of Bangladesh. Bangladesh Med Res Counc Bull 31.2 (2005): 75–82.

Shaw GM et al. Periconceptional intake of vitamin A among women and risk of neural tube defect-affected pregnancies. Teratology 55.2 (1997): 132–133.

Shearer MJ. Vitamin K metabolism and nutriture. Blood Reviews 6 (1992): 92–104.

Shehata HA, Nelson-Piercy C. Drugs to avoid in pregnancy, Curr Obstet & Gyneco, 10 (2000): 44–52.

Shrim A et al. Pregnancy outcome following use of large doses of vitamin B6 in the first trimester. J Obstet Gynaecol 26.8 (2006): 749–751.

Sills IN et al. Vitamin D deficiency rickets. Reports of its demise are exaggerated. Clin Pediatr (Phila) 33.8 (1994): 491–493.

Simpson M et al. Raspberry leaf in pregnancy: Its safety and efficacy in labor. Journal of Midwifery & Women's Health 46.2 (2001): 51–59.

Sontrop J et al. Depressive symptoms during pregnancy in relation to fish consumption and intake of n-3 polyunsaturated fatty acids. Paediatric and Perinatal Epidemiology 22.4 (2008): 389–399.

Soudamini KK et al. Mutagenicity and anti-mutagenicity of selected spices. Indian J Physiol Pharmacol 39.4 (1995): 347–353.

Specker BL. Do North American women need supplemental vitamin D during pregnancy or lactation? Am J Clin Nutr 59.2 (1994): 484S–490.

Sripramote M, Lekhyananda N. A randomized comparison of ginger and vitamin B6 in the treatment of nausea and vomiting of pregnancy. J Med Assoc Thai 86.9 (2003): 846–853.

Steen MT et al. Neural-tube defects are associated with low concentrations of cobalamin (vitamin B12) in amniotic fluid. Prenat Diagn 18.6 (1998): 545–555.

Steer C et al. THe Methylenetetrahydrofolate Reductase (MTHFR) C677T Polymorphism is Associated with Spinal BMD in Nine-Year-Old Children. J Bone Miner Res (2008).

Su KP et al. Omega-3 fatty acids for major depressive disorder during pregnancy: Results from a randomized, double-blind, placebo-controlled trial. Journal of Clinical Psychiatry 69.4 (2008): 644–651.

Suarez L et al. Maternal Serum B12 Levels and Risk for Neural Tube Defects in a Texas–Mexico Border Population. Annals of Epidemiology 13.2 (2003): 81–88.

Suharno D et al. Supplementation with vitamin A and iron for nutritional anaemia in pregnant women in West Java, Indonesia. Lancet 342.8883 (1993): 1325–1328.

Tannis MJ. Potential toxicities of herbal therapies in the developing fetus. Birth Defects Research Part B: Developmental and Reproductive Toxicology 68.6 (2003): 496–498.

Téllez-Rojo M et al. A randomized controlled trial of calcium supllementation to reduce blood lead levels (and fetal lead exposure) in pregnant women. Epidemiology 17.6 (2006): s123.

Thaver D et al. Pyridoxine (vitamin B6) supplementation in pregnancy. Cochrane Database Syst Rev 2 (2006): CD000179.

Thomas, KJ et al. Use and expenditure on complementary medicine in England: a population based survey. Complement Ther Med 9.1 (2001): 2–11.

Tindle HA et al. Trends in use of complementary and alternative medicine by US adults: 1997–2002. Altern Ther Health Med 11(1) (2005): 42–49.

Trotter M, Hixon BB. Sequential changes in weight, density, and percentage ash weight of human skeletons from an early fetal period through old age. Anat Rec 179.1 (1974): 1–18.

Tsui B et al. A survey of dietary supplement use during pregnancy at an academic medical center. Am J Obstet Gynecol 185.2 (2001): 433–437.

Tytgat GN et al. Contemporary understanding and management of reflux and constipation in the general population and pregnancy: a consensus meeting. Aliment Pharmacol Ther 18.3 (2003): 291–301.

Vaidya B et al. Detection of thyroid dysfunction in early pregnancy: universal screening or targeted high-risk case finding? J Clin Endocrinol Metab 92.1 (2007): 203–207.

Valsecchi L et al. Serum levels of alpha-tocopherol in hypertensive pregnancies. Hypertens Pregnancy 18.3 (1999): 189–195.

van den Broek N et al. Vitamin A supplementation during pregnancy for maternal and newborn outcomes. Cochrane Database Syst Rev, 2010 Issue 11:Art. No.: CD008666. DOI:10.1002/14651858.CD008666.pub2.

van der Meer IM et al. High prevalence of vitamin D deficiency in pregnant non-Western women in The Hague, Netherlands. Am J Clin Nutr 84(2) (2006): 350–353.

Velzing-Aarts FV et al. Umbilical vessels of preeclamptic women have low contents of both n-3 and n-6 long-chain polyunsaturated fatty acids. Am J Clin Nutrit 69.2 (1999): 293–298.

Vieth R et al. Wintertime vitamin D insufficiency is common in young Canadian women, and their vitamin D intake does not prevent it. Eur J Clin Nutr 55(12) (2001): 1091–1097.

Vieth R et al. Efficacy and safety of vitamin D3 intake exceeding the lowest observed adverse effect level. Am J Clin Nutr 73.2 (2001): 288–294.

Villar J, Belizan JM. Same nutrient, different hypotheses: disparities in trials of calcium supplementation during pregnancy. Am J Clin Nutr 71(5 Suppl) (2000): 1375S–1379S.

Villar J et al. Epidemiologic observations on the relationship between calcium intake and eclampsia. Int J Gynaecol Obstet 21.4 (1983): 271–278.

Villar J et al. Calcium supplementation reduces blood pressure during pregnancy: results of a randomized controlled clinical trial. Obstet Gynecol 70.3 (Pt 1) (1987): 317–322.

Villar J et al. Nutritional interventions during pregnancy for the prevention or treatment of maternal morbidity and preterm delivery: an overview of randomized controlled trials. J. Nutr. 133.5 (2003): 1606S–1625.

von Kries R et al. Assessment of vitamin K status of the newborn infant. J Pediatr Gastroenterol Nutr 16.3 (1993): 231–238.

Wacker WE, Parisi AF. Magnesium metabolism. N Engl J Med 278.12 (1968): 658–663.

Waller DP. et al. Lack of androgenicity of Siberian ginseng. JAMA 267.17 (1992): 2329.

Wang X et al. Vitamin C and vitamin E supplementation reduce oxidative stress-induced embryo toxicity and improve the blastocyst development rate. Fertility and Sterility 78.6 (2002): 1272–1277.

Webster WS, Freeman JAD. Is this drug safe in pregnancy? Reprod Toxicol 15.6 (2001): 619–629.

Weidner MS, Sigwart K. Investigation of the teratogenic potential of a zingiber officinale extract in the rat. Reprod Toxicol 15.1 (2001): 75–80.

Werler MM. et al. Maternal vitamin A supplementation in relation to selected birth defects. Teratology 42.5 (1990): 497–503.

West KP et al. Double blind, cluster randomised trial of low dose supplementation with vitamin A or beta carotene on mortality related to pregnancy in Nepal. BMJ 318.7183 (1999): 570–575.

Westney OE et al. Nutrition, genital tract infection, hematologic values, and premature rupture of membranes among African American Women. J Nutr 124.(6 Suppl) (1994): 987S–993S.

Whitehouse, B. Fragarine: an inhibitor of uterine action. BMJ 13 (1941): 370–371.

WHO. The prevalence of anaemia in women: a tabulation of available information, World Health Organization, Geneva, 1992.

WHO. WHO traditional medicine strategy 2002–2005, World Health Organization, Geneva 2002.

Woods SE et al. Serum chromium and gestational diabetes. J Am Board Fam Med 21.2 (2008): 153–157.

Wouters MG et al. Hyperhomocysteinemia: a risk factor in women with unexplained recurrent early pregnancy loss. Fertil Steril 60.5 (1993): 820–825.

Wright ME. A case-control study of maternal nutrition and neural tube defects in Northern Ireland. Midwifery 11.3 (1995): 146–152.

Xue CC et al. Complementary and alternative medicine use in Australia: a national population-based survey. J Altern Complement Med 13.6 (2007): 643–650.

Zeghoud F et al. Subclinical vitamin D deficiency in neonates: definition and response to vitamin D supplements. Am J Clin Nutr 65.3 (1997): 771–778.

Zeisel SH. Nutritional importance of choline for brain development. J Am Coll Nutr 23.(6 Suppl) (2004): 621S–626S.

Zhou SJ et al. Routine iron supplementation in pregnancy has no effect on iron status of children at six months and four years of age. J Pediat 151.4 (2007): 438–440.

Zimmermann MB. The adverse effects of mild-to-moderate iodine deficiency during pregnancy and childhood: a review. Thyroid 17.9 (2007): 829–835.

CHAPTER 12

INTRODUCTION TO WELLNESS

A NEW ACADEMIC DISCIPLINE — WELLNESS ONLINE

WHAT IS 'WELLNESS'?

'Wellness' is a concept that has gained popularity in recent years but still has no rigorously developed definition, theory or philosophy. At a very simple level, wellness can be equated with health which, according to the World Health Organization (WHO), is 'a state of complete physical, mental and social well-being and not merely the absence of disease or infirmity' (WHO 1948). Wellness, however, can also be seen as distinct from health, in that it is holistic and multidimensional. The notion of wellness includes not only physical, mental and social dimensions, but also emotional, cultural, spiritual, educational, sexual, occupational, financial, environmental, ethical and existential dimensions, with the assumption being that if any one of these dimensions is deficient, complete wellness cannot be achieved.

Wellness describes a quality of systems rather than isolated entities and, as such, it is dependent on relationships and must take into account both content and context. Because it describes systems, the notion of wellness can be applied to individuals as well as to communities, businesses and large-scale economies and requires an ecological perspective that can be expanded to include the concepts of human security, corporate social responsibility, social justice, environmental impact and sustainability, together with subjective fulfillment and physiological wellbeing.

In 1961, wellness pioneer Halbert Dunn defined wellness in his book *High-level wellness* as 'an integrated method of functioning which is oriented toward maximizing the potential of which the individual is capable' (Dunn 1961, p 4). He acknowledged that wellness is dependent on the relationship between individuals and their environment, stating that wellness 'requires that the individual maintain a continuum of balance and purposeful direction within the environment where he is functioning'. He also stated that 'wellness is a direction in progress toward an ever-higher potential of functioning' (p. 6).

More recently the (US) President's Council on Physical Fitness and Sports proposed a uniform definition of wellness as 'a multidimensional state of being describing the existence of positive health in an individual as exemplified by quality of life and a sense of well-being' (Corbin & Pangrazi 2001). Yet another definition suggests that wellness is an 'active process of becoming aware of and making choices toward a more successful existence' (US National Wellness Institute 2009). Another proposed definition is:

Wellness is the multidimensional state of being 'well', where inner and outer worlds are in harmony: a heightened state of consciousness enabling you to be fully present in the moment and respond authentically to any situation from the 'deep inner well of your being'. Wellness is dynamic and results in a continuous awakening and evolution of consciousness and is the state where you look, feel, perform, and stay 'well' and, therefore, experience the greatest fulfilment and enjoyment from life and achieve the greatest longevity (Cohen 2008a, p 8).

This definition implies that the state of wellness allows the greatest flexibility to respond to situations and therefore provides the greatest resilience to stress and disease. Wellness in this context can be seen as the best preventive medicine. In this definition wellness is also seen as a state of consciousness that guides the quality of our relationships with the world and therefore cannot be viewed separately from the environment in which it occurs. Thus, if 'health' is 'wholeness', then wellness is the experience of an ever-expanding realisation of what it means to be whole (Cohen 2008a).

Travis and Ryan suggest that wellness is never a static state, but rather a way of life, and that wellness and illness exist along a continuum: just as there are degrees of illness, there are also degrees of wellness. Travis and Ryan further see wellness as a choice, a process, a balanced channelling of energy, the integration of body, mind and spirit and the loving acceptance of self (Travis & Ryan 2004).

If health and disease are considered to be at opposite ends of a spectrum, then it is possible to classify health into three broad areas: ill health (illness), average health and enhanced health (wellness) (Fig 12.1). The divide between ill health and average health is generally defined in Western medical terms, which classify diseases based on symptom patterns or other diagnostic parameters. Western medicine uses a bottom–up approach that aims to define and understand illness, and develop interventions such as drugs and surgery to treat or prevent the disease and control factors that reduce wellbeing ('stressors').

The divide between average health and enhanced health is less distinct. Enhanced health is more than just being disease-free: it assumes high levels of physical strength, stamina and mental clarity, as well as physical beauty and maximal enjoyment and fulfilment from life. This requires the holistic integration of multiple factors that determine physical, psychological, emotional, social, economic, environmental and spiritual health. In many Eastern philosophies, the idea of enhanced health can be extended to the concept of 'perfect health' or 'enlightenment', whereby a person is 'at one with the universe' and hence in a state of perfect bliss or 'nirvana' (Cohen 2003).

Moving up the spectrum from illness to wellness allows for greater flexibility of response and hence greater resilience; the best form of prevention is therefore to be as high on the spectrum as possible. Thus, while 'stressors' tend to reduce the ability to respond and create downwards movement, upwards movement can be facilitated by 'blissors', which create greater wellbeing. Throughout the spectrum, however, there is also a central axis that represents the core of our being. This central core, which may be termed the 'soul' or the 'essence', is an eternal and immortal aspect of the self that is naturally and blissfully at one with the universe.

FIGURE 12.1 The illness–wellness spectrum (Cohen 2008a)

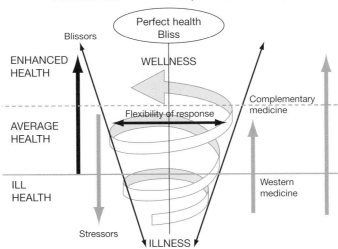

Bliss, or 'ananda' in Sanskrit, is considered by Vedic scholars to be the innermost level of the individual self, as well as the nature of the whole universe. It is the goal of the path to enlightenment and is found in the deepest experience of meditation and the innermost level of our being (Maharishi 1957–64). Bliss is also the ultimate aim of Eastern healing and spiritual practices, which adopt a top-down approach by attempting to elicit bliss through meditation and other practices that enhance wellbeing ('blissors') (Cohen 2008a).

The state of bliss can also be considered as the ultimate in achieving human potential. As the late anthropologist Joseph Campbell states:

I think that most people are looking for an experience that connects them to the ecstasy of what it could feel like to be totally alive. To know the unburdened state of total aliveness is the pinnacle of the human potential (Campbell 1988).

This 'state of total aliveness' is what many people may consider to be 'wellness'.

THE WORLD IN CRISIS

It seems that all people at some time have tried to tackle the question of how to live well in the world. This single question has driven human endeavour and led to innovations that have created new technologies and ways of living that have allowed human populations to expand exponentially (Meadows et al 1976).

Expanding human populations and exploitation of the natural environment has led to a series of global crises that are challenging the financial system, the climate and the environment leading to global terrorism and social unrest, pandemics, environmental pollution, general toxicity and natural disasters, which are breaching national boundaries and threatening human security. We also currently live in a world where one-third of the world's population is dying from diseases linked to malnutrition and starvation; another third is dying from obesity and diseases related to overconsumption; toxic chemicals are continuously being created and released into our environment and food supply; and people are becoming increasingly disconnected from their natural environment and one another.

Modern healthcare systems are also struggling to provide quality care to all in need, as the burden of illness-care reaches barely manageable proportions. It is becoming clear that the current illness-based medical model is not sustainable and is ill-equipped to meet the needs of the global population or deal with the consequences of an ageing population, increasing healthcare costs and an epidemic of lifestyle-related diseases such as obesity, diabetes, heart disease and cancer.

A disproportionate focus on illness has allowed unhealthy lifestyle practices to remain largely unchecked, thereby allowing them to expand across the globe to the point where they now represent the greatest threat to human health and survival. A 2005 report by WHO entitled *Preventing chronic disease: A vital investment* estimates that of the 58 million deaths in the world in 2005, 35 million (60%) were caused by chronic diseases such as heart disease, stroke, cancer, chronic respiratory diseases and diabetes. The report goes on to suggest that 80% of premature heart disease, stroke and type 2 diabetes and 40% of all cancers are preventable, concluding that the main modifiable risk factors for these diseases are lifestyle-related and include unhealthy diets, physical inactivity and tobacco use (WHO 2005).

It has been predicted that, as a result of unhealthy lifestyles, for the first time in history the lifespan of the next generation in the United States could be shorter than that of their parents (Olshansky et al 2005). In a PriceWaterhouseCoopers (PWC) report on the future of healthcare entitled *HealthCast 2020: Creating a sustainable future* (PWC 2005), it is suggested that 'There is growing evidence that the current health systems of nations around the world will be unsustainable if unchanged over the next 15 years' (PWC 2005, p 2), while 'preventive care and disease management programs have untapped potential to enhance health status and reduce costs' (PWC 2005, p 4).

IN SEARCH OF WELLNESS

It is becoming increasingly evident that the fate of all people on Earth is linked and that as a global species we must find sustainable ways to live well in the world together. Humanity has reached a 'tipping point', bringing the possibility of either substantial hardship or a breakthrough into new ways of living and a new phase in human evolution. This new phase represents a culmination of thousands of years of human history, during which different philosophies, traditions and technologies have attempted to address the questions of life, ageing, illness and death.

The search for wellness is a common goal for all people. It can be understood as a conscious extension of the basic animal instinct to avoid pain that has its origins at the dawn of humanity when consciousness first became self-reflective (Cohen 2000). This search has influenced the evolution of medicine, which has seen the elaboration of two distinct yet complementary approaches: Eastern medicine, which is based on holistic thinking that maintains a cosmological and systems perspective outlining a philosophy of life; and Western medicine, which is based on a reductionist approach, emphasising controlled scientific experimentation and mathematical analysis (Cohen 2002).

The different health paradigms that aim to improve health and wellness have attempted to address the same issues in different ways. The principle of consilience suggests that there is an underlying unity of knowledge whereby a small number of natural laws may underpin seemingly different conceptual frameworks (Wilson 1999). Indeed, there are general concepts and principles that seem to recur as themes across different healthcare paradigms.

THE THERMODYNAMICS OF WELLNESS

Perhaps the most ubiquitous principle in medical thought is the idea that life is dependent on energy. The science of energy is well described in the field of thermodynamics, which proposes universal laws that give rise to precise mathematical equations that form the foundation for modern science and technology. However, while the field of thermodynamics purports to describe all energetic processes, it is seldom applied directly to the fields of health and medicine, despite 'energy' being a basic principle in virtually every healing tradition.

The concept of energy is described in different traditions as 'life energy', 'vital force', 'prana', 'chi' (or 'Qi'), and is said to flow along defined pathways and support the functioning of living systems. Traditional Chinese medicine has developed a sophisticated framework for conceptualising this energy: it is seen to encompass the concept of 'flow' and to move according to the dynamic interplay of the opposite yet complementary forces of 'yin' and 'yang', which guide the process of transformation whereby non-living things become animate. In this view, pain and disease are said to result when the energetic flow is disrupted, and healing is aimed at restoring the natural balance and flow (Cohen 2002).

As science does not recognise a form of energy specific to living systems, many concepts underlying Eastern medicine have been criticised as unscientific. There are parallels, however, between Eastern and Western concepts, which can be seen to be linked through the concept of information. Information can be measured in terms of energy or 'joules/degree Kelvin' (Tribus & McIrvine 1971), and there is a congruence between the concepts of 'Qi' in Eastern medicine and 'information' in thermodynamics.

Thus the Eastern concept of disease arising from a blockage of 'Qi' can be seen to parallel the second law of thermodynamics, which describes a tendency towards disorder or entropy in an isolated system. Disease and the adverse effects of ageing, which include progressive degeneration of tissues together with loss of function, can therefore be related to an increase in entropy as a consequence of blockages or isolation of different systems. In contrast, the ability of living systems to grow, evolve and learn appears to defy the second law and can be related to an open exchange between organisms and the environment. This can be extended to the concept of 'nirvana', or perfect bliss, whereby a person is 'at one with the universe', and there is no distinction between self and non-self, thus creating an open system that is no longer prone to the increase in entropy that occurs in isolated systems (Cohen 2002).

WELLNESS AND FLOW

While it may be true that life depends on energy, living systems must remain 'open', as it is the flow of energy through them that maintains their integrity. The concept of 'flow' is a powerful one that provides a bridge between Eastern and Western thought. The concept of flow applies to both thermodynamic processes and systems theory, as well as to the cyclic thinking of Eastern medicine. The concept of flow has also been applied to subjective psychological states that involve the integrated functioning of mind and body. This concept has been developed by Mihalyi Csikszentmihalyi, who describes flow as 'a joyous, self-forgetful involvement through concentration, which in turn is made possible by a discipline of the body' (Csikszentmihalyi 1992).

The state of flow occurs when perceived challenges exactly match the skills and capacity to respond. Such a state is therefore a 'whole of consciousness' phenomenon that requires the integrated action of both physiological and psychological processes, and hence the involvement of the entire being. In requiring 'wholeness', the 'flow state' is aligned with health and wellness, and engenders positive feelings that include:

- being completely involved in what we are doing — focused, concentrated

- a sense of ecstasy — of being outside and beyond everyday reality

- great inner clarity — knowing what needs to be done and how well we are doing it (introspective, realistic feedback)

- knowing the activity is able to be done — that our skills are adequate to the task

- a sense of serenity — having no undue concerns or worries about oneself, and a feeling of growing beyond the boundaries of the ego

- timelessness — being thoroughly focused on the present so that hours seem to pass by in minutes

- intrinsic motivation — whatever produces flow becomes its own reward (Csikszentmihalyi 2004).

The idea that positive psychological states and wellbeing require 'open systems' is recognised in everyday common language in the phrases 'having an open heart' or 'open mind'. The concept of flow sustaining life is also a basic tenet of Chinese and other traditional medicine philosophies. A thermodynamic model that includes the concept of energy and flow can also be seen to include many parallels between Eastern and Western concepts, and thus provide links between different conceptual systems (Fig 12.2) (Cohen 2010).

For example, the process of flow leading to transformation and the maintenance of living systems parallels the concept of the five elements or phases of transformation that is common to Chinese medicine, Ayurvedic

FIGURE 12.2 Pictorial conceptualisation of wellness concepts from traditional Chinese medicine (Cohen 2008a)

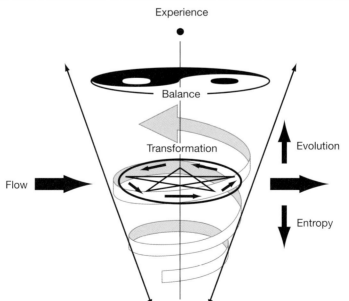

medicine and ancient Greek medicine (which considered quintessence as a fifth element in addition to air, water, fire and earth). The result of this transformation is represented by the concept of 'yin' and 'yang', which refers to interdependent yet mutually exclusive opposites and can be compared to the concept of 'complementarity' in quantum physics or the concept of homeostatic balance in physiology. The result of this balance leads to an increase or decrease in order as described by entropy or evolution, while the infinite nature of direct experience can be compared to the concept of 'Tao' or the mathematical concept of 'absolute infinity', both of which are defined as being inherently incomprehensible (Cohen 2002).

WELLNESS METRICS

Wellness is holistic and multidimensional, and involves content and context. As such it is both subjective and objective, and is difficult to quantify. As yet there are no agreed upon metrics by which wellness can be reliably measured, despite the existence of many potential indicators and proxy measures that may be applied to populations as well as individuals. Thus, it is now possible to measure subjective states such as 'quality of life', 'happiness' and 'wellbeing' through instruments such as the Australian Quality of Life Index (Cummins et al 2008), as well as to use more objective and physiological measures such as anthropometric and biometric data. Objective indicators of wellness can also be obtained from tissue sampling and measuring biochemical, hormonal, genetic, haematological and toxological data, as well as by testing functional capacity and performance. Further indicators for wellness can be obtained from demographic, socio-economic and epidemiological data, which can be used to appraise access to food, shelter, education, employment, healthcare and consumer goods, as well as to rate health risks, ecological footprint, morbidity, mortality and life expectancy (Cohen 2008a).

The multidimensional nature of wellness makes any single measure inadequate, and so attempts have been made to combine measures from the different domains. For example, the BankWest Quality of Life Index tracks Australian living standards across municipalities based on key indicators of the labour market, the housing market, the environment, education and health (BankWest 2008).

In attempting to measure 'full spectrum wellness', Travis and Ryan adopt the concept of a 'wellness energy system', which implies a thermodynamic model and measures wellness in terms of inputs and outputs. They acknowledge that 'we are all energy transformers, connected with the whole universe', and that 'all our life processes, including illness, depend on how we manage energy' (Travis & Ryan 2004). These authors further describe 12 aspects of wellness, which include inputs provided by breathing, eating and sensing, and outputs described as self-responsibility and love, transcending, finding meaning, intimacy, communicating, playing and working, thinking, feeling and moving. These 12 aspects of wellness are the basis for the wellness inventory, which evolved from early health-risk appraisal techniques to become the first computerised wellness assessment tool using a self-reported questionnaire.

Perhaps the most comprehensive attempt to create a metric for wellbeing is the 'Happy Planet Index', which uses both subjective and objective data in an attempt to measure the ecological efficiency with which countries achieve long and happy lives for their citizens. The Happy Planet Index is a composite measure that is calculated by multiplying life satisfaction by life expectancy and then dividing by ecological footprint. It therefore takes a thermodynamic approach to the wellness of populations by dividing outputs (the length and happiness of human life) by inputs (natural resources) (Marks et al 2014). The finding that the average scores across nations are low, that all nations could do better and that no country does well on all three indicators or achieves an overall high score on the index has led the Happy Planet Index to be currently renamed the '(Un) Happy Planet Index' (Marks et al 2014).

THE WELLNESS REVOLUTION

Since the emergence of self-reflective consciousness, every culture at every point in history has maintained various practices that aim at achieving and maintaining the wellbeing of individuals and the wider community. These practices invariably include the use of the local environment, food, water and plants, as well as various indigenous healing practices, such as massage and traditional cultural practices that are performed to focus the mind and anchor the experience of being well in ritual, routine and direct sensual experience.

While every culture throughout history has had its own wellness practices and philosophies, a culture that is global or sustainable has never existed before (Cohen 2008a). In the current millennium, however, there is a need for global solutions that provide an integrated response to the many world crises and an orientation towards wellness promises to provide such solutions. Thus, it is suggested that along with the current crises, the world is also experiencing the start of a 'wellness revolution' and the accompanying growth of a 'wellness industry'.

THE WELLNESS INDUSTRY

In his 2002 book *The wellness revolution*, economist Paul Zane Pilzer estimated that the value of existing items in the US wellness industry had reached approximately US$200 billion. This included US$70 billion for vitamins and US$25 billion for spas and fitness centres — about half the amount spent on automobiles in the United States (Pilzer 2002). Pilzer suggests that the US$200 billion is only the tip of the iceberg, and that wellness products and services represent the beginning of a new trillion-dollar sector of the US economy. In an updated edition of his book, Pilzer estimated that in 2007 the US wellness industry had expanded to over US$500 billion and that the untapped market for wellness had increased in size thanks to millions of new wellness consumers (Pilzer 2007).

The growth of the wellness industry is evidenced by the dramatic growth of the global spa industry (now considered by many to be the 'spa and wellness' industry), which has recently emerged as a global phenomenon through a convergence of industries, traditions and therapeutic practices. While spa therapies have been around since ancient times in many different forms that reflect the cultural, social and political milieu in which they are embedded, these practices are now being rediscovered, integrated and branded to create a new global industry that draws from a range of aligned industries, including beauty, massage, hospitality, tourism, architecture, property development, landscape design,

fashion, food and beverage, fitness and leisure, personal development, as well as complementary, conventional and traditional medicine (Cohen 2008a).

Fuelled by the merging of the travel dollar with the health dollar, spas are now springing up all over the world and have become a standard feature of luxury hotels and resorts. Spas are reported to be the fastest-growing leisure industry, and it was estimated that by 2001 revenues from spas had already overtaken revenues from amusement parks, box office receipts, vacation ownership and ski resorts (ISPA 2002). A 2008 report on the global spa economy suggests that global revenue from spas in 2007 was worth more than US$255 billion globally and that the wider wellness industry was worth an additional US$1.1 trillion (SRI International 2008). More recently, the wellness industry cluster was estimated to represent a $1.9 trillion global market, which included diverse but related industries including beauty and anti-ageing ($679 billion), fitness and mind–body ($390 billion), healthy eating and weight loss ($276 billion), personalised preventive health ($243 billion), complementary and alternative medicine ($133 billion), wellness tourism ($106 billion), spa ($60 billion), medical tourism ($50 billion) and workplace wellness ($31 billion) (SRI International 2010).

In offering to deliver on wellness, the spa industry is moving beyond luxury and pampering into the area of providing healthcare and, even further, raising consciousness. As such, the global spa industry is a melting pot for a whole host of products and services that encourage enhanced health and wellbeing and are drawn from a wide variety of traditions that include conventional, complementary and traditional medicine. Thus spas are adopting an integrative approach; they are taking holistic medical concepts out of clinics and combining them with the world of hospitality and leisure to place them in sustainable, enjoyable and nurturing environments.

Hotels certainly have a much greater appeal than hospitals. By combining hospitality with an integrative medicine model that emphasises lifestyle change and personal empowerment, the spa and wellness industry has the potential to transcend conventional medicine and create a globally sustainable health system. While most spas do not, as yet, create formal medical records, instigate diagnostic tests or perform medical procedures, these are all taking place in some medi-spas and destination spas, and some spas are beginning to integrate conventional and complementary medicine with hospitality to create hybrid hospital-spa-hotels ('hos–spa–tels'). As these are integrated into international hospitality chains, they create the potential for the delivery of a global integrated health service based on wellness principles (Cohen 2008a).

CONSCIOUS CONSUMPTION

The rise of the wellness industry is aligned with a move towards 'lifestyles of health and sustainability' (LOHAS). LOHAS is a demographic defining a particular market segment related to sustainable living and 'green' ecological initiatives, and is generally composed of a relatively upscale and well-educated population segment. In 2006 the LOHAS market segment was estimated to represent a US$209 billion market for goods and services focused on health, the environment, personal development and sustainable living. The focus of LOHAS is conscious consumption and covers diverse market segments such as personal health, natural lifestyles, green building, alternative energy and transportation, and ecotourism (for more information about LOHAS, see www.lohas.com).

A strong component of the LOHAS movement is the trend for consumers to choose more holistic, prevention-based models of healthcare, and this is evidenced by the increasing use of complementary and alternative medicine (Tindle et al 2005). This trend may reflect a growing disenchantment with the medical profession's seemingly one-sided emphasis on science and technology, as well as a growing demand for autonomy in healthcare decisions. Certainly, the general population is now better informed than ever and has better access to health information. The public is subsequently demanding more from healthcare providers and is not interested only in treating illness. Instead they want to maximise their health, prevent or slow down the ageing process and achieve higher levels of functioning (Cohen 2001).

The LOHAS movement has arisen out of a growing awareness that rampant consumerism seems to be taking over and destroying the planet. Certainly, unchecked and unconscious consumption can be seen to be at the root of many of the world's problems. Thus while we as consumers currently have access to a seemingly unlimited choice of goods in every size and colour, we remain disconnected from the products and services we purchase and often do not know where they come from, how they are produced, who produced them, what is in them, how they are disposed of or who benefits from their purchase.

In response to this, there is a growth in conscious consumer trends badged with different labels such as: green, natural, organic, fairtrade, corporate social responsibility, eco, ethical investment, sustainable, barefoot luxury. These have given rise to 'locovor' restaurants (those that source food within 160 kilometres/100 miles), carbon offset programs, green buildings, carbon neutral businesses, ecotourism, ethnotourism, voluntourism, downsizing, compacting, tree-change, social capital and triple and quadruple bottom-line reporting.

It is suggested that this range of conscious consumer trends can be integrated under the banner of 'conshumanism', which is a term that defines 'conscious and humane consumption' or 'consumption with maximal awareness, efficiency and enjoyment and minimal pain, energy, waste and pollution' (Cohen 2008a). Conshumanism embraces an overarching concept that can integrate multiple consumer trends towards greater transparency, equity, accountability, social responsibility, environmental sustainability and ethics. The common feature of these trends is increasing information and consciousness about consumption as well as incorporating an awareness of wellness into everyday lifestyle decisions.

TOWARDS A WELLNESS POLICY AGENDA

While treating illness has traditionally been the domain of the medical system, there is a growing realisation that wellness is holistic and multifaceted, and that implementing a wellness agenda requires wellness to become part of the fabric of our society, so that it infiltrates the education system, workplaces and the consciousness of every individual. This will require concerted action from multiple sectors, including civil society, governments, corporations and individuals.

GOVERNMENT INITIATIVES

The year 2008 seems to have been a watershed year for Australian government wellness initiatives. The Australia 2020 Summit called for the development of a 'whole-of-life wellness model' and a 'wellness footprint' to evaluate, measure and resource services across portfolios (Good & Roxon 2008), while the National Health and Hospitals Reform Commission, the National Preventative Health Task Force, the Primary Health Care Strategy Reference Group and the Indigenous Health Equity Council were established, all with a mandate for health reform (Moodie et al 2008).

The National Preventative Health Task Force subsequently produced a discussion paper entitled 'Australia, the healthiest country by 2020', which acknowledged the need for a coordinated approach to wellness, stating that:

> Our health is not only determined by our physical and psychological make-up and health behaviours, but also by our education, income and employment; our access to services; the place in which we live in [sic] and its culture; the advertising we are exposed to; and the laws and other regulations in place in our society (Preventative Health Task Force 2008).

These initiatives led to the establishment of the Australian National Preventive Health Agency in 2011, which now serves to support the development and implementation of evidence-based approaches to preventive health initiatives targeting obesity, harmful alcohol consumption and tobacco.

WORKING TOWARDS WELLNESS

In addition to the above government initiatives there are widespread calls for a more proactive, wellness-oriented approach to be taken by the corporate sector. Illness places a huge burden not only on government health systems and communities, but also on industry, with the potential for catastrophic effects. While the costs to industry from illness due to absenteeism are clear, it is only recently that the costs of 'presenteeism' have been assessed. It has been estimated that presenteeism — when workers turn up for work but are unproductive because of an ongoing illness — involves a greater cost than absenteeism, and may represent up to 60% of an employee's total lost

productivity and medical costs (Goetzel et al 2004). Presenteeism may also pose serious threats to workplace safety, lead to dissemination of infectious diseases and have hidden long-term costs, as well as compounding other lifestyle and social issues.

There is therefore a clear advantage in addressing wellness in the workplace, as this may have a positive impact on a company's productivity, recruitment, retention and ultimate profitability. As many employees spend a significant portion of their life at work, workplace wellness programs are also well positioned to address the growing burden of chronic lifestyle-related disease.

At the 2008 World Economic Forum Annual Meeting in Davos, Switzerland, there was a call for action to raise the issue of employee health on the corporate agenda. At the meeting, the results of a collaboration between the World Economic Forum and the WHO were released, suggesting that workplace wellness programs are a real but under-exploited opportunity to tackle the growing worldwide epidemic of chronic disease. This coincided with a PriceWaterhouseCoopers report, *Working towards wellness: accelerating the prevention of chronic disease*, which suggested that large multinational corporations are now looking for wellness strategies to implement in their workplaces and the communities in which they operate, and are rolling out comprehensive wellness programs in multiple countries, even though there are challenges in the implementation, evaluation and monitoring of such programs (PWC 2007).

As yet there is still no robust accounting for wellness, despite the evolution of triple and quadruple bottom-line reporting; however, the corporate sector appears to be taking workplace wellness programs beyond health screening and occupational health and safety programs, and there are moves to engage employees and the wider community in wellness and lifestyle initiatives through corporate social responsibility, environmental sustainability and community development agendas.

LIFESTYLE MEDICINE

Wellness impacts on every aspect of our lives, and experiencing wellness requires the holistic integration of multiple factors that determine physical, psychological, emotional, social, economic, environmental and spiritual health. Wellness is therefore ultimately an issue of lifestyle. In order to embrace wellness or enhanced health, the key 'life activities' that determine our health must be addressed. These life activities are summarised by the SENSE approach (see Chapter 1). We all need to manage stress, move, eat, interact with other people, interact with the world and learn. If we improve the way we do these activities, we will naturally improve our wellbeing. Wellness therefore involves the following:

- **stress management** — managing stressors (e.g. effective time management strategies and priority setting), and including everyday activities that enhance our ability to cope with stressors (e.g. meditation, breathing exercises and hobbies, and infusing life with creativity, humour and fun)
- **exercise** — engaging in regular physical activity that improves our aerobic capacity (e.g. walking), physical strength (e.g. resistance training) and flexibility (e.g. yoga)
- **nutrition** — receiving adequate nutrition through the consumption of a wide variety of fresh, seasonal, whole foods that are stored and prepared appropriately; minimising our exposure to toxins by using organic produce; and avoiding tobacco smoke and environmental toxins
- **social and spiritual interaction** — devoting ourselves to quality time with others and fostering love and intimacy in all our personal relationships; developing an ethic of service to others and a sense of social responsibility (e.g. volunteering and community work); giving to charities (e.g. time, effort, money); ethical investing and purchasing
- **education** — learning about ourselves and others, our environment and our place in it, and attempting to avoid obvious hazards while living sustainable, ecological lifestyles.

In recognition of the impact that lifestyle has on illness, developments in health funding in Australia have enabled allied health professionals to become part of a team that can address lifestyle issues. This has led to the emergence of 'lifestyle medicine', which is deemed to be a new discipline that attempts to bridge the gap between health promotion and conventional medicine by applying 'environmental, behavioural, medical and motivational principles to the management of lifestyle-related health problems in a clinical setting' (Egger et al 2008).

Managing lifestyle issues changes the emphasis from conventional treatment to one where patients need to be more involved in their own care, and which therefore requires the clinician to have considerable motivational knowledge and skills. It involves the therapeutic use of lifestyle interventions in the management of disease (Egger et al 2009). Lifestyle medicine may also involve health coaching, a practice in which health professionals apply evidence-based psychological, counselling and coaching principles and techniques to assist their patients to achieve positive health and lifestyle outcomes through cognitive and behaviour change (Gale 2014).

A NEW ACADEMIC DISCIPLINE

It appears that the wellness revolution has created the opportunity for wellness to be framed as a new academic discipline. The multidimensional and holistic nature of wellness, however, suggests that wellness is in fact a 'transdiscipline' requiring extensive collaboration and communication across diverse discipline areas to work on wellness-oriented teaching, learning and research projects.

Wellness seems to have an emerging research agenda, with one of the four Australian Government National Research Priorities being 'Promoting and maintaining good health'. This priority area aims to support preventive healthcare and enable people to make healthy choices, and includes the following key research themes: a healthy start to life, ageing well, ageing productively and preventive healthcare (Department of Education, Employment and Workplace Relations 2009). While this research priority area seems to target wellness-related research, wellness underpins many disparate research areas, ranging from theoretical and bench-top science to clinical research as well as social and policy research. A wellness agenda is therefore also inherent in other research priority areas, such as sustainability, frontier technologies and safeguarding Australia from terrorism, crime, invasive diseases and pests.

While a wellness research agenda is emerging, significant hurdles remain. Specific research into wellness and disease prevention is hindered by a lack of discrete outcome measures with which to measure wellness. Additional challenges include the design of programs that monitor and promote adherence, novel delivery models and the training, regulation and accreditation of suitable practitioners.

Although training and regulation pose challenges, wellness is a growing area in education and training and is increasingly becoming the focus of academic programs at undergraduate and postgraduate levels. International demand for a wellness-oriented academic program is located in three principal healthcare sectors: the conventional healthcare disciplines, which have an increasing emphasis on health promotion; the complementary and allied health sector including fitness, sports science, nutrition and psychology; and the rapidly growing hospitality, leisure and spa sector.

The need for wellness-related education is demonstrated by current health workforce shortages, the lack of experienced managers and therapists to work in spas, hospitality and leisure and the need for business professionals to embrace workplace wellness. A Productivity Commission report on Australia's health workforce suggested four broad approaches to overcome current health workforce shortages and distribution problems, and to address the future pressures facing the system. The first of these approaches involves strategies aimed at reducing the underlying demand for healthcare through 'wellness' and preventive strategies. This report also commented on the need for a health workforce with increased skills in health promotion (Productivity Commission 2006).

Creating a new academic (trans)discipline around wellness is a challenge, as there is a need to align the wellness industry with the professional and educational standards of the healthcare and business sectors. Such an alignment is evident in the continual increase in the provision and standard of education programs in wellness-related areas such as naturopathy, massage, fitness, yoga and spa therapies. This has led to calls for wellness-education-related accreditation and standards. In answering this call, the US National Wellness Institute recently set up an Academic Accreditation Committee and developed a set of baccalaureate-degree-level standards and processes that will lead to accreditation of academic programs and graduate certification (US National Wellness Institute 2008).

In Australia, RMIT University took on a leadership role and established the world's first postgraduate Master of Wellness program. Vocational outcomes from these programs, however, are currently unclear and potentially diverse as no position descriptions currently require applicants to have a postgraduate wellness degree. Thus, the program was designed to provide graduate students from diverse backgrounds, including both health science and business graduates, with a holistic overview of wellness principles and practices. The program also aimed to have a positive impact on students' personal health and wellbeing, and uses cutting-edge educational technology and the latest understanding about adult teaching and learning to deliver a fully online program with a global reach.

WELLNESS ONLINE

Wellness is a product of consciousness and it is said that 'the currency of wellness is connection' (Travis & Ryan 2004). With the advent of the internet as well as the development of information and communications technology (ICT), the world is certainly becoming more connected. Over the past two decades the development of the internet and ICT has progressed so rapidly that it is now possible for everyone on the globe to be linked via mobile communications technology that infiltrates almost every aspect of society.

It is clear that wellness-related technologies are converging in an online environment. Already ICT is used to support healthcare delivery, and electronic health-information systems promise to improve efficacy, safety and quality of care through the provision of alerts and reminders, diagnostic support, therapy critiquing and planning, prescribing decision support, information retrieval, image recognition and interpretation, as well as through the discovery of new phenomena and the creation of medical knowledge (Coiera 2003).

The advent of personal computing and modern consumer electronics has made technologies that were once accessible only to technical specialists available to the general population via home-based and mobile platforms. For example, online risk calculators can provide the basis for lifestyle advice and motivation for implementing positive lifestyle changes, and online tools can provide assessments via subjective questionnaires, as well as by the direct testing of cognitive and other functional status.

Biometric monitors further allow remote wellness monitoring by uploading data on various physiological parameters such as activity and sleep. These devices are being integrated into other personal electronic devices such as phones and digital music players. For example, Apple and Nike offer a kit in which a shoe sensor communicates with a wireless iPod receiver to transmit workout information such as elapsed time, distance travelled and calories burned (Cohen 2008b).

Online data collection allows personal information to be analysed and interpreted with the assistance of online experts, who in turn have access to sophisticated knowledge-management technologies, including bibliographic databases and decision support systems. Furthermore, online education offers unprecedented opportunities to deliver education across the planet, and develop knowledge and skills wherever they are required.

THE FUTURE OF WELLNESS

While the worldwide web is still young, when considered as a single machine it represents the largest and most reliable machine ever built with information-processing power approaching the same order as a human brain. The size and power of the web is now doubling every two years, and it is expected that its future evolution will lead to services and opportunities that are yet to be imagined (Kelly 2007). Its global reach provides a unique platform for connecting people, ideas and practices, essential parts of the wellness equation. Yet, how best to harness the web's capabilities to improve individual and global wellness remains unclear.

Many questions remain. Will the harnessing of global connectivity be able to enhance how we experience our environment and avert the many crises we are facing? Will online environments facilitate therapeutic and health enhancing experiences? Will initiatives such as electronic personal health records provide everyone with an online health record that will enhance continuity of care and provide opportunities for epidemiological research and public health initiatives? Will online access provide everyone access to education and the wealth of the world's knowledge? Will 'augmented reality' become the norm and 'virtual reality' become indistinguishable from 'reality'? Will video games become better than real life? Will social networking provide a forum for meaningful connection and provide an end to loneliness and social isolation?

It seems clear that over the next few decades changing global demographics, accompanied by major societal changes brought about by climate change, and technological innovations will have an impact on personal, community and global wellbeing and will forever change how humans live. The development of wellness as a key focus for research, education, healthcare, government policy and industry can only improve the outlook for present and future generations.

REFERENCES

BankWest. Quality of life index 2008. Available: www.bankwest.com.au/media-centre/financial-indicator-series/bankwest-quality-of-life-index-2008-1269940008245; 6 Aug 2014.

Campbell J. The power of myth. New York: Doubleday, 1988.

Cohen M. The evolution of holistic medicine. In: Cohen M (ed). Pathways to holistic health. Clayton, Vic: Monash Institute of Public Health, 2000, pp 11–24.

Cohen M. From complementary to integrative and holistic medicine. In: Cohen M (ed). Perspectives on holistic health. Clayton, Vic: Monash Institute of Public Health, 2001, pp 33–42.

Cohen M. Energy medicine from an ancient and modern perspective. In: Cohen M (ed). Prescriptions for holistic health. Clayton, Vic: Monash Institute of Health Services Research, 2002, pp 97–108.

Cohen M. Integrative medicine, principles of practice. In: Cohen M (ed). Holistic healthcare in practice. Clayton, Vic: Australian Integrative Medicine Association, 2003, pp 39–56.

Cohen M. Spa, wellness and human evolution. In: Cohen M & Bodeker G (eds), Understanding the global spa industry. Oxford: Butterworth–Heinemann, 2008a, pp 3–25.

Cohen M. Wellness technologies. In: Cohen M & Bodeker G (eds), Understanding the global spa industry. Oxford: Butterworth–Heinemann, 2008b, pp 237–257.

Cohen, M. Wellness and the Thermodynamics of a Healthy Lifestyle, Asia-Pacific Journal of Health, Sport and Physical Education 1.2 (2010): 5–12.

Coiera E. Clinical decision support systems. Guide to health informatics, 2nd edn. London: Arnold, 2003, Ch 25.

Corbin C, Pangrazi R. Toward a uniform definition of wellness: a commentary. Research Digest. President's Council on Physical Fitness and Sports 3.15 (2001): 1–8.

Csikszentmihalyi M. Flow: The psychology of happiness. London: Rider, 1992.

Csikszentmihalyi M. Talks Mihaly Csikszentmihalyi: Creativity, fulfillment and flow. TED talks, 2004. Available: www.ted.com/index.php/talks/mihaly_csikszentmihalyi_on_flow.html; 6 Aug 2014.

Cummins B et al. The wellbeing of Australians — differences between statistical sub-divisions, towns and cities. Australian Unity Wellbeing Index Report 19.1. Melbourne, Australian Centre on Quality of Life (Deakin University), 2008.

Department of Education, Employment and Workplace Relations. Australia's national research priorities: Promoting and maintaining good health, DEST, 2009.

Dunn HL. High-level wellness. Arlington, VA: Beatty Press, 1961.

Egger G et al. Lifestyle medicine. Sydney: McGraw-Hill, 2008.

Egger GJ et al. The emergence of 'lifestyle medicine' as a structured approach for management of chronic disease. Med J Aust 190.3 (2009): 143–145.

Gale J. Health Coaching Australia (HCA). Health coaching model for chronic condition prevention and self-management CCPSM. Available: www.healthcoachingaustralia.com/health-coaching/about-health-coaching.htm; 6 Aug 2014.

Goetzel RZ et al. Health, absence, disability, and presenteeism: Cost estimates of certain physical and mental health conditions affecting U.S. employers. J Occup Environ Med 46.4 (2004): 398–412.

Good M, Roxon N. A long-term national health strategy. Australia 2020 Summit Final Report, 2008. Available: http://www.ias.uwa.edu.au/__data/assets/pdf_file/0004/69232/A_long-term_national_health_strategy_Australia_2020_summit.pdf; 6 Aug 2014.

ISPA. The International Spa Association 2002 Spa Industry Study. Lexington, KY: International Spa Association, 2002.

Kelly K. Predicting the next 5,000 days of the web. TED talks 2007. Available: www.ted.com/talks/kevin_kelly_on_the_next_5_000_days_of_the_web.html; accessed 6 Aug 2014.

Maharishi, Mahesh Yogi. Thirty years around the world — dawn of the age of enlightenment, vol 1. Vlodrop: Maharishi Vedic University Press, 1957–1964.

Marks N et al. The happy planet index. Available: www.happyplanetindex.org/; accessed 6 Aug 2014.

Meadows DH et al. The limits to growth: a report for the Club of Rome's project on the predicament of mankind. London: Earth Island, 1976.

Moodie R et al. A national agency for promoting health and preventing illness. An options paper commissioned by the National Health and Hospitals Reform Commission (2008).

Olshansky SJ et al. A potential decline in life expectancy in the United States in the 21st century. N Engl J Med 352 (2005): 1138–1145.

Pilzer PZ. The wellness revolution: How to make a fortune in the next trillion dollar industry. Hoboken, NJ: John Wiley, 2002.

Pilzer PZ. The new wellness revolution: How to make a fortune in the next trillion dollar industry. Hoboken, NJ: John Wiley, 2007.

Preventative Health Task Force. Australia, the healthiest country by 2020: A discussion paper. 2008. Available: www.preventativehealth.org.au/internet/preventativehealth/publishing.nsf/Content/discussion-technical-1; 6 Aug 2014.

Productivity Commission. Australia's health workforce. Research Report. 2006. Available: www.pc.gov.au/projects/study/healthworkforce/docs/finalreport; 6 Aug 2014.

PWC (PriceWaterhouseCoopers). HealthCast 2020: Creating a sustainable future. (2005). Available: http://www.pwc.com/gx/en/healthcare/healthcast-series-future-trends/creating-a-sustainable-future.jhtml; accessed 6 Aug 2014.

PWC (PriceWaterhouseCoopers). Working towards wellness: Accelerating the prevention of chronic disease. World Economic Forum, 2007. Available: http://www.weforum.org/pdf/Wellness/report.pdf; 6 Aug 2014.

SRI (Stanford Research Institute) International. The global spa economy 2007. New York: Global Spa Summit, 2008.

SRI International. Spas and the global wellness market: Synergies and opportunities, New York: Global Spa Summit (2010). Retrieved from http://www.globalspasummit.org Accessed 07/07/2010.

Tindle HA et al. Trends in use of complementary and alternative medicine by US adults: 1997–2002. Altern Ther Health Med 11.1 (2005): 42–49.

Travis JW, Ryan RS. Wellness workbook: How to achieve enduring health and vitality, 3rd edn, Berkeley CA: Celestial Arts, 2004.

Tribus M, McIrvine EC. Energy and information. Scientific American 9 (1971): 179–84.

US National Wellness Institute. Academic program accreditation, 2008. Available: http://www.nationalwellness.org/?page=Accredited_Programs; 6 Aug 2014.

US National Wellness Institute. Defining Wellness, 2009. Available online: http://welltacc.org/index.php/wellness.html; 6 Aug 2014.

WHO. Preamble to the Constitution of the World Health Organization as adopted by the International Health Conference, New York, 19–22 June, 1946. New York: Official Records of the World Health Organization, 1948, p 100.

WHO. Preventing chronic diseases: A vital investment. WHO global report, 2005. Available: www.who.int/chp/chronic_disease_report/en/index.html; 6 Aug 2014.

Wilson EO. Consilience: The unity of knowledge. New York: Vintage, 1999.

INDEX

Page numbers followed by "f" indicate figures, "t" indicate tables, and "b" indicate boxes.